CONTROL of VIRUS DISEASES

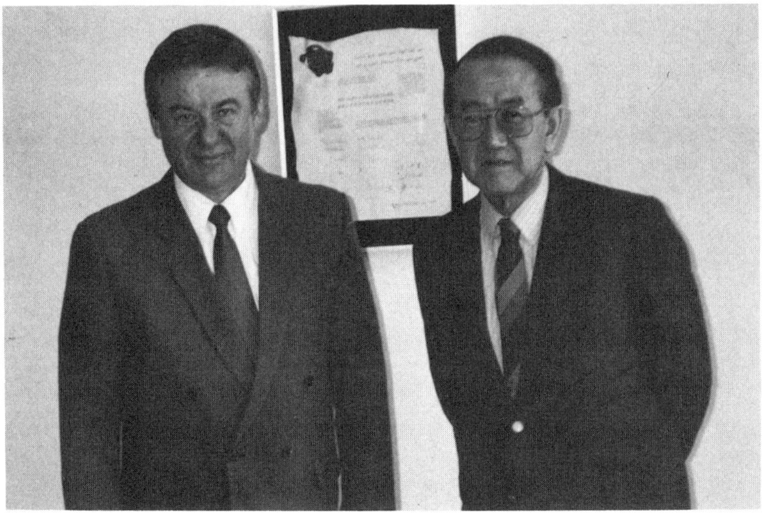

The control of virus diseases, which is actively promoted through the scientific activities of the International Comparative Virology Organization (ICVO), is a high-priority goal of the World Health Organization (WHO), as proven by numerous achievements. Doctor Hiroshi Nakajima (right), Director-General of WHO, and Professor Edouard Kurstak, President of ICVO, at WHO headquarters in Geneva. Between them is the WHO certification of the eradication of smallpox disease, considered a major success.

CONTROL of VIRUS DISEASES

Second Edition, Revised and Expanded

edited by

Edouard Kurstak

Faculty of Medicine
University of Montreal
Montreal, Quebec, Canada

Marcel Dekker, Inc. **New York • Basel • Hong Kong**

Library of Congress Cataloging-in-Publication Data

Control of virus diseases / edited by Edouard Kurstak. -- 2nd ed., rev. and expanded.
p. cm.
Includes bibliographical references and index.
ISBN 0-8247-8683-1 (alk. paper)
1. Viral vaccines. 2. Virus diseases--Prevention. I. Kurstak, Edouard.
[DNLM: 1. Virus Diseases--prevention & control. WC 500 C764]
QR189.5.V5C66 1992
614.5'75--dc20
DNLM/DLC
for Library of Congress 92-49728
CIP

This book is printed on acid-free paper.

MARCEL DEKKER, INC.
270 Madison Avenue, New York, New York 10016

Current printing (last digit):
10 9 8 7 6 5 4 3 2 1

PRINTED IN THE UNITED STATES OF AMERICA

Preface

The second edition of *Control of Virus Diseases* is devoted entirely to the major human viruses and related diseases, which remain a worldwide unresolved problem. Special attention is given to AIDS, hepatitis, measles, poliomyelitis, rabies, Japanese encephalitis, dengue, and respiratory and diarrheal viruses, all of which are responsible for millions of cases of death annually as well as untold human disability and suffering.

In seventeen well-documented chapters, internationally renowned experts in infectious diseases and immunization provide a state-of-the-art treatment of human virus infections. This single, comprehensive volume offers a wide range of new findings and references on the latest advances against highly infectious viruses, with emphasis on biotechnology and improved conventional vaccines, development of immunization programs, the role of molecular epidemiology surveillance strategy, and viral chemotherapy. Recent findings on genome organization and on genetic variability of viruses, especially for human immunodeficiency virus (HIV), are related directly to the attempts to produce safe and immunogenic vaccines and to the strategies to control virus diseases. These aspects are also discussed and documented in this book. In fact, since the emergence of AIDS, the development of a safe and effective HIV vaccine has become an international public health priority.

The AIDS virus kills many fewer patients annually than hepatitis B virus (HBV) or measles virus. However, so-called HIV exit disease continues to exercise special effects on patients, their families and the public at large. No other infectious disease in modern medical history has generated the concerns and efforts that AIDS has. The research to find an effective vaccine and drug against AIDS will also generate progress for the development of vaccines and chemotherapy against other viruses.

The importance of AIDS, with a World Health Organization–estimated 6 to 8 million persons presently infected and 40 million HIV seropositive cases expected by the year 2000, is well recognized. However, the carriers of HBV today represent a worldwide population of 200 to 300 million. It is estimated that 20% to 30% of them will die of chronic cirrhosis or primary hepatocellular carcinoma. The major goal of immunization strategies against hepatitis B virus is the prevention of chronic HBV infection and its sequelae. As explained in this volume, the objective of immunization in the areas of HBV endemicity is to prevent infancy and childhood infections through universal vaccination at birth or early in the first year of life.

Despite effective vaccines, measles virus kills 1 to 2 million children annually in developing countries, and poliomyelitis continues to exercise its crippling effects on children. For these reasons, special attention is given in the second edition to the development of virus vaccines and to worldwide immunization programs based on WHO recommendations. In five chapters, WHO experts describe vaccines and immunization programs and strategies for hepatitis B, measles, poliomyelitis, influenza viruses, and other acute respiratory viral infections. A possible eradication of wild poliovirus and the global control of measles virus by the year 2000 are presented as goals.

It should be stressed that before the introduction of the WHO Expanded Programme on Immunization (EPI), nearly 130 million measles cases and about 16 million deaths of children annually were the result of this virus infection. Today, with 80% of children vaccinated against measles, millions of deaths are prevented each year. These figures give an idea of the magnitude of the problem and what it is possible to achieve through well-designed, coordinated, and global immunization programs to control virus diseases.

New concepts of modern biotechnology and the use of viral vectors to immunize against rabies, Japanese encephalitis, and dengue, as well as the current approaches in vaccinology including the rotavirus vaccine development, are described in four chapters. Prevention of rotavirus infections is one of the public health services' priorities in developing countries, where 2–3 million children die from this disease. Finally, a chapter is devoted to the viral vaccines produced by biotechnology. It is predicted that this technology will replace conventional methods and that the vaccines produced will be safe and efficacious immunogens, available worldwide during the next decade.

This second edition of *Control of Virus Diseases* is addressed mainly to all public health professionals concerned with viral diseases, particularly in hospitals, clinics, centers of infectious diseases, governmental health services, research institutes, and medical schools, as well as to vaccine producers and experts in immunization strategies. It is my hope that this book will be a useful tool for those involved in the control of viral diseases and a source of the latest information on vaccine development and immunization programs.

My sincere thanks and gratitude are conveyed to the contributors, for the effort and care with which they prepared their well-documented and updated chapters, and to the staff of Marcel Dekker, Inc., for their cooperation in the production of this volume.

Edouard Kurstak

Contents

PART VII: VIRUS VACCINES AND BIOTECHNOLOGY

CONTRIBUTORS

Lorne A. Babiuk Veterinary Infectious Disease Organization, Saskatoon, Saskatchewan, Canada

James B. Campbell Department of Microbiology, University of Toronto, Toronto, Ontario, Canada

Gillian Chaloner-Larsson* Plasma Derivatives Section, Blood Products Division, Bureau of Biologics, Drugs Directorate, Health Protection Branch, Health and Welfare Canada, Ottawa, Ontario, Canada

Christopher John Clements Expanded Programme on Immunization, World Health Organization, Geneva, Switzerland

Guillermo Contreras Bureau of Biologics, Drugs Directorate, Health Protection Branch, Health and Welfare Canada, Ottawa, Ontario, Canada

Felicity T. Cutts Communicable Disease Epidemiology Unit, London School of Hygiene and Tropical Medicine, London, England

Edson da Silva Departamento de Virologia, Fundação Oswaldo Cruz, Rio de Janeiro, Brazil

Lina De Division of Viral and Rickettsial Diseases, Center for Infectious Diseases, Centers for Disease Control, Atlanta, Georgia

Ciro de Quadros Expanded Programme on Immunization, Pan American Health Organization, Washington, D.C.

*Retired

Kenneth H. Eckels Department of Biologics Research, Division of Communicable Disease and Immunology, Walter Reed Army Medical Center, Walter Reed Army Institute of Research, Washington, D.C.

John Furesz Bureau of Biologics, Drugs Directorate, Health Protection Branch, Health and Welfare Canada, Ottawa, Ontario, Canada

Yuri Ghendon Microbiology and Immunology Support Services, World Health Organization, Geneva, Switzerland

Matthew A. Gonda Laboratory of Cell and Molecular Structure, Program Resources, Inc./DynCorp, National Cancer Institute—Frederick Cancer Research and Development Center, Frederick, Maryland

Daniel Hazlett Viral Products Division, Bureau of Biologics, Drugs Directorate, Health Protection Branch, Health and Welfare Canada, Ottawa, Ontario, Canada

A. Hossain Department of Microbiology and Immunology, Faculty of Medicine, University of Montreal, and International Comparative Virology Organization, Montreal, Quebec, Canada

Harry F. Hull Expanded Programme on Immunization, World Health Organization, Geneva, Switzerland

Akira Igarashi Department of Virology, Institute of Tropical Medicine, Nagasaki University, Nagasaki City, Japan

Olen Kew Division of Viral and Rickettsial Diseases, Center for Infectious Diseases, Centers for Disease Control, Atlanta, Georgia

Robert J. Kim-Farley Expanded Programme on Immunization, World Health Organization, Geneva, Switzerland

Christine Kurstak Department of Microbiology and Immunology, Faculty of Medicine, University of Montreal, and International Comparative Virology Organization, Montreal, Quebec, Canada

Edouard Kurstak Department of Microbiology and Immunology, Faculty of Medicine, University of Montreal, and International Comparative Virology Organization, Montreal, Quebec, Canada

Raymond G. Marusyk Provincial Laboratory of Public Health, University of Alberta, Edmonton, Alberta, Canada

Julie B. Milstien Biologicals Unit, World Health Organization, Geneva, Switzerland

Baldev Nottay Division of Viral and Rickettsial Diseases, Center for Infectious Diseases, Centers for Disease Control, Atlanta, Georgia

M. Steven Oberste Laboratory of Cell and Molecular Structure, Program Resources, Inc./Dyncorp, National Cancer Institute—Frederick Cancer Research and Development Center, Frederick, Maryland

Laszlo Palkonyay Viral Products Division, Bureau of Biologics, Drugs Directorate, Health Protection Branch, Health and Welfare Canada, Ottawa, Ontario, Canada

Mark Pallansch Division of Viral and Rickettsial Diseases, Center for Infectious Diseases, Centers for Disease Control, Atlanta, Georgia

Yuri Pervikov Microbiology and Immunology Support Services, World Health Organization, Geneva, Switzerland

Mark J. Redmond Veterinary Infectious Disease Organization, Saskatoon, Saskatchewan, Canada

Marta I. Sabara* Praxis Biologics Inc., Rochester, New York

M. Strassburg Data Collection and Analysis, Los Angeles County Department of Health Services, Los Angeles, California

Carole Torel Expanded Programme on Immunization, World Health Organization, Geneva, Switzerland

A. Al Tuwaijri Department of Microbiology and Immunology, Faculty of Medicine, University of Montreal, and International Comparative Virology Organization, Montreal, Quebec, Canada

---

**Present affiliation*: SmithKline Beecham Animal Health, Lincoln, Nebraska.

Nicholas A. Ward Expanded Programme on Immunization, World Health Organization, Geneva, Switzerland

Owen S. Weislow Anti-AIDS Virus Drug Screening Laboratories, Program Resources, Inc./DynCorp, and National Cancer Institute—Frederick Cancer Research and Development Center, National Institutes of Health, Frederick, Maryland

Changgao Yang Viral Products Division, Bureau of Biologics, Drugs Directorate, Health Protection Branch, Health and Welfare Canada, Ottawa, Ontario, Canada

Chen-Fu Yang Division of Viral and Rickettsial Diseases, Center for Infectious Diseases, Centers for Disease Control, Atlanta, Georgia

Ying Zhang* Department of Microbiology, University of Toronto, Toronto, Ontario, Canada

*_Present affiliation_: Department of Epidemiology, Dalian Medical College, Dalian, People's Republic of China.

PART I

AIDS AND HUMAN IMMUNODEFICIENCY VIRUSES

1

AIDS—The Human Immunodeficiency Virus

Molecular and Structural Aspects of Its Biology

Matthew A. Gonda and M. Steven Oberste *Program Resources, Inc./DynCorp, National Cancer Institute—Frederick Cancer Research and Development Center, Frederick, Maryland*

I. HISTORICAL PERSPECTIVE

The human immunodeficiency virus type 1 (HIV-1) is the causative agent of acquired immunodeficiency syndrome (AIDS). AIDS is a disease characterized by a slow, progressive impairment of the immune system, opportunistic infections, and encephalopathy. Since AIDS was first recognized in 1981 (Gottlieb et al., 1981), remarkable progress has been made in defining the cause of this new disease. Foremost was the identification and isolation of the causative agent, HIV-1 (Barre-Sinoussi et al., 1983; Gallo et al., 1984), a member of the lentivirus subfamily of retroviruses (Gonda et al., 1985, 1986). More recently, a second human immunodeficiency virus (HIV-2), which is more closely related to the simian immunodeficiency viruses (SIVs), was discovered in humans in West Africa (Clavel et al., 1986; Guyader et al., 1987). HIV-2 appears to be less pathogenic than HIV-1 and is infrequently associated with AIDS-like syndromes. HIV-1 has a worldwide distribution, whereas HIV-2 infections are geographically restricted, occurring primarily in western African nations (Romieu et al., 1990).

HIV-1 is spread through the exchange of body fluids, primarily blood and blood products, but also through sexual intercourse. HIV-1 infects cells of the immune system; lymphocytes bearing the CD4 molecule on their surface are the main targets (Klatzmann et al., 1984; Dalgleish et al., 1984), although macrophages are also infectible and may play a significant role as a virus reservoir and in the progression of the disease (Gendelman et al., 1989; Gartner and Popovic, 1990; Meltzer et al., 1990). Direct infection of CD4+ lymphocytes, primarily T-helper cells, results in their depletion from the peripheral blood. The depletion of CD4+ lymphocytes produces immune dysfunction that, in time, cripples the immune system's ability to combat effectively opportunistic infections and cancers; other hematopoietic abnormalities may also exist that exacerbate the disease (Zon et al., 1987; Steinberg et al., 1991). HIV-1 also infects brain macrophages and microglial cells and can induce central nervous system disorders (Shaw et al., 1985; Watkins et al., 1990; Jordan et al., 1991). The HIV-1 infection may be clinically quiescent for a long period of time before the AIDS-related complex (ARC) or frank AIDS becomes apparent; this latent period may last up to a decade (Bachetti and Moss, 1989). Despite the long lag between the initial infection and the onset of clinical symptoms of AIDS, the virus is constantly replicating in some tissues of the body.

The rapid and extensive virologic, immunologic, and molecular characterizations of HIV-1 have allowed for progress in several major areas in understanding and combating the spread of this inexorable disease. The first was the growth of the AIDS virus in tissue culture cells, which enabled the large-scale propagation and purification of virus for the development of sensitive antigen-based immunologic assays to screen infected blood for HIV-1 antibodies. This has helped to prevent the spread of infection in the population by eliminating HIV-1-contaminated blood. Intravenous drug abuse now accounts for the largest number of HIV-infected blood transmissions in most parts of the world. The use of these diagnostic methods in seroepidemiologic surveys also provided knowledge of the global extent of HIV-1 infection; it is now known that the HIV-1 infection has reached pandemic proportions (Mann, 1990; Piot et al., 1990). This information emphasizes the desperate need for an effective vaccine and antiviral drugs to curtail the worldwide progression of HIV-1 infections. The second major area of progress was the discoveries that led to a detailed definition of the structure, and identification of the protein subunits, of the virus particle. The major structural proteins encoded by the *gag*, *pol*, and *env* genes of HIV-1 have been immunologically identified and functionally studied (Allan et al., 1985; Robey et al., 1985; Lillehoj et al., 1988; Mervis et al., 1988; Putney et al., 1990). This information has permitted the targeting of viral proteins for use in the development of candidate vaccines for HIV-1. Finally, the molecular cloning and nucleotide sequencing of HIV-1 proviruses have provided a complete "blueprint" of the genome organization of the virus. This blueprint has shown that HIV-1 is a very complex virus with a number of nonstructural/accessory genes that are involved in the regulation of virus expression and infectivity during its life cycle, and may also play an important role in the pathogenesis of the virus (Cullen and Greene, 1990; Kieny, 1990; Haseltine, 1990; Cullen, 1991). A better understanding of the HIV-1 genetic blueprint and how the virus and host regulate virus expression may provide additional insight for the development of novel prophylactic or therapeutic agents to control HIV-1 infections.

This chapter will focus on summarizing what is known about the structure of the virus particle, virus life cycle, virus–host interactions, molecular organization of the virus genome, genome variability, evolutionary relationships, and mechanisms of replication of HIV-1. Details of the biology of HIV-2 will be provided for comparison but will not be discussed extensively. The main purpose of this overview of the molecular and structural aspects of HIV-1 is to provide a basis for understanding the complexity of this virus and the difficulties that will be encountered in developing vaccines and treatments for HIV-1 infection and AIDS, and to point to areas of HIV-1 biology that may be exploited in the development of these agents.

II. HIV-1 EVOLUTIONARY RELATIONSHIPS AND RETROVIRUS PHYLOGENY

Retroviruses are complex parasitic biomolecules that can develop nonpathogenic as well as pathogenic relationships with their hosts. Retroviruses are classified based on their morphology or ultrastructure, pathobiology, and nucleotide sequence and genome organization. There are three subfamilies of retroviruses: oncoviruses, lentiviruses, and spumaviruses. HIV, like all other retroviruses, encodes the unifying and unique enzyme reverse transcriptase (RT), which catalyzes the flow of genetic information from RNA→DNA, counter to that (DNA→RNA) of most conventional biological systems. Retroviruses can be grouped broadly as being endogenous or exogenous. The endogenous viruses are transmitted vertically in the germ line while the exogenous viruses are transmitted horizontally. HIV-1 is an exogenous retrovirus since its sequences can only be found in the DNA of HIV-1-infected individuals.

The first indications that HIV-1 was a lentivirus came from the observations that it shared both morphologic similarities and sequence homology with the lentiviruses of domesticated animals (Gonda et al., 1985, 1986). The complete nucleotide sequences of HIV-1 and HIV-2 have been determined (Ratner et al., 1985; Muesing et al., 1985; Sanchez-Pescador et al., 1985; Wain-Hobson et al., 1985; Guyader et al., 1987), which has allowed for a more extensive and exacting comparison of the evolutionary relationship of the HIVs to other retroviruses. Overall, the genomes of retroviruses are quite divergent. Nevertheless, the RT domain of the *pol* gene is one region of the genome that is relatively well conserved in all retroviruses. Figure 1A shows 90 consecutive amino acids from the amino terminus of the RT domains of a series of retroviruses, including representatives of the oncovirus, spumavirus, and lentivirus subfamilies. Pairwise comparisons between these amino acid sequences show that the known lentiviruses, HIV-1, HIV-2, several SIVs, bovine immunodeficiency-like virus (BIV), feline immunodeficiency virus, equine infectious anemia virus, caprine arthritis encephalitis virus, visna virus, and ovine progressive pneumonia virus, contain 60% or more of their residues in common over this stretch of RT. A Fitch-Margoliash phylogenetic tree (Fig. 1B) was developed for the amino acid alignments of RT shown in Figure 1A. This phylogenetic tree gives a relative estimate of the relatedness of the retrovirus family. There are two main branches in the retrovirus phylogenetic tree: one for the retroviruses whose RTs have a preference for Mn^{2+} and one for those with a preference for Mg^{2+}. There are two subbranches for the retroviruses whose RTs have a preference for Mg^{2+} cation: one of these leads to the oncoviruses and the other to the lentiviruses. It is clear from this analysis that HIV-1 clusters with the lentiviruses. The closest lentivirus relatives to HIV-1 and HIV-2 are the SIVs; however, HIV-2 is more closely related to the SIVs in this analysis. The lentivirus evolutionary relationship has been of predictive value in understanding much about the pathobiology of HIV-1, viral mechanisms for evading the host immune response, and infection parameters of the AIDS process. Moreover, it highlights the use of members of the lentivirus subfamily of retroviruses for the development of relevant animal models for HIV-like infections for antiviral therapy and vaccine studies.

III. LIFE CYCLE OF VIRUS IN HIV-1 INFECTIONS

The life cycle of retroviruses, and therefore that of HIV-1, can be divided into two major phases: infection and expression (Fig. 2). In the first phase, free virus attaches to the cell receptor (CD4 molecule) via the envelope glycoproteins. Attached virus penetrates the host cell membrane by a mechanism that is not clearly understood but is believed to be

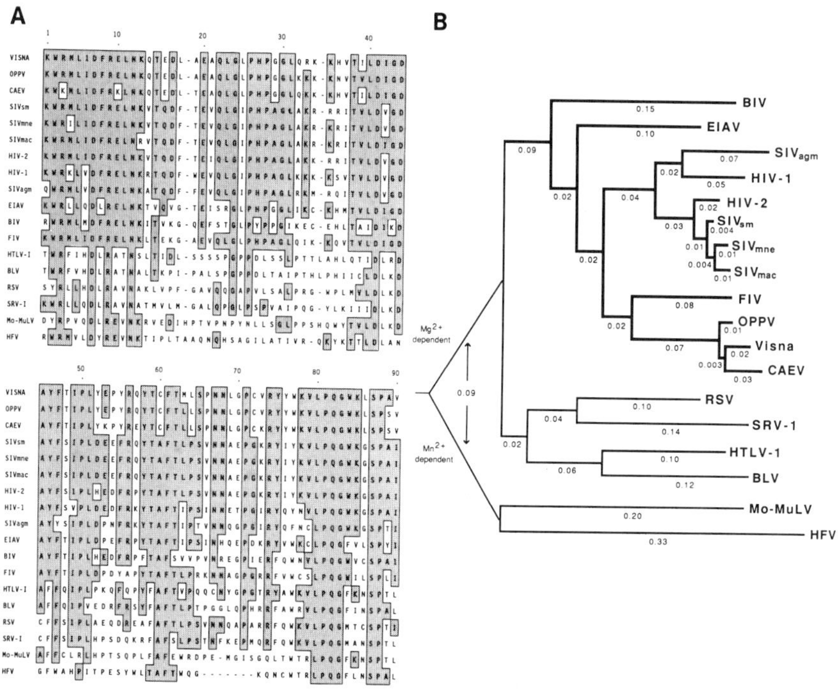

FIGURE 1 Evolutionary relationship of HIV-1 and HIV-2 to other retroviruses. (A) Alignment of 90 consecutive amino acids in the conserved RT domain of the *pol* genes from lentiviruses with those of other retroviruses. Retroviruses used are visna virus, OPPV, SIVsm, SIVmne, SIVmac, HIV-2, HIV-1, SIVagm, EIAV, BIV, FIV, HTLV-1, BLV, RSV, SRV-1, Mo-MuLV, and HFV. The alignment shown is generally that found to be optimal with visna virus; slight improvements in the other pairwise alignment scores can be made by minor shifts in the placement of gaps. Shaded boxes are drawn around identical residues when seven or more lentiviruses share that residue. (B) Fitch-Margoliash phylogenetic tree based on analysis of the 90 amino acids from the highly conserved RT domain of Pol of lentiviruses and, for comparison, those of other retroviruses, as presented in Garvey et al. (1990). Branch lengths are in units of -logM where M is the frequency of matching residues. The tree was rooted with HFV (human spumavirus) and Mo-MuLV (mouse oncovirus) as the outgroup taxa because they consistently had the lowest alignment scores and because their RTs preferentially use Mn^{2+} cations as cofactor. The average standard deviation of the tree was 5.17%. (From Garvey et al., 1990. Reprinted with permission of the editors and Academic Press, Inc.)

receptor-mediated endocytosis (Haseltine, 1990). Regardless of the exact mechanism, the virus is uncoated and the genome-length RNA is released into the cytoplasm with virus-specific enzymes, which include the viral RT and the integrase/endonuclease (IN). The single-stranded viral RNA is reverse-transcribed into double-stranded DNA by the action of these two enzymes. The double-stranded linear viral DNA, called the provirus, is transported to the nucleus. The provirus can circularize and integrate into the host DNA with the aid of the IN (Bushman et al., 1990). In the integrated state, the virus can remain transcriptionally inactive, or latent, and the viral genetic information remains in the cell as long as it survives. The proviral DNA replicates every time the infected-cell DNA is replicated. For all practical purposes, the viral DNA has become a permanent part of the infected cell until it dies or is removed by the virus-specific activity of the immune system.

In the second stage of the life cycle, the integrated provirus is transcribed by a cellular RNA polymerase into genome-length RNA. The primary transcript is spliced by cellular enzymes into the subgenomic mRNAs (discussed below). The primary transcript and subgenomic

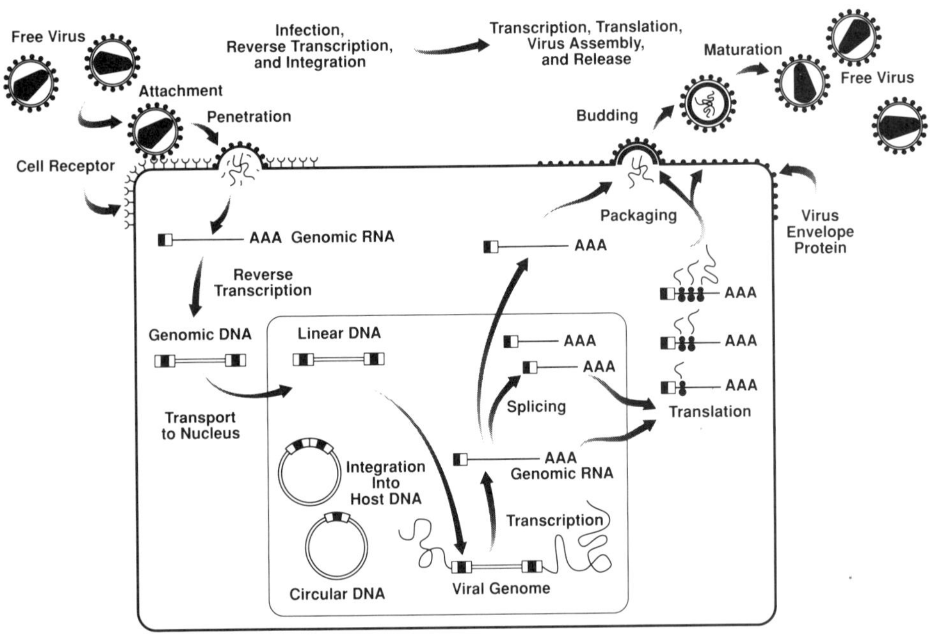

FIGURE 2 Life cycle of HIV-1.

mRNAs are translated on the cellular ribosomes, producing the structural and accessory gene products. The structural proteins make their way to the plasma membrane where they are assembled, incorporating the full-length transcript, into virus particles. The virus particles are released from the cell by a process called budding. The core structures mature in the extracellular milieu. Maturation of the virus particle is necessary for it to become infectious. The free virus can then go on to infect another cell, thus reinitiating the replication cycle.

IV. ULTRASTRUCTURE OF THE VIRUS PARTICLE

The morphogenesis of the HIV-1 virus particle reflects its relationship to the lentivirus subfamily of retroviruses (Gonda et al., 1985, 1989; Gonda, 1988; Gelderblom et al., 1990) and can be evaluated by electron microscopic examination in thin sections of HIV-1-infected cells (Fig. 3). For comparison, the primate lentivirus SIV and nonprimate lentivirus BIV are included in Figure 3. In HIV-1, there is no intracellular form of the virus particle, as seen with some other types of retroviruses (Gonda et al., 1989). Viral core proteins initially assemble beneath the envelope-glycoprotein-studded plasma membrane where they coalesce. The first evidence of virus particle formation is the appearance of a crescent-shaped nucleoid beneath the plasma membrane. The viral nucleoid continues to form by incorporation of additional Gag precursor and Gag-Pol polyproteins and the genomic RNA. Particle morphogenesis continues until a circular nucleoid is reached. At this stage, the immature virus particles are released from the plasma membrane by budding. These immature extracellular virus particles are believed not to be fully infectious. The final stage in the morphogenesis of the particle occurs after cleavage of the Gag precursor and Gag-Pol polyproteins into their respective functional units (discussed below). This is presumed to occur concomitantly with condensation of the circular nucleoid into a bar or cone shape and correlates with infectivity of the virus particle.

V. NUCLEOTIDE SEQUENCE AND GENOME ORGANIZATION

The nucleotide sequences for the genomes and subgenomic messages for many diverse isolates of HIV-1 and HIV-2 have been determined and are available through various sequence databases, including Genbank. The HIV-1 and HIV-2 genomes, in the form of the viral RNA, are approximately 9,200 and 9,700 base pairs (bp), respectively (Ratner et al., 1985; Wain-Hobson et al., 1985; Sanchez-Pescador et al., 1985; Guyader et al.,

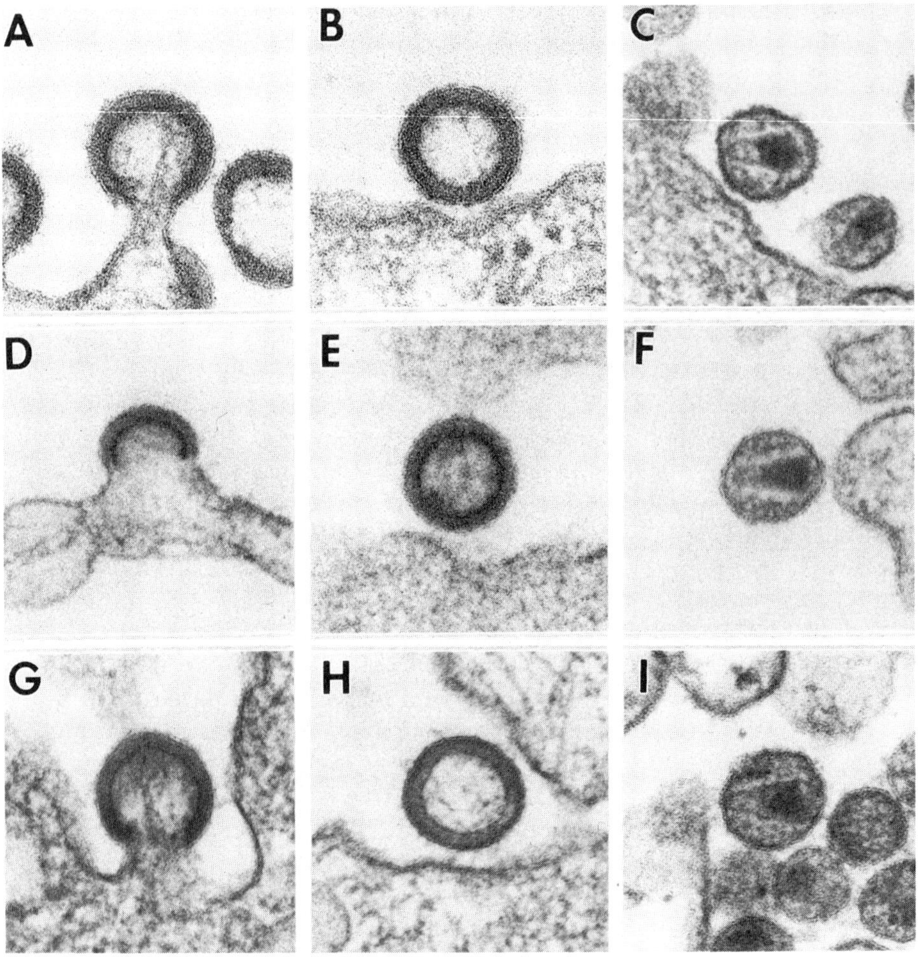

FIGURE 3 Ultrastructure and morphogenesis of HIV-1 (A–C), SIV (D–F), and BIV (G–I). Early bud (A, D, and G). Immature extracellular virion (B, E, and H). Mature extracellular virion (C, F, and I).

1987). Open reading frame (ORF) analysis of the DNA sequences of HIV-1 and HIV-2 has revealed their genetic organization. The translations of identified ORFs have given some insight into the predicted protein products of the virus. The salient features of this analysis are presented below. The accepted nomenclature for retroviruses and the HIV-1 and HIV-2 genes and their products has been standardized (Leis et al., 1988;

Gallo et al., 1988; Laurence, 1988); the HIV-1 and HIV-2 structural and accessory gene products are presented in Table 1.

A. Genome Organization

The genomes of all replication-competent retroviruses contain the obligatory *gag*, *pol*, and *env* genes, flanked on the 5′ and 3′ ends by the long terminal repeats (LTRs); the HIV-1 and HIV-2 genomes are no exception (Fig. 4; Table 1). The *gag* and *pol* genes are in different reading frames and overlap. The *env* gene is found in the 3′ end of the genome separated from the *pol* sequences by the complex "central region," which is the hallmark of lentiviruses (Cullen and Greene, 1990; Garvey et al., 1990; Haseltine, 1990; Cullen, 1991). In the central region, between and overlapping the *pol* and *env* genes, are a series of five ORFs that have been identified as *vif*, *tat* exon 1, *rev* exon 1, *vpr*, and either *vpu* or *vpx*. As shown in Figure 4, the *tat* and *rev* genes are comprised of two exons; the second exons of *tat* and *rev* are found in the 3′ end of the *env* region but are in different reading frames from *env* and each other. The *vpu* gene is exclusive to HIV-1, whereas *vpx* is present only in HIV-2 and SIV. Both HIV-1 and HIV-2 have an ORF overlapping sequences in the 3′ end of the *env* ORF and the LTR, termed *nef*, that does not appear to be present in nonprimate lentiviruses (Garvey et al., 1990).

B. Complexities of the Transcription Map

The transcription map of HIV-1 reflects the intricacy of the genome. Based on Northern analyses and characterization of cDNAs, at least five size classes of mRNA encode the various structural and accessory genes of the virus (Rabson et al., 1985; Muesing et al., 1985; Kieny, 1990; Haseltine, 1990). An abbreviated summary of the transcripts identified for HIV is shown in Figure 5. All viral transcripts contain a common 5′ leader consisting of sequences derived from the R and U5 regions of the LTR and the region immediately preceding *gag*. This segment of the genome also contains the encapsidation or ψ signals for incorporation of RNA into the virus particle. It appears that additional sequence information is required for RNA packaging, since only the genome length RNA appears in the virus particle and removal of the ψ sequences does not completely abolish particle formation or RNA encapsidation (Clavel and Orenstein, 1990).

The genome length transcript is the virion RNA and is also used as the mRNA for the translation of both Gag and Pol proteins. The *env* mRNA is derived from the primary transcript by removal of a single intron between the common leader sequence and a splice acceptor site before the beginning of the *env* ORF. The *vif*, *vpu*, *vpr*, and *nef* transcripts are also singly

TABLE 1 Structural and Accessory Gene Products of HIV-1 and HIV-2

ORF	Protein(s)	Function
gag	MA-CA-NC	Encodes the Gag precursor. Contains the minimal information necessary for virus particle formation. Cleaved by virus-encoded protease into matrix (MA), capsid (CA), nucleocapsid (NC), and p6 (associated with virion assembly) proteins found in the core of the mature virion.
pol	PR-RT-IN	Encodes the polymerase precursor. Cleavage products are protease (PR), reverse transcriptase (RT), and integrase–endonuclease (IN). Pol products are responsible for the enzymatic functions of the virus.
env	SU-TM	Encodes the envelope precursor containing the surface membrane (SU) and the transmembrane (TM) glycoproteins. SU is the virus receptor which interacts with the CD4 molecule; the TM anchors SU to the viral membrane.
vif	Vif	Viral infectivity factor. Modulates the infectivity of cell-free virus.
tat	Tat	*trans*-Activator of transcription. Increases the steady-state level of viral RNA in infected cells and increases translational efficiency.
rev	Rev	Regulator of expression of virion proteins. Facilitates the transport of unspliced and singly spliced mRNAs to the cytoplasm.
nef	Nef	Negative factor. May downregulate virus expression in some lymphoid cell types.
R	Vpr	Viral protein R. A virion-associated, second *trans*-activator of transcription.
U	Vpu	Viral protein U. May affect the release of virus particles from infected cells (HIV-1 only).
X	Vpx	Viral protein X. Sometimes found in virion. Function is unknown (HIV-2 and SIV only).

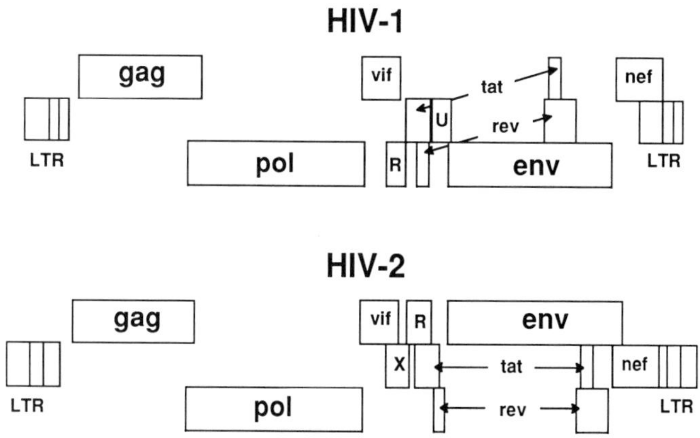

FIGURE 4 Genome organization of HIV-1 and HIV-2.

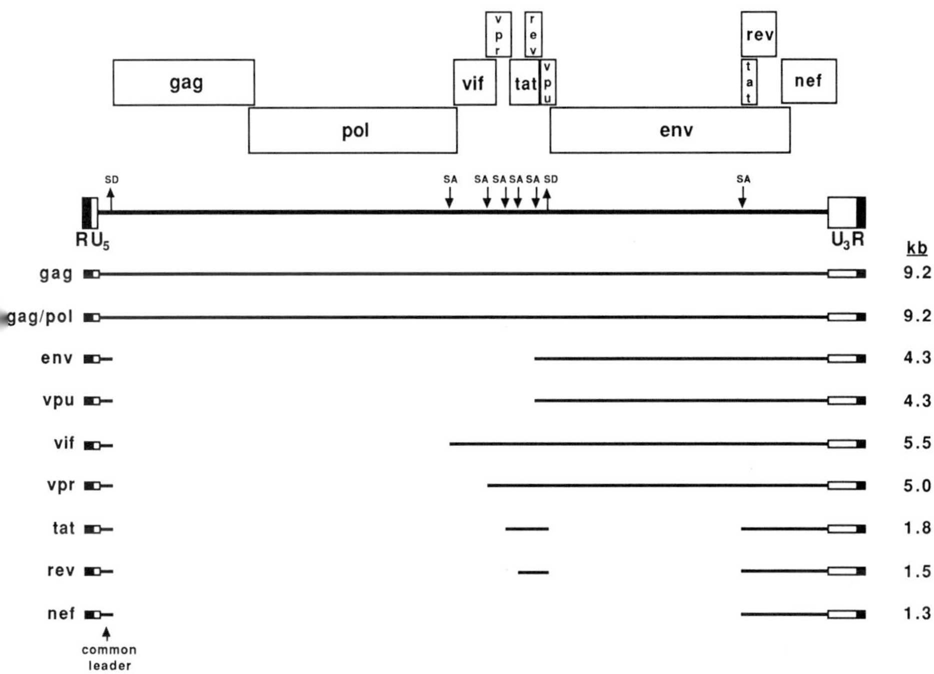

FIGURE 5 Transcriptional map of HIV-1.

spliced in a manner similar to the *env* mRNA using splice acceptors immediately preceding each of these genes. The *tat* and *rev* genes are derived from the primary transcript by multiple splicing of the primary transcript (Kieny, 1990; Haseltine, 1990). In their simplest form, the *tat* mRNAs are doubly spliced, although some *tat* mRNAs have been shown to contain additional untranslated sequences preceding *tat* exon 1, indicating that some *tat* messages are triply spliced; singly spliced forms are also present in small amounts. The additional upstream sequences do not appear to contribute to the coding capacity of the triply spliced *tat* mRNAs since they precede the first initiation codon in the message. Alternative splicing patterns for *vpu* and *vif*, other than those shown in Figure 5, have been obtained, but these variations do not affect the outcome of the translated product. The alternative mRNAs for the accessory genes are not unexpected considering the large repertoire of splice acceptor and donor sites available near each of the ORFs of the central region.

C. Structure and Function of the Viral LTRs

In all retroviruses, the proviral DNA contains two copies of the viral LTR, one at each end of the genome (Fig. 4). In the 5′ to 3′ direction, the LTR can be dissected into U3, R, and U5 regions. The U3 sequences are derived from the 3′ end and U5 sequences from the 5′ end of the viral RNA; the R sequences are present at both ends. The HIV-1 LTR contains a number of *cis*-acting sequences whose functions are to initiate, enhance, and terminate transcription. Transcriptional activation of HIV-1's LTR can occur by various mechanisms including cellular lymphoid triggering signals, endogenous viral *trans*-activators, and heterologous viral *trans*-activators that have been discussed in great detail by others (Tong-Starksen and Peterlin, 1990).

VI. PROCESSING, FUNCTION, AND LOCATION OF VIRION PROTEINS

A. Gag and Pol

The HIV-1 Gag precursor and Gag–Pol polyprotein are both translated from the primary transcript (Figs. 5 and 6). Since the *gag* and *pol* genes overlap and are in different reading frames, the synthesis of the Gag-Pol polyprotein requires a –1 frameshift in the translation of its mRNA (Jacks et al., 1988; Varmus, 1988). Figure 6 shows the proposed cleavage pattern of HIV-1 Gag and Pol proteins. The viral protease (PR) resides in the amino proximal region of the Pol precursor and is required for the correct processing of Gag and Pol proteins into functional units in the virion. The

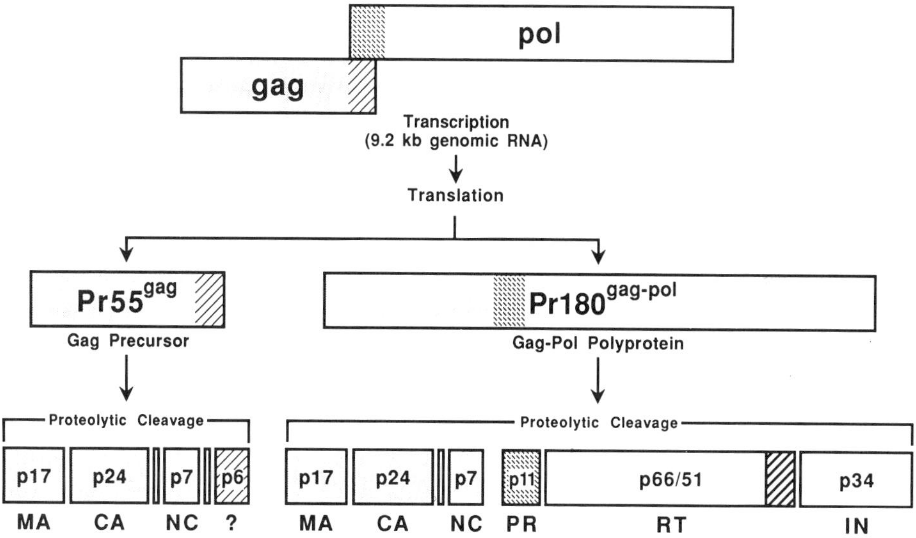

FIGURE 6 Processing of HIV-1 Gag and Pol proteins.

viral PR becomes active soon after budding of the virus particle from the plasma membrane. It specifically cleaves sites between the Gag and Pol regions of the Gag–Pol polyprotein and within the Gag and Pol precursors.

The Gag precursor ($Pr55^{gag}$) is cleaved into the matrix (MA), capsid (CA), and a complex of proteins initially linked to the nucleocapsid (NC) protein (Swanstrom et al., 1990). In HIV-1, the MA, CA, and NC proteins are designated, based on their observed molecular weights, p17, p24, and p7, respectively (Casey et al., 1985; Robey et al., 1985; di Marzo Veronese et al., 1987; Henderson et al., 1988a; Mervis et al., 1988; Swanstrom et al., 1990). A 6 kD protein (p6) is found at the carboxy-terminus of the NC protein and is believed to be involved in virus particle assembly, since mutations in this region affect virus morphology and release. Two smaller peptides have been identified that result from the cleavage of the p7 from CA and p6; the functions of the two smaller peptides are unknown (Henderson et al., 1988a; Henderson, personal communication). The function of the MA protein is to direct insertion of the Gag precursor into the plasma membrane; at its amino terminus, the MA protein of the HIV-1 Gag precursor contains myristic acid, which is believed to facilitate insertion into the plasma membrane (Schultz et al., 1988; Gottlinger et al., 1989).

The CA protein is the major core protein, while the NC protein is involved in packaging the viral RNA (Gorelick et al., 1990), and may also be an important component in facilitating virus particle assembly.

The Gag–Pol polyprotein ($Pr180^{gag-pol}$) contains both Gag and Pol peptides (Fig. 6). The Gag–Pol polyprotein represents approximately 5% of the core of HIV-1 and, because of the –1 frameshift, the carboxy-terminal Gag amino acid sequences (p6) are not present in $Pr180^{gag-pol}$ (Henderson, personal communication). However, the –1 frameshift allows for translation of the overlapping PR sequences in *pol*. The Pol precursor is composed of three major domains: PR, RT, and IN (Lightfoote et al., 1986; Swanstrom et al., 1990). It is believed that the viral PR cleaves itself free of the amino proximal Gag proteins and the RT domain and then further cleaves the IN from the RT (Swanstrom et al., 1990). The PR and RT proteins appear to function as dimers (Miller et al., 1989; Barber et al., 1990). In the RT dimer, one of the molecules is proteolytically processed at its carboxyl end by the viral PR; the dimer structure is believed to be p66/p51 (Hizi et al., 1988; Ferris et al., 1990). The PR, RT, and IN proteins are designated p11, p66/51, and p34, respectively.

Recent work on the expression of lentivirus Gag precursors in the baculovirus–insect cell expression system has shown that the Gag precursor is the minimal subgenomic element necessary for production of particles resembling naturally occurring virions; the virus-like particles produced in this system have the typical morphology of immature extracellular virus and lack virion RNA (Gheysen et al., 1989; Delchambre et al., 1989; Rasmussen et al., 1990). Recombinant vaccinia virus constructs expressing the HIV-1 *gag* and *pol* genes have also been shown to form virus-like particles; however, because both Gag and Pol proteins are produced, the viral PR is present and active (Karacostas et al., 1989). Thus, virus-like particles produced in this system can resemble either immature or mature extracellular virus, as observed in HIV-1 infected lymphocytes (Gonda et al., 1985; Karacostas et al., 1989). These results further support the role of the viral PR in the maturation of the virus particle.

B. Env

The HIV-1 envelope (Env) proteins are large glycoproteins (Allan et al., 1985; Robey et al., 1985; Willey et al., 1988; Darr and Ho, 1990). The nascent Env precursor is synthesized as an 88 kD protein from its own subgenomic mRNA, glycosylated, and subsequently cleaved into the mature surface (SU) and transmembrane (TM) glycoproteins by a cellular protease (Allan et al., 1985; Robey et al., 1985; Walker et al., 1987; Sodroski et al.,

1990) (Fig. 7). A signal peptide near the amino terminus of the nascent Env precursor directs it into the endoplasmic reticulum. In the endoplasmic reticulum, the Env polypeptide chain is heavily modified by the addition of complex sugar side chains that are high in mannose content. The carbohydrate side chains on the newly synthesized Env polypeptide are terminally modified in the Golgi complex before being expressed on the cell surface (Willey et al., 1988). There are 27 potential N-linked glycosylation sites on the HIV-1 Env precursor (gp160); most of these (21) reside on the SU glycoprotein, while the remainder (6) are found on the TM protein. As much as 40% of the empirically derived molecular weight of the Env precursor and SU protein (gp120) can be attributed to N-linked glycosylation. The function of the SU protein is to act as the viral receptor. The TM protein (gp41) has three functional domains: extracellular, transmembrane, and cytoplasmic. The primary structural function of the TM protein is to anchor the SU protein to the cell surface; it also participates in the fusigenic process of virus entry and syncytium induction.

C. Virion Location of Structural Gene Products

The virus particle can be dissected into two major components: the viral envelope and the core (Fig. 8). The viral envelope is comprised structurally of a lipid bilayer membrane, cellular proteins, and gp120 and gp41; some gp160 may be present in the viral envelope since it is detected in Western blots of cell-free virus. The heavily glycosylated gp120 is on the outside of the virus particle, which makes it accessible to the cell receptor (CD4) (discussed below). The gp120 also interacts with gp41, which is embedded in the viral envelope at its hydrophobic domain and partly exposed to the outside at its lightly glycosylated amino-terminal end. The TM protein has a large cytoplasmic tail that directs its external–internal cellular orientation. The Env glycoproteins are believed to interact as oligomers, most likely dimers (Pinter et al., 1989; Schawaller et al., 1989; Chakrabarti et al., 1990; Earl et al., 1990; Weiss et al., 1990; Moss et al., 1991). Also included in the viral envelope is the MA protein, p17. It is unclear whether the MA protein is exposed to the extracellular milieu, but recent data on the development of neutralizing antibodies and cytotoxic T-cells to p17 and a peptide corresponding to the amino-terminus of p17 suggest that it may be accessible to immune surveillance (Naylor et al., 1987; Papsidero et al., 1989; Achour et al., 1990). While drawings of viral envelopes are static images, the interaction of viral envelope proteins, including p17, with each other and with cellular proteins are probably very dynamic, allowing for

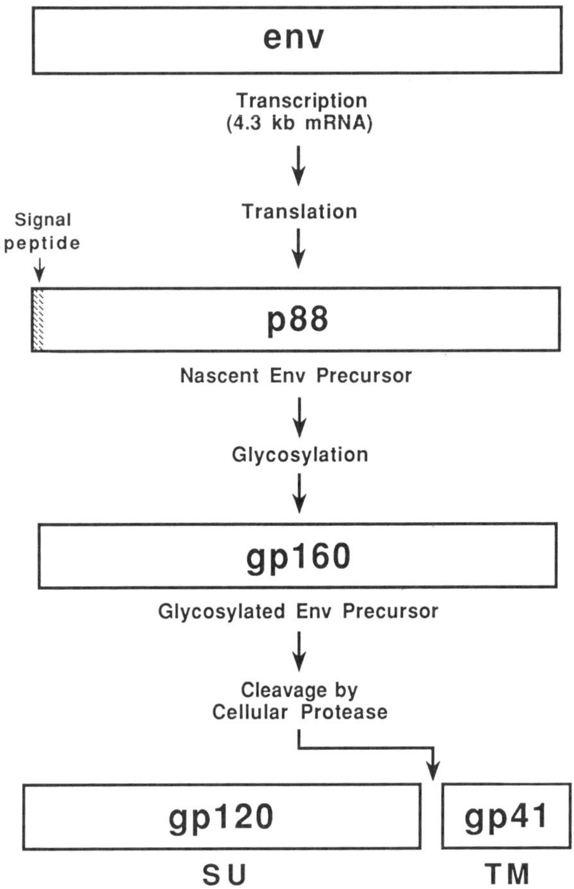

FIGURE 7 Processing of HIV-1 Env proteins.

the transmembrane mobility of p17, which may result in its unexpected surface expression.

The cores of mature HIV-1 particles are bar or cone shaped (Figs. 3 and 8). The major constituent of the core is the CA protein, p24. It makes up the outside of the core structure. Encapsulated inside the core is the genomic RNA. Several of the other Gag and Pol proteins are also believed to reside within the core; these include the NC (p7), p6, PR, RT, and IN. There may be an association with the viral RNA for some of these proteins; little else is known of the assembly of the inner core structure.

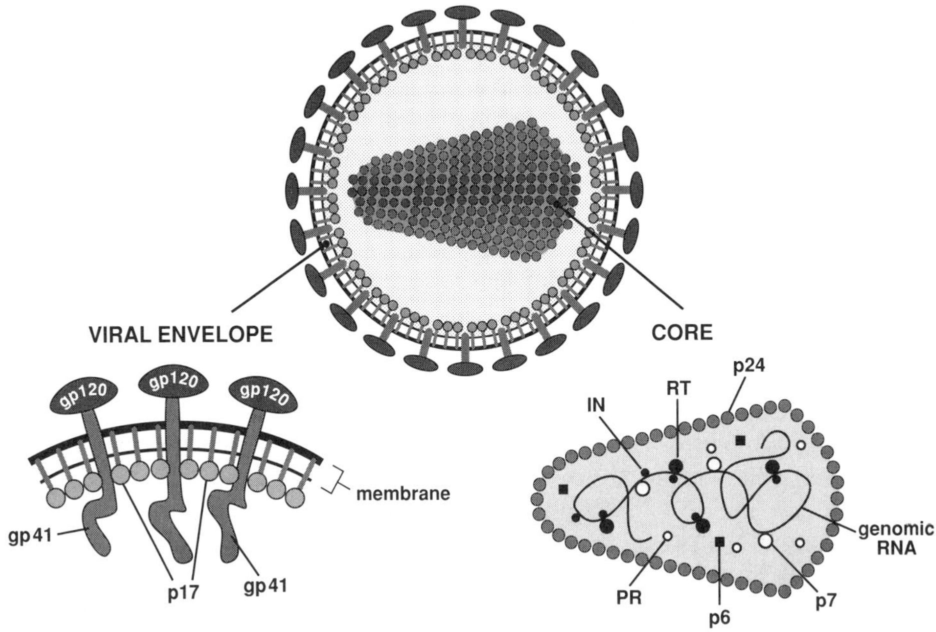

FIGURE 8 Schematic representation of the HIV-1 virion.

VII. FUNCTIONS OF NONSTRUCTURAL/ACCESSORY GENE PRODUCTS

The genomes of HIV-1 and HIV-2 are very complex, encoding six accessory gene products (Fig. 4; Table 1). The proteins encoded by the accessory genes have been shown to regulate viral gene expression and infectivity (Cullen and Greene, 1990; Kieny, 1990; Haseltine, 1990; Cullen, 1991). The genes found in the central region of HIV-1 are *vif* (virion infectivity factor), *tat* (transactivator of transcription), *rev* (regulator of expression of virion proteins), *vpr*, and *vpu*. HIV-2 and the SIVs contain the *vpx* ORF, instead of *vpu*, which is a distinguishing feature of the primate lentiviruses. All the human and primate lentiviruses also contain an ORF known as *nef* (negative regulatory factor) near the 3′ end of the genome. The *tat, rev,* and *nef* genes are all expressed early, whereas, in the case of HIV-1 at least, the remaining regulatory genes and the structural genes are expressed later in the infection, under the control of the *rev* gene product (see below).

A. Tat

The Tat protein of HIV-1 activates transcription from the viral LTR, increasing the steady-state level of viral RNA in infected cells (Arya et al., 1985; Sodroski et al., 1985; Peterlin et al., 1986; Gendelman et al., 1986). Tat also appears to enhance translation of viral mRNAs through interaction with viral RNA at the "TAR" (transactivation region) site, a region of conserved secondary structure at the 5′ end of all viral RNAs. Tat proteins with a similar function have been identified in other lentiviruses. In HIV-1, Tat is a 14 kD protein, composed of at least two functional domains. A cysteine-rich region, highly conserved among most lentiviruses, is involved in the formation of metal-linked Tat homodimers (Frankel et al., 1988). This domain has been shown to be required for maintenance of a replication-competent phenotype in HIV-1 (Ruben et al., 1989; Rice and Carlotti, 1990). A second domain, rich in basic amino acids, is located in the carboxy portion of the protein and is required for localization of Tat to the nucleoli of infected cells (Hauber et al., 1987; Ruben et al., 1989). A *trans*-dominant HIV-1 *tat* mutant, which truncates the basic domain, is capable of inhibiting *tat*-induced gene expression from the HIV-1 LTR (Pearson et al., 1990). The inhibitory interaction of partially defective regulatory proteins suggests a role for them in antiviral strategies.

B. Rev

The HIV-1 Rev protein enhances production of viral structural proteins by facilitating the transport of unspliced and singly spliced viral RNAs from the nucleus to the cytoplasm (Felber et al., 1989; Malim et al., 1989b; Emerman et al., 1989). The functional expression of Rev is essential for HIV-1 structural gene expression. The 19 kD Rev protein interacts with a structured RNA target (RRE, rev-responsive element) present only in incompletely spliced messages (Malim et al., 1989b; Cullen and Greene, 1990; Cullen, 1991); this interaction overcomes a block in mRNA transport. The mechanism by which Rev facilitates transport of RRE-containing RNAs to the cytoplasm is not well-understood, but it may involve the displacement of cellular splicing factors that hold RNAs containing RRE sequences in the nucleus or the cooperative interaction of Rev with a component of the RNA transport pathway (Chang and Sharp, 1990; Malim et al., 1989b; Felber et al., 1989; Cullen and Greene, 1990; Cullen, 1991). Rev is a phosphoprotein phosphorylated at one or more serine residues, presumably by protein kinase C (Hauber et al., 1988). *Trans*-dominant HIV-1 *rev* mutants that interfere with the function of the wild-type Rev protein were recently described (Malim et al., 1989a; Mermer et al., 1990). Like Tat, Rev contains a basic domain that is required for nuclear (Malim et al., 1989a) and nucleolar (Felber et al., 1989; Cochrane et al., 1990) localization of the protein. This basic domain may also play a role in sequence-specific recognition of the RRE.

C. Vif

The *vif* gene is the largest of the lentiviral central region ORFs, encoding a protein of 192 amino acids in HIV-1 and 215 amino acids in HIV-2. A 23 kD protein has been identified as Vif in HIV-1-infected cells. In HIV-1, the infectivity of cell-free virus derived from *vif* mutants is greatly reduced and fewer viral particles are produced, but the precise nature of the defect remains unknown (Fisher et al., 1987; Strebel et al., 1987). Since viral transcription and protein synthesis appear to be normal in the absence of functional Vif, it was proposed that Vif may play a role in the morphogenesis or maturation of virus particles (Cullen and Greene, 1990). Based on limited amino acid sequence similarity between the HIV-1 and HIV-2 Vif proteins and a family of thiol proteases, it has been suggested that HIV-1 Vif may be a cysteine protease whose function is to modify the gp41 protein (Guy et al., 1991), but a direct role for Vif in HIV infection or pathogenesis has yet to be demonstrated. Vif proteins are poorly conserved among diverse primate lentiviruses, but they contain two short, highly conserved sequence motifs, $SL(I/V)X_4YX_9Y$ (amino-proximal) and SLQXLA (carboxyl-proximal), which are also found in some nonprimate lentiviruses (Oberste and Gonda, 1992). The functional significance of these two short motifs has not been determined, but they demonstrate that the *vif* locus is conserved among divergent lentiviruses. A better understanding of Vif function may come from the study of the products of the *vif* loci present in other lentiviruses.

D. Vpr, Vpu, and Vpx

The functions of Vpr, Vpu, and Vpx remain largely undefined and all three are dispensable for virus replication in vitro. HIV-1 Vpr is a 13 kD protein that has recently been shown to be virion-associated and to interact in *trans* with HIV-1 promoter sequences in the LTR to enhance expression of viral proteins (Yuan et al., 1990; Cohen et al., 1990b). Although Vpr is not required for viral infectivity, there is disagreement over whether it affects the kinetics of viral replication (Dedera et al., 1989; Ogawa et al., 1989).

The 16 kD Vpu protein increases the efficiency of virus maturation and release from infected cells, and may play a role in modulating the cytopathic effect of HIV-1 in culture (Strebel et al., 1989; Terwilliger et al., 1989; Klimkait et al., 1990). In addition, there is evidence that Vpu is phosphorylated and may interact with the membrane of infected cells.

Vpx, a protein of 14–16 kD, appears to be dispensable for HIV-2 replication in culture (Yu et al., 1988; Hu et al., 1989), but Guyader et al. (1989) have reported a 10-fold reduction in virus output by a *vpx* mutant grown in primary lymphocytes. The Vpx is a minor component of HIV-2 and SIV virions (Henderson et al., 1988b), but its function remains obscure. It may have a role in in vivo pathogenesis, which has not yet been discovered in cell culture systems.

E. Nef

The Nef protein of HIV-1 is a 27 kD myristoylated phosphoprotein that is not required for virus replication. Although it has several features in common with the G-protein family of signal transduction proteins, its role in HIV replication and pathogenesis remains controversial. While several investigators have reported that Nef inhibits gene expression from the HIV-1 LTR (Ahmad and Venkatesan, 1988; Niederman et al., 1989), others claim that Nef has no effect on viral gene expression or replication (Kim et al., 1989; Hammes et al., 1989). One must assume that differences in cell types or culture systems must be responsible for these conflicting results. In rhesus macaques experimentally infected with an SIV strain containing a premature stop codon in the *nef* reading frame, there is strong selection for the presence of a functional *nef* ORF (Kestler et al., 1991). The Nef^{+} phenotype may be important in maintaining high virus loads in these animals, which suggests a role for *nef* in the in vivo pathogenesis of primate lentiviruses.

F. Other Accessory Genes

An additional ORF, termed *vpt*, is present in the central region of HIV-1, partially overlapping *tat, rev,* and *vpu* (Sonigo et al., 1985). Since *vpt* lacks an initiator codon, it has been proposed that expression of the putative 17 kD Vpt protein involves a −1 frameshift similar to that required for *pol* ORF translation (Cohen et al., 1990a). Vpt protein has not, however, been detected in HIV-1 infected cells, so its importance in viral replication and/or pathogenesis requires further investigation.

A novel 26–28 kD accessory protein with a tripartite structure has been identified in HIV-1-infected cells. Designated Tnv (Salfeld et al., 1990) or Tev (Benko et al., 1990), this protein incorporates portions of Tat, Env, and Rev and is recognized by monospecific antisera to both Tat and Rev. *tnv/tev*-Specific cDNAs have been described that contain *tat* coding exon 1, a small portion of *env*, and the second coding exon of *rev*. Tnv reportedly has Tat, but not Rev, activity, while Tev has both Tat and Rev activities. While a specific function for Tnv/Tev in HIV infection has not yet been demonstrated, its existence underscores the complexity of lentivirus gene organization and expression strategies.

VIII. ENVELOPE GLYCOPROTEINS AND CELL RECEPTOR

Lentiviruses, and HIV-1 in particular, infect cells of the immune system, most notably lymphocytes and monocytes/macrophages (Gendelman et al., 1986, 1989; Haase, 1986; Gartner and Popovic, 1990). The CD4 molecule is the main portal of entry of HIV-1 (and HIV-2) into the host cell; the interaction of HIV-1 gp120 with CD4 initiates the infection process (Sattentau and Weiss, 1988). HIV-1 gp120 has developed a strong affinity (10^9 M^{-1}) for CD4, and CD4 is the prime cellular determinant in the tropism of this virus (Lasky et al., 1987). In HIV-1 infected cell cultures, anti-CD4 antibodies have been shown to coprecipitate CD4 and gp120 because of this high affinity. The destruction or suppression of CD4+ cells in HIV-1 infections is responsible for the severe immunodeficiency observed in patients with AIDS (Gallo, 1990). Lymphocyte subsets, particularly T-helper cells and monocytes/macrophages, and some bone marrow cells express the CD4 molecule, although there are differences in the concentrations of CD4 on each of these cell types, with CD4+ T lymphocytes having the largest number of molecules.

The HIV-1 Env glycoproteins serve two main functions for the virus. The first is to recognize the cell receptor and the second is to mediate membrane-to-membrane fusion between the virus particle and the uninfected cell. The fusigenic potential of the viral Env proteins also mediates cell-to-cell fusion, probably by a mechanism analogous to that of virus entry, and the formation of multinucleated giant cells (syncytia). The gp41 molecule carries the main determinant for cell fusion. The fusigenic process most likely involves at least two steps: the interaction of gp120 with CD4, followed by interaction of gp41 with the opposing cell membrane. The formation of syncytia may be one explanation for the detection of CD4+ cells in patients with AIDS (Haseltine, 1990). Another possible explanation for the destruction of CD4+ cells may be that free gp120 binds to uninfected cells and a primed immune response destroys these cells. The gp120 and gp41 may also have some immunosuppressive effects by causing the abnormal up- or downregulation of cytokines and an imbalance in their normal pathways.

The host responds to the HIV-1 infection by developing both humoral and cellular immune responses (Javaherian et al., 1989; Lyerly et al., 1990; Walker, 1990). Functional and antigenic maps of the HIV-1 SU and TM proteins have been made and various functional domains, including those involved in CD4 recognition, cytotoxic T-lymphocyte recognition, neutralization, variability, and fusion, have been mapped (Putney et al., 1990). Sera from patients with AIDS contain antibodies that can neutralize the infectivity of HIV-1; the main neutralizing epitope has been mapped to a region of gp120 called the PND (primary neutralizing determinant) or V3 loop (Javaherian et al., 1989), although other domains may also elicit a neutralizing response.

IX. GENOMIC DIVERSITY AND VIRUS PERSISTENCE

Genomic variability is a striking feature of lentivirus biology. Sequence comparisons of the genomes of various isolates of HIV-1 have shown that the greatest sequence divergence exists in the *env* gene (Alizon et al., 1986; Hahn et al., 1986; Starcich et al., 1986; Fisher et al., 1988; Saag et al., 1988). The ability of the virus to mutate rapidly in the face of a strong immune response and create escape variants may be one mechanism the virus uses to ensure its spread within the host, and possibly within populations. However, the major mechanism by which lentiviruses persist in their host is not through virus variability but through the integration of the provirus into the host DNA. Cell tropism is determined by two areas of the virus genome: the Env proteins and the viral LTR (Sodroski et al., 1990; Tong-Starksen and Peterlin, 1990). Each of these regions is very complex in HIV-1. It is conceivable that mutations in either of these two areas could affect the replication capacity of the virus and create variants that differ in cell tropism, replication capacity, or virulence.

X. CONCLUDING REMARKS

The AIDS virus is a complex retrovirus of the lentivirus subfamily that has evolved various strategies to ensure its survival in humans. Most devastating is HIV-1's ability to infect the very cells necessary to defend the host. Nevertheless, because of its complexity, there are stages in its life cycle that may be exploited in attempting to understand its pathogenesis and devise means to eradicate it.

The AIDS epidemic continues to spread worldwide. At the time of this writing, the World Health Organization forecasts that 15 million adults will be infected with HIV-1 by 1995. Although we have amassed considerable knowledge about the molecular biology and structure of HIV-1 and HIV-2, there still are several paradoxes that remain to be solved. First, patients with AIDS develop a strong immune response to the HIV-1 infection in terms of binding and neutralizing antibodies (Allan et al., 1985;

Robey et al., 1985; Javaherian et al., 1989) and cytotoxic T cells are also present (Lyerly et al., 1990; Walker, 1990). Despite this strong response, the patient with AIDS ultimately succumbs to the fatal virus infection. Since there is a long delay between contracting the infection and the onset of clinically apparent AIDS, it is assumed that during this period the immune system is providing adequate protection. We need to define better the protective features of this immune response and try to mimic it. Second, the ability of the virus to mutate rapidly suggests that it can continue to provide a repertoire of mutants to overcome both an antiviral immune response and antiviral drugs. This has already been documented for AIDS patients given AZT (Larder et al., 1989). These two parameters will be the major challenges in developing novel strategies for vaccines and treatments for HIV-1. At the moment, education about AIDS and how it is spread is our best defense against HIV-1 infection.

ACKNOWLEDGMENTS

We thank K. Nagashima for electron microscopy, L. Henderson for thoughtful discussion on HIV proteins, K. Garvey for assistance with computer graphics, L. Pallansch for critical reading of the manuscript, and G. Serig for assistance in preparing the manuscript. This project has been funded in part with Federal funds from the Department of Health and Human Services under contract number NO1-CO-74102 with Program Resources, Inc. The content of this publication does not necessarily reflect the views or policies of the Department of Health and Human Services, nor does mention of trade names, commercial products, or organizations imply endorsement by the U.S. Government.

REFERENCES

Achour, A., Picard, O., Zagury, D., Sarin, P. S., Gallo, R. C., Naylor, P. H., and Goldstein, A. L. (1990). *Proc. Natl. Acad. Sci. USA 87*:7045–7049.

Ahmad, N., and Venkatesan, S. (1988). *Science 241*:1481–1485.

Alizon, M., Wain-Hobson, S., Montagnier, L., and Sonigo, P. (1986). *Cell 46*:63–74.

Allan, J. S., Coligan, J. E., Lee, T.-H., McLane, M. F., Kanki, P. J., Groopman, J. E., and Essex, M. (1985). *Science 230*:810–813.

Arya, S. K., Guo, C., Josephs, S. F., and Wong-Staal, F. (1985). *Science 229*:69–73.

Bachetti, P., and Moss, A. R. (1989). *Nature (London) 338*:251–253.

Barber, A. M., Hizi, A., Maizel, J. V., Jr., and Hughes, S. H. (1990). *AIDS Res. Hum. Retroviruses 6*:1061–1072.

Barre-Sinoussi, F., Chermann, J. C., Rey, F., Nugeyre, M. T., Chamaret, S., Gruest, J., Dauguet, C., Axler-Blin, C., Vézinet-Brun, F., Rouzioux, C., Rozenbaum, W., and Montagnier, L. (1983). *Science 220*:868–871.

Benko, D. M., Schwartz, S., Pavlakis, G. N., and Felber, B. K. (1990). *J. Virol. 64*:2505–2518.

Bushman, F. D., Fujiwara, T., and Craigie, R. (1990). *Science 249*:1555–1558.

Casey, J. M., Kim, Y., Andersen, P. R., Watson, K. F., Fox, J. L., and Devare, S. G. (1985). *J. Virol. 55*:417–423.

Chakrabarti, S., Mizukami, T., Franchini, G., and Moss, B. (1990). *Virology 178*: 134–142.

Chang, D. D., and Sharp, P. A. (1990). *Science 249*:614–615.

Clavel, F., Guétard, D., Brun-Vézinet, F., Chamaret, S., Rey, M.-A., Santos-Ferreira, M. O., Laurent, A. G., Dauguet, C., Katlama, C., Rouzioux, C., Klatzmann, D., Champalimaud, J. L., and Montagnier, L. (1986). *Science 233*:343–346.

Clavel, F., and Orenstein, J. M. (1990). *J. Virol. 64*:5230–5234.

Cochrane, A. W., Perkins, A., and Rosen, C. A. (1990). *J. Virol. 64*:881–885.

Cohen, E. A., Lu, Y., Göttlinger, H., Dehni, G., Jalinoos, Y., Sodroski, J. G., and Haseltine, W. A. (1990a). *J. Acquired Immune Defic. Syndr. 3*:601–608.

Cohen, E. A., Terwilliger, E. F., Jalinoos, Y., Proulx, J., Sodroski, J. G., and Haseltine, W. A. (1990b). *J. Acquired Immune Defic. Syndr. 3*:11–18.

Cullen, B. R. (1991). *J. Virol. 65*:1053–1056.

Cullen, B. R., and Greene, W. C. (1990). *Virology 178*:1–5.

Dalgleish, A. G., Beverley, P. C. L., Clapham, P. R., Crawford, D. H., Greaves, M. F., and Weiss, R. A. (1984). *Nature* (London) *312*:763–766.

Darr, E. S., and Ho, D. D. (1990). *Semin. Virol. 1*:105–214.

Dedera, D., Hu, W., Vander Heyden, N., and Ratner, L. (1989). *J. Virol. 63*:3205–3208.

Delchambre, M., Gheysen, D., Thines, D., Thiriart, C., Jacobs, E., Verdin, E., Horth, M., Burny, A., and Bex, F. (1989). *EMBO J. 8*:2653–2660.

di Marzo Veronese, F. D., Rahman, R., Copeland, T. D., Oroszlan, S., Gallo, R. C., and Sarngadharan, M. G. (1987). *AIDS Res. Hum. Retroviruses 3*:253–264.

Earl, P. L., Doms, R. W., and Moss, B. (1990). *Proc. Natl. Acad. Sci. USA 87*:648–652.

Emerman, M., Vazeux, R., and Peden, K. (1989). *Cell 57*:1155–1165.

Felber, B. K., Hadzopoulou-Cladaras, M., Cladaras, C., Copeland, T., and Pavlakis, G. N. (1989). *Proc. Natl. Acad. Sci. USA 86*:1495–1499.

Ferris, A. L., Hizi, A., Showalter, S. D., Pichuantes, S., Babe, L., Craik, C. S., and Hughes, S. H. (1990). *Virology 175*:456–464.

Fisher, A. G., Ensoli, B., Ivanoff, L., Chamberlain, M., Petteway, S., Ratner, L., Gallo, R. C., and Wong-Staal, F. (1987). *Science 237*:888–893.

Fisher, A. G., Ensoli, B., Looney, D., Rose, A., Gallo, R. C., Saag, M. S., Shaw, G. M., Hahn, B. H., and Wong-Staal, F. (1988). *Nature (London) 334*:444–447.

Frankel, A. D., Bredt, D. S., and Pabo, C. O. (1988). *Science 240*:70–73.

Gallo, R. C., Salahuddin, S. Z., Popovic, M., Shearer, G. M., Kaplan, M., Haynes, B. F., Palker, T. J., Redfield, R., Oleske, J., Safai, B., White, G., Foster, P., and Markham, P. D. (1984). *Science 224*:500–503.

Gallo, R., Wong-Staal, F., Montagnier, L., Haseltine, W. A., and Yoshida, M. (1988). *Nature* (London) *333*:504.
Gallo, R. C. (1990). *J. Acquired Immune Defic. Syndr. 3*:380–389.
Gartner, S., and Popovic, M. (1990). *AIDS Res. Hum. Retroviruses 6*:1017–1021.
Garvey, K. J., Oberste, M. S., Elser, J. E., Braun, M. J., and Gonda, M. A. (1990). *Virology 175*:391–409.
Gelderblom, H. R., Özel, M., Gheysen, D., Reupke, H., Winkel, T., Herz, U., Grund, C., and Pauli, G. (1990). In *Animal Models in AIDS*, H. Schellekens and M. C. Horzinek (Eds.), Elsevier, Amsterdam, pp. 1–26.
Gendelman, H. E., Phelps, W., Feigenbaum, L., Ostrove, J. M., Adachi, A., Howley, P. M., Khoury, G., Ginsberg, H. S., and Martin, M. A. (1986). *Proc. Natl. Acad. Sci. USA 83*:9759–9763.
Gendelman, H. E., Orenstein, J. M., Baca, L. M., Weiser, B., Burger, H., Kalter, D. C., and Meltzer, M. S. (1989). *AIDS 3*:475–495.
Gheysen, D., Jacobs, E., De Foresta, F., Thiriart, C., Francotte, M., Thines, D., and De Wilde, M. (1989). *Cell 59*:103–112.
Gonda, M. A. (1988). *J. Electron Microsc. Tech. 8*:17–40.
Gonda, M. A., Wong-Staal, F., Gallo, R. C., Clements, J. E., Narayan, O., and Gilden, R. V. (1985). *Science 227*:173–177.
Gonda, M. A., Braun, M. J., Clements, J. E., Pyper, J. M., Gallo, R. C., Wong-Staal, F., and Gilden, R. V. (1986). *Proc. Natl. Acad. Sci. USA 83*:4007–4011.
Gonda, M. A., Boyd, A. L., Nagashima, K., and Gilden, R. V. (1989). *Arch. AIDS Res. 3*:1–42.
Gorelick, R. J., Nigida, S. M., Jr., Bess, J. W., Jr., Arthur, L. O., Henderson, L. E., and Rein, A. (1990). *J. Virol. 64*:3207–3211.
Gottlieb, M. S., Schroff, R., Schanker, H. M., Weisman, J. D., Pan, P. T., Wolf, R. A., and Saxon, A. (1981). *N. Engl. J. Med. 305*:1425–1431.
Gottlinger, H. G., Sodroski, J. G., and Haseltine, W. A. (1989). *Proc. Natl. Acad. Sci. USA 86*:5781–5785.
Guy, B., Geist, M., Dott, K., Spehner, D., Kieny, M.-P., and Lecocq, J.-P. (1991). *J. Virol. 65*:1325–1331.
Guyader, M., Emerman, M., Sonigo, P., Clavel, F., Montagnier, L., and Alizon, M. (1987). *Nature* (London) *326*:662–669.
Guyader, M., Emerman, M., Montagnier, L., and Peden, K. (1989). *EMBO J. 8*:1169–1175.
Haase, A. T. (1986). *Nature* (London) *322*:130–136.
Hahn, B. H., Shaw, G. M., Taylor, M. E., Redfield, R. R., Markham, P. D., Salahuddin, S. Z., Wong-Staal, F., Gallo, R. C., Parks, E. S., and Parks, W. P. (1986). *Science 232*:1548–1553.
Hammes, S. R., Dixon, E. P., Malim, M. H., Cullen, B. R., and Greene, W. C. (1989). *Proc. Natl. Acad. Sci. USA 86*:9549–9533.
Haseltine, W. A. (1990). In *AIDS and the New Viruses*, A. G. Dalgleish and R. A. Weiss (Eds.). Academic Press, San Diego, CA, pp. 11–40.
Hauber, J., Perkins, A., Heimer, E. P., and Cullen, B. R. (1987). *Proc. Natl. Acad. Sci. USA 84*:6364–6368.

Hauber, J., Bouvier, M., Malim, M. H., and Cullen, B. R. (1988). *J. Virol. 62*: 4801–4804.
Henderson, L. E., Copeland, T. D., Sowder, R. C., Schultz, A. M., and Oroszlan, S. (1988a). In *Human Retroviruses, Cancer, and AIDS: Approaches to Prevention and Therapy*. D. Bolognesi (Ed.). Alan R. Liss, New York, pp. 135–147.
Henderson, L. E., Sowder, R. C., Copeland, T. D., Benveniste, R. E., and Oroszlan, S. (1988b). *Science 241*:199–201.
Hizi, A., McGill, C., and Hughes, S. H. (1988). *Proc. Natl. Acad. Sci. USA 85*:1218–1222.
Hu, W., Heyden, N. V., and Ratner, L. (1989). *Virology 173*:624–630.
Jacks, T., Power, M. D., Masiarz, F. R., Luciw, P. A., Barr, P. J., and Varmus, H. E. (1988). *Nature* (London) *331*:280–283.
Javaherian, K., Langlois, A. J., McDanal, C., Ross, K. L., Eckler, L. I., Jellis, C. L., Profy, A. T., Rusche, J. R., Bolognesi, D. P., Putney, S. D., and Matthews, T. J. (1989). *Proc. Natl. Acad. Sci. USA 86*:6768–6772.
Jordan, C. A., Watkins, B. A., Kufta, C., and Dubois-Dalcq, M. (1991). *J. Virol. 65*:736–742.
Karacostas, V., Nagashima, K., Gonda, M. A., and Moss, B. (1989). *Proc. Natl. Acad. Sci. USA 86*:8964–8967.
Kestler, H. W., III, Ringler, D. J., Mori, K., Panicali, D. L., Sehgal, P. K., Daniel, M. D., and Desrosiers, R. C. (1991). *Cell 65*:651–662.
Kieny, M. P. (1990). *J. Acquired Immune Defic. Syndr. 3*:395–402.
Kim, S., Ikeuchi, K., Bryn, R., Groopman, J., and Baltimore, D. (1989). *Proc. Natl. Acad. Sci. USA 86*:9544–9548.
Klatzmann, D., Champagne, E., Chamaret, S., Gruest, J., Guetard, D., Hercend, T., Gluckman, J. C., and Montagnier, L. (1984). *Nature* (London) *312*:767–768.
Klimkait, T., Strebel, K., Hoggan, M. D., Martin, M. A., and Orenstein, J. M. (1990). *J. Virol. 64*:621–629.
Larder, B. A., Darby, G., and Richman, D. D. (1989). *Science 243*:1731–1734.
Lasky, L. A., Nakamura, G., Smith, D. H., Fennie, C., Shimasaki, C., Patzer, E., Berman, P., Gregory, T., and Capon, D. J. (1987). *Cell 50*:975–85.
Laurence, J. (1988). *AIDS Res. Hum. Retroviruses 4*:vii–viii.
Leis, J., Baltimore, D., Bishop, J. M., Coffin, J., Fleissner, E., Goff, S. P., Oroszlan, S., Robinson, H., Skalka, A. M., Temin, H. M., and Vogt, V. (1988). *J. Virol. 62*:1808–1809.
Lightfoote, M. M., Coligan, J. E., Folks, T. M., Fauci, A. S., Martin, M. A., and Venkatesan, S. (1986). *J. Virol. 60*:771–775.
Lillehoj, E. P., Salazar, F. H. R., Mervis, R. J., Raum, M. G., Chan, H. W., Ahmad, N., and Venkatesan, S. (1988). *J. Virol. 62*:3053–3058.
Lyerly, H. K., Tyler, D. S., Nastala, C. L., and Weinhold, K. J. (1990). In *AIDS Vaccine Research and Clinical Trials*, S. D. Putney and D. P. Bolognesi (Eds.). Marcel Dekker, New York, pp. 157–177.
Malim, M. H., Böhnlein, S., Hauber, J., and Cullen, B. R. (1989a). *Cell 58*:205–214.
Malim, M. H., Hauber, J., Le, S.-Y., Maizel, J. V., and Cullen, B. R. (1989b). *Nature* (London) *338*:254–257.

Mann, J. M. (1990). *J. Acquired Immune Defic. Syndr. 3*:438–442.
Meltzer, M. S., Nakamura, M., Hansen, B. D., Turpin, J. A., Kalter, D. C., and Gendelman, H. E. (1990). *AIDS Res. Hum. Retroviruses 6*:967–971.
Mermer, B., Felber, B. K., Campbell, M., and Pavlakis, G. N. (1990). *Nucleic Acids Res. 18*:2037–2044.
Mervis, R. J., Ahmad, N., Lillehoj, E. P., Raum, M. G., Salazar, F. H. R., Chan, H. W., and Venkatesan, S. (1988). *J. Virol. 62*:3993–4002.
Miller, M., Jaskolski, M., Rao, J. K. M., Leis, J., and Wlodawer, A. (1989). *Nature* (London) *337*:576–579.
Moss, B., Earl, P. L., and Doms, R. W. (1991). In *Retroviruses of Human AIDS and Related Animal Diseases*. M. Girard and L. Valette (Eds.). Pasteur Mérieux, Paris, France, pp. 177–180.
Muesing, M. A., Smith, D. H., Cabradilla, C. D., Benton, C. V., Lasky, L. A., and Capon, D. J. (1985). *Nature* (London) *313*:450–458.
Naylor, P. H., Naylor, C. W., Badamchian, M., Wada, S., Goldstein, A. L., Wang, S.-S., Sun, D. K., Thornton, A. H., and Sarin, P. S. (1987). *Proc. Natl. Acad. Sci. USA 84*:2951–2955.
Niederman, T. M. J., Thielan, B. J., and Ratner, L. (1989). *Proc. Natl. Acad. Sci. USA 86*:1128–1132.
Oberste, M. S., and Gonda, M. A. (1992). *Virus Genes 6*:95–102.
Ogawa, K., Shibata, R., Kiyomasu, T., Higuchi, I., Kishida, Y., Ishimoto, A., and Adachi, A. (1989). *J. Virol. 63*:4110–4114.
Papsidero, L. D., Sheu, M., and Ruscetti, F. W. (1989). *J. Virol. 63*:267–272.
Pearson, L., Garcia, J., Wu, F., Modesti, N., Nelson, J., and Gaynor, R. (1990). *Proc. Natl. Acad. Sci. USA 87*:5079–5083.
Peterlin, B. M., Luciw, P. A., Barr, P. J., and Walker, M. D. (1986). *Proc. Natl. Acad. Sci. USA 83*:9734–9738.
Pinter, A., Honnen, W. J., Tilley, S. A., Bona, C., Zaghouani, H., Gorny, M. K., and Zolla-Pazner, S. (1989). *J. Virol. 63*:2674–2679.
Piot, P., Laga, M., Ryder, R., Perriens, J., Temmerman, M., Heyward, W., and Curran, J. W. (1990). *J. Acquired Immune Defic. Syndr. 3*:403–412.
Putney, S. D., Javaherian, K., Rusche, J., Matthews, T., and Bolognesi, D. P. (1990). In *AIDS Vaccine Research and Clinical Trials*. S. D. Putney and D. P. Bolognesi (Eds.). Marcel Dekker, New York, pp. 3–61.
Rabson, A. B., Daugherty, D. F., Venkatesan, S., Boulukos, K. E., Been, S. I., Folks, T. M., Feorino, P., and Martin, M. A. (1985). *Science 229*: 1388–1390.
Rasmussen, L., Battles, J. K., Ennis, W. H., Nagashima, K., and Gonda, M. A. (1990). *Virology 178*:435–451.
Ratner, L., Haseltine, W., Patarca, R., Livak, K. J., Starcich, B., Josephs, S. F., Doran, E. R., Rafalski, J. A., Whitehorn, E. A., Baumeister, K., Ivanoff, L., Petteway, S. R., Jr., Pearson, M. L., Lautenberger, J. A., Papas, T. S., Ghrayeb, J., Chang, N. T., Gallo, R. C., and Wong-Staal, F. (1985). *Nature* (London) *313*:277–284.
Rice, A. P., and Carlotti, F. (1990). *J. Virol. 64*:1864–1868.
Robey, W. G., Safai, B., Oroszlan, S., Arthur, L. O., Gonda, M. A., Gallo, R. C., and Fischinger, P. J. (1985). *Science 228*:593–595.

Romieu, I., Marlink, R., Kanki, P., M'Boup, S., and Essex, M. (1990). *J. Acquired Immune Defic. Syndr.* *3*:220–230.
Ruben, S., Perkins, A., Purcell, R., Joung, K., Sia, R., Burghoff, R., Haseltine, W. A., and Rosen, C. A. (1989). *J. Virol.* *63*:1–8.
Saag, M. S., Hahn, B. H., Gibbons, J., Li, Y., Parks, E. S., Parks, W. P., and Shaw, G. M. (1988). *Nature* (London) *334*:440–444.
Salfeld, J., Göttlinger, H. G., Sia, R. A., Park, R. E., Sodroski, J. G., and Haseltine, W. A. (1990). *EMBO J.* *9*:965–970.
Sanchez-Pescador, R., Power, M. D., Barr, P. J., Steimer, K. S., Stempien, M. M., Brown-Shimer, S. L., Gee, W. W., Renard, A., Randolph, A., Levy, J. A., Dina, D., and Luciw, P. A. (1985). *Science* *227*: 484–492.
Sattentau, Q. J., and Weiss, R. A. (1988). *Cell* *52*:631–633.
Schawaller, M., Smith, G. E., Skehel, J. J., and Wiley, D. C. (1989). *Virology* *172*:367–369.
Schultz, A. M., Henderson, L. E., and Oroszlan, S. (1988). *Annu. Rev. Cell Biol.* *4*:611–647.
Shaw, G. M., Harper, M. E., Hahn, B. H., Epstein, L. G., Gajdusek, D. C., Price, R. W., Navia, B. A., Petito, C. K., O'Hara, C. J., Groopman, J. E., Cho, E.-S., Oleske, J. M., Wong-Staal, F., and Gallo, R. C. (1985). *Science* *227*:177–182.
Sodroski, J., Rosen, C., Wong-Staal, F., Salahuddin, S. Z., Popovic, M., Arya, S., Gallo, R. C., and Haseltine, W. A. (1985). *Science* *227*:171–173.
Sodroski, J., Kowalski, M., and Haseltine, W. (1990). In *AIDS Vaccine Research and Clinical Trials*. S. D. Putney and D. P. Bolognesi (Eds.). Marcel Dekker, New York, pp. 93–106.
Sonigo, P., Alizon, M., Staskus, K., Klatzmann, D., Cole, S., Danos, O., Retzel, E., Tiollais, P., Haase, A., and Wain-Hobson, S. (1985). *Cell* *42*:369–382.
Starcich, B. R., Hahn, B. H., Shaw, G. M., McNeely, P. D., Modrow, S., Wolf, H., Parks, E. S., Parks, W. P., Josephs, S. F., Gallo, R. C., and Wong-Staal, F. (1986). *Cell* *45*:637–648.
Steinberg, H. N., Crumpacker, C. S., and Chatis, P. A. (1991). *J. Virol.* *65*: 1765–1769.
Strebel, K., Daugherty, D., Clouse, K., Cohen, D., Folks, T., and Martin, M. A. (1987). *Nature* (London) *328*:728–730.
Strebel, K., Klimkait, T., Maldarelli, F., and Martin, M. A. (1989). *J. Virol.* *63*:3784–3791.
Swanstrom, R., Kaplan, A. H., and Manchester, M. (1990). *Semin. Virol.* *1*:175–186.
Terwilliger, E. F., Cohen, E. A., Lu, Y., Sodroski, J. G., and Haseltine, W. A. (1989). *Proc. Natl. Acad. Sci. USA* *86*:5163–5167.
Tong-Starksen, S., and Peterlin, B. M. (1990). *Semin. Virol.* *1*:215–227.
Varmus, H. (1988). *Science* *240*:1427–1435.
Wain-Hobson, S., Sonigo, P., Danos, O., Cole, S., and Alizon, M. (1985). *Cell* *40*:9–17.
Walker, B. D. (1990). In *AIDS Vaccine Research and Clinical Trials*. S. D. Putney and D. P. Bolognesi (Eds.). Marcel Dekker, New York, pp. 179–194.

Walker, B. D., Chakrabarti, S., Moss, B., Paradis, T. J., Flynn, T., Durno, A. G., Blumberg, R. S., Kaplan, J. C., Hirsch, M. S., and Schooley, R. T. (1987). *Nature* (London) *328*:345–348.

Watkins, B. A., Dorn, H. H., Kelly, W. B., Armstrong, R. C., Potts, B. J., Michaels, F., Kufta, C. V., and Dubois-Dalcq, M. (1990). *Science* *249*:549–553.

Weiss, C. D., Levy, J. A., and White, J. M. (1990). *J. Virol.* *64*:5674–5677.

Willey, R. L., Bonifacino, J. S., Potts, B. J., Martin, M. A., and Klausner, R. D. (1988). *Proc. Natl. Acad. Sci. USA* *85*:9580–9584.

Yu, X.-F., Ito, S., Essex, M., and Lee, T.-H. (1988). *Nature* (London) *335*:262–265.

Yuan, X., Matsuda, Z., Matsuda, M., Essex, M., and Lee, T. H. (1990). *AIDS Res. Hum. Retroviruses* *6*:1265–1271.

Zon, L. I., Arkin, C., and Groopman, J. E. (1987). *Br. J. Haematol.* *66*:251–257.

2

AIDS

Drug Discovery and Targets for Anti-HIV Therapy

Matthew A. Gonda and Owen S. Weislow *Program Resources, Inc./ DynCorp, National Cancer Institute—Frederick Cancer Research and Development Center, Frederick, Maryland*

I. INTRODUCTION

The human immunodeficiency virus (HIV) is the causative agent of the acquired immunodeficiency syndrome (AIDS). HIV-induced AIDS is characterized as a progressively debilitating disease with clinical manifestations that include lymphadenopathy, immunodeficiency, opportunistic infections, encephalopathy, emaciation, and cancers. The worldwide prevalence of HIV infections and AIDS is indicative of a pandemic; moreover, the number of new cases of HIV infection and AIDS continues to rise. Despite the fact that HIV-infected individuals mount a strong humoral and probably also a cellular immune response to the virus, the infection remains recalcitrant and persists for the patient's life. It appears that most, if not all, HIV-infected individuals eventually succumb to the disease and die within 10 years of acquiring the virus. The large "at risk" population, lack of an "effective" naturally acquired protective immunity to HIV, and the long duration over which a patient with AIDS survives highlight the urgent need for vaccines and the discovery of novel antiviral drugs.

HIV is a sophisticated retrovirus with a complex life cycle. This, coupled with the fact that it takes nearly a decade from the initial infection for the acute stages of disease to occur, suggests that the development of therapeutic approaches to control HIV replication and disease and prolong survival are both feasible and warranted. The practicality of therapy has recently been demonstrated with the dideoxynucleoside drugs 3′-azido-2′,3′-dideoxythymidine (AZT, or zidovudine) (Mitsuya et al., 1985; Yarchoan et al., 1986; Richman et al., 1987) and 2′,3′-dideoxyinosine (ddI) (Mitsuya and Broder, 1986), which were shown to bestow significant clinical benefits to patients with AIDS in both early and advanced stages of HIV infection.

The discussion in this chapter focuses on three topics. The first is to provide a brief overview of the structure and molecular biology of HIV and point to some salient stages in the virus–cell interaction that could be exploited in the development of therapeutic agents. A detailed review of the evolutionary, molecular, and structural aspects of the biology of HIV is found in Chapter 1, by Gonda and Oberste. The second charge is to describe the rationale behind, approaches to, and utility of in vitro antiviral screens in HIV drug discovery programs. The final aspect is a description of relevant lentivirus-animal models that may provide useful in vivo systems to test the pharmacokinetics, toxicity, and efficacy of therapeutic agents for HIV before they are used in humans. The reader is also referred to several excellent recent reviews that detail targeted therapy and advances in antiviral drug development for HIV (Mitsuya et al., 1990, 1991; Richman, 1990).

A. HIV Is a Pathogenic Retrovirus

To date, two distinct types of HIV have been discovered. The first is HIV type 1 (HIV-1), which is responsible for almost all of the clinical cases of AIDS reported. The other is HIV type 2 (HIV-2). Both HIV-1 and HIV-2 are infectious, cytopathic, and pathogenic members of the lentivirus subfamily of retroviruses (Gonda et al., 1985, 1986; Guyader et al., 1987). However, HIV-2 is more closely related to the simian immunodeficiency viruses (SIVs) and is seldom the cause of severe clinical illness. Most of the discussion of HIV will center on HIV-1 because of its prominence in the AIDS epidemic.

B. Overview of HIV Structure and Genome Organization

HIV-1 and HIV-2 are examples of organizationally complex retroviruses. Nevertheless, the HIV particle shares many structural traits with other exogenously transmitted retroviruses. HIVs are protein-encapsulated, plus-stranded RNA viruses that contain a unique enzyme, reverse transcriptase, which catalyzes the flow of genetic information from RNA to DNA, counter to most biological systems. The mature extracellular virus particle of HIV-1 can be subdivided into two major components: the viral core and envelope. The core is composed of *gag* and *pol* gene products, the major component being the capsid protein, p24; the minor components of the core are the nucleocapsid (p7), a small Gag protein (p6), and Pol proteins. A Pol derivative, the viral protease, is responsible for cleaving the Gag precursor (Pr55) and Gag–Pol polyproteins into their individual subunits. Two copies of the viral RNA genome, believed to be in the form of a dimer, are also found in the core of the virion. The viral envelope is derived from the plasma membrane and is comprised of the viral surface (gp120) and transmembrane (gp41) proteins and cellular proteins and lipids; the viral envelope proteins are highly glycosylated (Robey et al., 1985). In addition, the matrix protein (p17) of the *gag* gene is probably inserted in the viral envelope, which helps to localize the Gag precursor in the cell membrane during virus assembly. HIV is released from the cell membrane by budding.

Retroviruses replicate via a double-stranded DNA intermediate (called the provirus) formed through the activity of reverse transcriptase during transcription of the viral RNA. RNase H activity is also localized on the reverse transcriptase molecule and is utilized in degrading the viral RNA during second-strand DNA synthesis. The genome of HIV-1 is comprised of *gag, pol,* and *env* structural genes flanked on the 5′ and 3′ termini by the long terminal repeats (LTRs); the LTRs contain the regulatory sequences for the initiation, enhancement, and termination of transcription. In addition to the structural genes, there are six nonstructural/regulatory genes, often referred to as accessory genes. Five of these accessory genes are found in the central region of the genome between and overlapping the *pol* and *env* genes. The five accessory genes in the central region are called *vif* (viral infectivity factor), *tat* (trans-activator of transcription), *rev* (regulator of expression of virion proteins), *vpu,* and *vpr.* The *vpu* and *vpr* genes are believed to be involved in enhancing virus release and *trans*-activating the LTR, respectively. The sixth accessory gene, *nef* (negative regulatory factor), is located near the 3′ end of the genome; its role in up- and/or downregulating virus expression is controversial. As their names indicate, the products of several of the accessory genes are involved in regulating virus expression and infectivity. These proteins, as targets for therapy, will be discussed further below.

C. Significance of the Virus Life Cycle in Antiviral Strategies

The life cycle of HIV-1 is intricate and provides numerous opportunities for virus-specific therapeutic intervention. This intervention can be through stimulation of the immune response to the virus (immunotherapy) or by the introduction of inhibitory compounds (antiviral drugs). To date, however, neither approach has provided a definitive solution. The HIV life cycle can be divided into two phases: attachment, penetration, uncoating, reverse transcription, and integration; and transcription, translation, virus assembly, and release. The first interaction of the virus with its host cell (CD4+ lymphocyte or monocyte/macrophage) is accomplished through the specific binding (attachment) of viral (gp120) and cell (CD4) receptor. The viral envelope is believed to fuse with the cell membrane at the site of attachment, probably through the activity of the fusigenic domain of the transmembrane protein (gp41), thus permitting penetration. Penetration and uncoating of the virus particle occur next, releasing the naked RNA into the cytoplasm where it is transcribed by virion-associated reverse transcriptase into the double-stranded proviral DNA genome. The provirus migrates to the nucleus, where integration takes place with the help of the integrase protein (Varmus, 1988). The genome can remain transcriptionally silent until regulatory sequences in the LTR are activated by physical or physiological (host cell or heterologous virus) factors. Once activated, cellular RNA polymerases transcribe the DNA into genomic- and subgenomic-length viral transcripts that are translated into viral proteins. At this stage in the replication cycle, the accessory proteins are believed to orchestrate the correct expression, assembly, and release of immature virus particles by budding. The viral protease is believed to act in the late phase of replication, probably after release of the immature virions, by cleaving the Gag and Gag–Pol precursors into their individual functional subunits. Cleavage of the precursors by the activity of the viral protease is believed to be necessary for achieving infectivity by the virion (Kohl et al., 1988).

II. TARGETS FOR THE DISCOVERY AND DESIGN OF ANTIVIRAL DRUGS

A. Structural Proteins in the Virus

Env

The binding between viral (gp120) and cell (CD4) receptors provides the first interaction in the virus life cycle that is amenable to antiviral intervention. Disruption of the viral–cell receptor interaction has been accomplished in vitro by the use of soluble recombinant CD4 molecules (Capon et al., 1989; Clapham et al., 1989; Daar et al., 1990). In natural infections, antibodies that bind to the viral glycoproteins may also offer some protection by neutralizing the penetration and spread of the virus (Javaherian et al., 1989) or targeting infected cells for destruction by the cellular arm of the immune response (Lyerly et al., 1990; Walker, 1990). Such antibodies may naturally act to slow the progression of AIDS since HIV-infected individuals remain healthy for long periods before succumbing to the advanced stages of AIDS. It may be possible to improve on this immune response by genetically engineering specific epitopes that are functionally deficient in CD4-receptor binding for use in postinfection vaccination (van Kuyk et al., 1990). There are two possible drawbacks to this approach. One is the significant variability between different isolates of the AIDS virus. Such variability will make it difficult to find a set of epitopes that will be useful for all variants. Perhaps a cocktail of gp120 epitopes will be necessary. The other negative factor is that certain antibodies in sera from HIV-1-infected individuals may enhance infection by the use of the immunoglobulin Fc receptor in concert with CD4 (Takeda and Ennis, 1990; Takeda et al., 1990). Polyanionic polysaccharides, such as dextran sulfate, that interfere with virus–cell receptor binding may also be used (Veno and Kuno, 1987; Callahan et al., 1991). To date, however, these have not proven clinically useful (Abrams et al., 1989). The second event in virus attachment is the fusion of viral envelope and cell membrane at the site of virus attachment. Antibodies that inhibit fusion by gp41 may also be important in preventing virus entry. Perhaps fusigenic epitopes of gp41 in combination with a cocktail of gp120 epitopes, as mentioned above, could be employed. Moreover, this approach may also inhibit the cell-to-cell spread of the virus. A novel agent, oxathiin caboxanilide, recently described by Bader et al. (1991), may act by inhibiting viral–cell or cell–cell fusion.

Gag

The Gag precursor (Pr55) is myristoylated at its amino terminus and is the major protein found in immature virions. The Gag precursor is cleaved by the viral protease into the functional subunits, p17, p24, p7, and p6, the matrix, capsid, nucleocapsid, and a small protein believed to be involved in viral core assembly beneath the plasma membrane, respectively. Inhibition of Gag processing by the viral protease will be discussed below. The matrix protein, p17, interacts with the cell membrane and thus may be accessible to neutralizing antibodies and a target for cytotoxic lymphocytes (Sarin et al., 1986; Papsidero et al., 1989; Achour et al., 1990), as with the gp120 and gp41 proteins. The p24, p7, and p6 proteins are internal to the cell membrane and are inaccessible to antibodies. The p7 is the HIV-1 nucleoprotein that functions as a homodimer and is involved in encapsidation of the viral RNA; it may also be involved in assembly of Gag precursor molecules into the functional core structure beneath the plasma membrane. Perhaps the rational design of inhibitors of nucleoprotein function may be possible.

B. Viral Proteins with Enzymatic Function

The Pol precursor is synthesized along with Gag sequences by a –1 frameshift in the translation of the genomic length mRNA to yield a Gag–Pol polyprotein (Jacks et al., 1988; Varmus, 1988). The Gag and Pol portions of the Gag–Pol polyproteins are cleaved from one another by the viral protease. The protease further cleaves the Gag and Pol precursors into their functional active subunit forms. The Pol precursor in the HIV-1 Gag–Pol polyprotein is comprised of three proteins with enzymatic function: the viral protease, reverse transcriptase, and integrase. The reverse transcriptase and protease proteins have proven the most promising targets for antiviral therapy.

Protease

The viral protease of HIV-1 is structurally related to the family of aspartyl-type proteases (Swanstrom et al., 1990). Its homodimeric structure has been determined by x-ray crystallography (Meek et al., 1989; Wlodawer et al., 1989). The data from this analysis, in part, have provided the catalyst for the rational design of specific inhibitors of the HIV-1 protease (Dreyer et al., 1989; DesJarlais et al., 1990; Erikson et al., 1990; Kempf et al., 1990). Based on the three-dimensional structure of the protease active site, twofold (C2) symmetrical inhibitors have been successfully synthesized that are 10,000 times more potent in vitro against the HIV-1 protease than against related cellular aspartyl-type proteases (Erikson et al., 1990; Kempf et al., 1990). This avenue of research may lead to the rational design of additional compounds effective against the viral protease.

Reverse Transcriptase

By far the most progress in anti-HIV therapy has come from compounds that inhibit the viral reverse transcriptase. The viral reverse transcriptase is a heterodimer made up of a p66 and p51 molecule; the carboxyl terminus of the p66 molecule contains the RNase H activity. Several nucleoside analogues including AZT and ddI are potent reverse transcriptase inhibitors, as mentioned above, and are currently being used clinically to treat HIV-1 infections; several more are in various stages of clinical testing (Mitsuya et al., 1990, 1991). The high error rate of the HIV-1 reverse transcriptase is believed to be the main source of genetic variability in the HIV-1 genome (Roberts et al., 1988). Such variability may lead to HIV-1 variants that are drug resistant; in the case of AZT, drug-resistant strains already have been described (Larder et al., 1989; Larder and Kemp, 1989). A new class of reverse transcriptase inhibitors specific for HIV-1, tetra-imidazo [4,5,1-jk][1,4]-benzodiazepine-2(IH)-one and -thrione derivatives of benzodiazepine (TIBO) was recently described (Pauwels et al., 1990). These nonnucleoside reverse transcriptase inhibitors appear to act through mechanisms other than chain termination. Specific inhibitors of RNase H function may also be forthcoming.

Integrase

The integrase protein is responsible for inserting the provirus into the host genome. This is accomplished by modifying the terminal nucleotides from the 3′ ends of each DNA strand in the proviral genome before splicing it to host sequences. Once this is accomplished, the virus becomes part of the host genome, replicating every time the host DNA replicates, until the infected cell dies or is removed by the host's immune response. Little more is known of the integrase protein. Nevertheless, because of its enzymatic function, purified HIV-1 integrase protein would be an important target for crystallization studies and may provide some clues to the rational design of integrase inhibitors.

C. Viral Accessory/Regulatory Gene Products

The accessory genes of HIV-1 are involved in regulating virus expression and the infectivity of the virus particle. The activities of the Tat and Rev proteins are fairly well understood (Cullen and Greene, 1990; Cullen, 1991; Haseltine, 1990). Tat binds to specific sequences in the *trans*-activating region (TAR) of the LTR to enhance transcription and translation. Rev binds to the rev responsive element (RRE) found in the 5′ portion of the transmembrane region of *env* in unspliced or singly spliced messages to facilitate their transport to the cytoplasm. Cellular factors may cooperate in the activity of these two proteins. The activities of Vif, Vpu, and Vpr are less well understood. Since the nonstructural/accessory proteins are intracellular proteins, accessibility to interventive strategies become problematic. As yet unidentified diffusible inhibitors that interfere with Tat or Rev function by blocking their interaction with TAR or RRE target sequences, respectively, may be one approach. The use of antisense DNA to inhibit the translation of *tat* and *rev*, or any other genes, may be another approach (Agrawal et al., 1989; Graham and Maio, 1990; Rhodes and James, 1990; Agrawal, 1991; Sczakiel and Pawlita, 1991).

III. IN VITRO VIRAL SCREENS IN DRUG DISCOVERY PROGRAMS

A. Approaches to the In Vitro Identification of Anti-HIV Drugs

Several excellent reviews of general approaches to in vitro and in vivo testing of antiviral drugs and discussions of specific HIV antiviral agents already exist in the literature (see for example, Kern, 1990; Richman, 1990; Mitsuya et al., 1991). We will try, in this discussion, to review techniques that have found general acceptance in drug discovery efforts aimed specifically at HIV and point the reader to references with sufficient technical detail for further study. The emphasis in this discussion will be focused more on the technology of in vitro screening than on specific agents. Only two compounds (AZT and ddl) have actually been approved for clinical use, both of them nucleoside analogs that are antagonists of the viral reverse transcriptase (Yarchoan et al., 1986, 1988; Ahluwalia et al., 1987; Mitsuya et al., 1991). The techniques described here will, we hope, provide a stimulus for the identification of agents with alternative mechanisms of action.

Investigators may choose between rational or empirical approaches to identify antiviral agents (Prusoff et al., 1990). Rational or target-specific protocols can be used effectively where biochemical events, specific to viral replication, have been identified. Enzymes, macromolecules, regulatory proteins, and virus-specific receptors are useful targets for this approach. Contrary to empirical or "blind screening" approaches, which detect a broader range of drug specificities, target-specific rational methods depend on a detailed understanding of a target's structure or biochemistry. HIV's complex replicative cycle, including its viral-specific regulatory pathways, makes it a prime target for rational studies. Advances in x-ray crystallography and nuclear magnetic resonance have provided three-dimensional structures for several important HIV-associated enzymes and structural components (for a review, see Prusoff et al., 1990). Such structural information permits the design of inhibitors that are active against specific viral functions (e.g., the HIV viral protease). Thus, the rational approach lends itself to the development of viral-specific therapies that can be identified only by chance in "blind screening." However, the rational approach is not a useful procedure for large-scale drug discovery. Typically, rational studies use molecular or biochemical assays or unusual cellular or molecular constructs created using contemporary recombinant DNA technologies. Most are target-specific, in vitro systems that do not directly provide quantitative information on drug toxicity. For this and other reasons, rational assays require follow-up testing in cell-based systems. Finally, one would require a great deal of information about both the virus replicative cycle and multiple-target systems to cover the entire virus life cycle. Thus, where economy is an issue, large-scale drug discovery programs should not be restricted to the rational approach.

Untargeted assay methodologies support empirical or "blind screening" of materials for antiviral activity. Contrary to target-specific rational techniques, empirical approaches are typically cell-based and measure the end result of virus infection such as the development of cytopathic effects (CPE), release of viral structural or enzymatic components, and the production of infectious virions. One need not have a keen understanding of virus-specific targets to use such strategies, and a single assay will usually suffice as a primary screen for agents acting in any portion of the virus replicative cycle. In addition, assuming one chooses the appropriate assay endpoint, cell-based systems can provide effective drug concentration and toxicity data in a single assay. The final choice as to the type of assay used must take many other factors into account, including types of materials to be tested (pure synthetics, natural product extracts, or colored compounds) and whether they will require additional purification (e.g., bioassay-guided fractionation of natural product extracts). Some of the general features that are considered a prerequisite for an ideal anti-HIV drug screen are listed in Table 1, and serve as a useful starting point.

B. The Ideal Antiviral Screen

To be truly useful, an empirical screen must be able to handle very large numbers of samples. The National Cancer Institute's anti-AIDS virus primary screen, for example, is geared to handle 20,000–40,000 samples yearly (Boyd, 1988; Weislow et al., 1989). Such capacity increases the

TABLE 1 The Ideal Anti-HIV Screen

Safe
Simple
Rapid turnaround
Reproducible
Adaptable to automated or semiautomated technologies
Handle large numbers of samples
Handle microliter aliquots
Duplicate in vivo events
Yield effective and cytotoxic doses
Identify actives regardless of mechanism
Inexpensive

potential for exposure of technical staff to HIV. Thus, assay systems must incorporate safety features that minimize opportunities for such exposure. An easily implemented screen with a simple protocol capable of handling microliter aliquots contributes to laboratory safety by reducing the number of unnecessary manipulations; it also encourages the use of automated or semiautomated technologies, preserves test materials, and promotes rapid sample turnaround. This latter benefit is particularly useful where the primary screening assay supports bioassay-guided fractionation of natural product extracts. Likewise, by reducing or eliminating manual handling of infectious materials, automation fosters laboratory safety while reducing assay variability, which, in turn, enhances assay reproducibility and sensitivity.

The assay chosen should duplicate viral in vivo cytopathogenicity. The cellular target(s) for virus infection and the mechanism(s) used by the virus to spread from cell to cell and to kill the target should be mimicked wherever possible. Moreover, the virus life cycle should be complete and fully infectious virions produced. These factors should ensure development of a system to identify antivirals regardless of mechanism of action. An assay chosen to serve in a primary screen should also provide data to rank test compounds based on the difference between cytotoxic and effective drug concentrations, also known as the selectivity (SI) or therapeutic indexes (TI). Cell-based systems capable of quantitating cytopathic effects can measure drug-induced toxicity and provide data for SI or TI rankings, a process critical to the evaluation, selection, and ultimate development of active agents. Utilization of economical approaches to antiviral screening and the acquisition of as much information as possible before resources are committed are vital to cost-effective drug development.

C. Empirical Approach Methodology: Cell-Based Assays

The criteria listed above suggest that to be efficient and cost-effective, antiviral drug discovery programs should use cell-based assays as primary screens. Some typical assay systems and their endpoints are summarized in Table 2. Cell-based assays for HIV typically use suspensions of CD4+ T-lymphoblastoid cells as the targets of choice. This stems from HIV's preferential replication in, and isolation from, CD4+ lymphocytes in vivo. In addition, depletion of the CD4+ cell plays a major role in AIDS pathogenesis, and leukemic clones of CD4+ lymphocytes, sensitive to HIV infection and cytopathogenicity, are readily available. However, the CD4+ lymphocyte is not the only cell that supports HIV replication. Care should be exercised to include a secondary drug screen to confirm antiviral

TABLE 2 Cell-Based Assays and Endpoints for Anti-HIV Activity

- Inhibition of HIV replication
  - Inhibition of viral protein synthesis (p24 ELISA)
  - Inhibition of viral enzyme synthesis (RT)
  - Inhibition of infectious virion production (syncytial analysis)
- Inhibition of HIV-induced CPE
  - Determination of cell viability
    - Vital dyes
    - BCECF fluorescence
    - Metabolic assays (MTT/XTT)
  - Plaque reduction assays
  - Inhibition of giant cell (syncytium) formation

activity in other known target cells (e.g., monocyte/macrophages and cells of the central nervous system or colon).

There are two general methods for the quantitation of cell-based assays when used in drug discovery. The first measures the effect of potential antiviral agents on the products of infection, including viral structural components (di Marzo Veronese et al., 1985; Nara et al., 1987c; Schinazi et al., 1989), enzymes (Popovic et al., 1984; Vrang et al., 1987), or infectious virions (Dalgleish et al., 1984; Harada et al., 1985; Nara et al., 1987a). The second quantitates antiviral effects indirectly by making a determination of virus-induced CPE (Ito et al., 1978; Mitsuya et al., 1984; Dalgleish et al., 1984; Harada et al., 1985; Karpas et al., 1985; Nakashima et al., 1986; Hamamoto et al., 1987; Nara et al., 1987a). The capsid (p24) internal core protein of HIV-1 or HIV-2 can be quantitated using one of several commercially available antigen capture kits. The antigen capture assays are easy to perform, handle large numbers of samples, and can be adapted to automated systems. The same is true for assays of the viral reverse transcriptase. However, p24 and reverse transcriptase assays provide no toxicity data; this may lead to the confusion of drug toxicity with apparent antiviral activity and does not permit one to rank compounds on the basis of their therapeutic index. Moreover, quantitation of viral structural components provides no information on the infectivity of virions produced in the presence of drug, and, therefore, certain classes of compounds may not be recognized. Finally, commercial kits can be fairly expensive when used in large-scale systems. However, this approach has been used with good results by many laboratories and is required when using cells insensitive to HIV's acute cytolytic effects (monocyte/

macrophages, peripheral blood mononuclear cells, etc.) or to confirm a drug's antiviral activities.

Other assays that measure the effects of agents on HIV replication directly include focal plaque or syncytium protocols (Harada et al., 1985; Nara et al., 1987a; Montefiori et al., 1988; Pincus et al., 1991). These assays take advantage of HIV's pronounced CPE including virus-induced cytolysis and cell fusion. They also provide a direct determination of drug effects on residual virus infectivity following treatment, but yield only subjective drug toxicity data. An example of this approach is the quantitation of HIV-induced multinucleated giant cell (syncytium) formation (Nara et al., 1987a). This assay has been used in many studies of virus neutralization and has found a niche in vaccine development. Although sensitive, plaque or syncytium assay data are collected using labor-intensive macroscopic or microscopic approaches that are not suitable for large-scale screening. However, as is the case for determinations of viral structural components or enzymes, infectivity assays serve as important adjuncts to cytoprotection studies by confirming antiviral effects.

Suppression of HIV-induced CPE, as noted above, represents an indirect measure of an agent's antiviral activity. Macroscopic and microscopic HIV-CPE endpoints were used in the initial studies of AZT's anti-HIV activity (for a review, see Mitsuya et al., 1987). A subjective determination was first made of AZT inhibition of virus replication by observing differences in the pellet sizes of HIV-infected vs. uninfected lymphoblastoid cells in round-bottomed microculture dishes. A more quantitative estimation of HIV-CPE can be made by determining cell viability using the vital dye trypan blue. Endpoints in vital dye assays can usually be determined microscopically or colorimetrically. Biscarboxyethyl carboxyfluorescein (BCECF) is a vital dye that fluoresces when metabolized by cellular esterases (Rink et al., 1982). Like the vital stains described above, the fluorescent product of BCECF is retained by cells with intact plasma membranes. Although the determination of endpoints microscopically using compounds such as trypan blue can be labor intensive and inconvenient, the colorimetric and fluorescence endpoints of neutral red (Montefiori et al., 1988) and BCECF, respectively, can be automated and are applicable to large-scale screening (Gulakowski et al., 1991).

A novel approach for determining cell viability uses measurements of cellular metabolic activity as an endpoint (Pauwels et al., 1988; Schwartz et al., 1988; Weislow et al., 1989). In particular, tetrazolium salts have proven useful in the identification of antiviral agents. Cellular dehydrogenases reduce tetrazoliums to colored products or formazans that can be measured using simple colorimetric techniques. Both 3-(4,5-dimethylthiazol-2-yl)-2,5-diphenyltetrazolium bromide (MTT) and 2,3-bis[2-methoxy-4-nitro-5-sulfophenyl] (XTT) have been used in the search for anti-HIV agents. Viable, metabolically active cells reduce MTT to a crystallized formazan that must be dissolved before being read. Reduction of XTT, on the other hand, produces a soluble product whose measurement is easily accomplished without many of the aspiration, solubilization, and centrifugation steps usually associated with MTT use. The result is a shorter, simpler, safer assay when XTT is used.

D. Factors Influencing Cell-Based Assays

One of the authors (OSW) has operated a cell-based assay with a metabolic endpoint (XTT reduction) as part of a primary screen for anti-HIV agents for more than 4 years. This experience has provided much information concerning the factors that have an impact on an assay's sensitivity and reproducibility. These are summarized in Table 3 and are discussed in greater detail below.

Increasing the multiplicity of infection (moi) increases both cell death and the amount of drug required to protect a given fraction of target cells. That is, assay sensitivity may be compromised by too much input virus. Likewise, virus infectivity (the ratio of infectious virions to noninfectious viral structural components or enzymes) must be controlled. Keeping the moi constant, while increasing infectivity, effectively decreases assay sensitivity. The rapidity with which infectious virions are produced and spread through the culture has a similar depressing effect on assay sensitivity. The impact of virus infectivity and growth rate can be controlled by using consistent virus stock preparation methods to ensure maximum infectivity and by carefully titrating all virus stocks against known antiviral agents, such as AZT, before use.

TABLE 3 Factors that Influence Cell-Based Assays

Virus concentration
Virus infectivity
Route of infection
Temperature of infection
Interval between infection and drug addition
Method of virus spread
Virus growth rate
Cell number
Length of assay
Sample color, solvent, toxicity

The method or route used to infect cells in vitro can restrict control of the moi and the interval between infection and drug exposure. For example, cultures routinely infected by cocultivating chronically infected cells with uninfected target cells provide variable results in drug assays due to inconsistencies in cell killing, which arise from the lack of control of the moi. However, cell–cell fusion may represent a major route of HIV spread in vivo and should be included as a screen in the secondary testing of all active compounds. Due to the finer control over moi, cell-free virus should be utilized in initial screening wherever possible. Again, cell-free virus or chronically infected cells should always be titrated in the presence of known antiviral standards (e.g., AZT) whenever new virus, virus-infected cells, or target-cell stocks are introduced. This point cannot be overemphasized.

Under what conditions and at what time interval after inoculation with virus should test drugs be introduced to the infected culture? Studies using various temperatures and intervals during and following infection have shown that assay sensitivity is enhanced and a broader range of compounds with antiviral activity identified if one treats early after inoculation or infects at low temperature (4°C) (Weislow et al., unpublished observations). Shortening the incubation period following virus introduction or decreasing the temperature of incubation increases sensitivity by preventing the virus from rapidly proceeding into its replicative cycle. This effect can also be obtained by allowing virus and target cell to interact in the presence of a test agent. This "in-well" infection strategy is easily adapted to microculture vessels and eases the path to automation.

Cell-based assay systems do suffer from a number of disadvantages, including host-cell restriction to virus-induced killing and resistance to antiviral drug effects. Some CPE assays, as noted above, can be quite labor intensive or may miss some compounds that have direct effects on virions, and all require secondary confirmation of antiviral activity. These difficulties may be overcome by the use of proper endpoints, judicious use of confirmatory testing, employment of multiple cell lines in the primary screen, and/or by careful observation of cell line sensitivity to antiviral effects. Despite these problems, cell-based assays represent the single most cost-effective use of resources to screen for antiviral agents.

E. Confirmatory Second-Stage Evaluation

We suggested above that many primary assays fail to deliver the complete picture of a compound's activity. Either drug toxicity data are lacking (as is the case for assays of viral structural components or enzymes) or antiviral activity, determined indirectly (as in cell-based, metabolic assays, for example), requires confirmation. Moreover, if a test system misses some portion of the HIV life cycle, it may fail to detect a compound's activity. Toxicity data can, of course, be obtained by subsequent analysis in cell-based assay systems. Confirmation of antiviral activity, obtained indirectly in cytoprotection assays, can be acquired by syncytium analysis and/or p24 enzyme-linked immunosorbent assay (ELISA) of residual virus production. Some deficiencies in test systems may be circumvented by appropriate modification of the primary screen. For example, employing low levels of input virus, separate preincubations of uninfected target cells and input virus with test compounds, and the use of controls to verify multiple rounds of infection, ensure complete coverage of the HIV replicative cycle.

In addition to a confirmation of activity, much useful information is to be gained by cell tropism and mode-of-action studies. HIV infects a variety of target cells and has demonstrated cytopathogenicity for physiological systems such as the central nervous system. Moreover, variants of HIV, with specific cellular tropisms and resistance to existing therapies, arise constantly (Larder et al., 1989; Larder and Kemp, 1989). Laboratory strains of HIV are not representative of most patient isolates and the T-lymphoblastoid cell lines serving as preclinical in vitro screens can differ markedly in their sensitivity to antiviral agents. Thus, it is vital that promising compounds have demonstrable activity against as many cellular targets (including normal peripheral mononuclear cells) and HIV variants as possible. Finally, testing against multiple cellular variants and virus strains (i.e., simian, bovine, or feline lentiviruses) can provide a bridge to the requisite in vivo assessments of toxicity and efficacy.

Future HIV chemotherapy will almost certainly use regimens of combination drug treatment (Groopman, 1991). This approach is ordained by existing treatment-induced toxicities (Richman et al., 1987), drug resistance (Larder et al., 1989), ethical considerations, dwindling naive test patient populations, and competition for other limited resources. Thus, consideration should always be given to extensive in vitro combinational analysis such as with AZT, ddC, or ddI. These studies may also help to clarify mechanisms of drug action (e.g., by pointing toward additive or synergistic behavior). This leads to one final consideration for preclinical in vitro evaluation. Although not required for clinical use, a clear understanding of a drug's mode or mechanism of action, in addition to being intellectually satisfying, can be of immense value in the design of more potent and less toxic analogues. Moreover, knowing how an agent works assists in identifying drugs that could be expected to augment existing therapeutic agents and highlights critical components of virus replication.

Thus, studies of the mechanism(s) of virus–drug interactions can have a significant impact on our understanding of HIV biology.

IV. ANIMAL MODELS FOR IN VIVO DRUG TESTING

Animal models are useful as preclinical intermediates for assessing the pharmacokinetics, toxicity, and in vivo efficacy of potentially useful antiviral drugs before they are used in humans. The WHO Global Program on AIDS has reviewed the present data on animal models for HIV and derived a hypothetical "ideal" HIV–animal model for the evaluation of candidate drugs (Esparza and Osmanov, 1989). The WHO "ideal" model for drugs recommends the following: HIV itself should be used; testing should be on a small animal with well-known genetics, immunology, and metabolism; the target cells should be CD4+ lymphocytes and macrophages; the target organs should include blood, lymphoid tissues, and the brain; the mode of transmission should mimic that of HIV, including perinatal transmission; and the induced disease should have a short incubation period and resemble AIDS in humans.

Such an ideal model does not exist; therefore, various retrovirus–animal models have been substituted for the in vivo testing of promising anti-HIV drugs. The ultimate selection of the most appropriate retrovirus–animal model for obtaining preclinical data will depend on the parameters of the study design. Because HIV is an exogenous lentivirus and shares many of the features of lentivirus biology, including persistent infections of the immune system (Table 4), it is thought that the lentivirus subfamily of retroviruses will offer the most promising models (Desrosiers and Ringler, 1989; Letvin, 1990). However, all retrovirus–animal models will no doubt contribute useful information, depending on the viral protein, function, or facet of the life cycle targeted by the test drug (Gardner and Luciw, 1989). Table 5 outlines some general criteria that should be considered in selecting an animal model of HIV-like infection for drug studies. A brief discussion of some of the potential lentivirus–animal models that are under development or are currently available for antiviral testing follows.

HIV can infect chimpanzees (Alter et al., 1984; Fultz et al., 1986; Nara et al., 1987b), gibbons (Lusso et al., 1988), rabbits (Filice et al., 1988; Kulaga et al., 1989), and chimeric mice containing reconstituted human immune tissues (McCune, 1990; Kaneshima et al., 1991; Mosier et al., 1991). Transgenic mice carrying a functional HIV proviral genome have also been constructed (Leonard et al., 1988). However, none of these animals progress to an AIDS-like disease as observed in humans, and the scarcity

TABLE 4 Clinical Manifestations of Lentivirus Infections in Natural Hosts

Lentivirus	Disease Description
Ovine visna, maedi, and progressive pneumonia virus	Progressive lethal pneumonia, chronic encephalomyelitis, spasticitiy, paralysis, lymphadenopathy, mastitis, generalized wasting, opportunistic infections
Caprine arthritis encephalitis virus	Generalized wasting, chronic leukoencephalomyelitis, progressive arthritis, osteoporosis, paralysis
Equine infectious anemia virus	Fever, persistent viremia, hemolytic anemia, lymphoproliferation, immune-complex glomerulonephritis, bone marrow depression, central nervous system lesions
Bovine immunodeficiency-like virus	Persistent lymphocytosis, lymphadenopathy, central nervous system lesions, weakness, emaciation
Feline immunodeficiency virus	Immunodeficiency-like syndrome, generalized lymphadenopathy, leukopenia, fever, anemia, emaciation, opportunistic infections
Simian immunodeficiency virus	Immunodeficiency, neuropathologic changes, wasting, opportunistic infections
Human immunodeficiency virus	Immunodeficiency, lymphadenopathy, opportunistic infections, encephalopathy, emaciation, Kaposi's sarcoma, and other cancers

Source: Adapted from Gonda (1988). *J. Electron Microsc. Tech.* *8*:17–40, with permission of the editors and Wiley-Liss, a division of John Wiley and Sons, Inc..

and/or size of primates susceptible to HIV infection excludes them from all but the most crucial drug testing. Rabbits are the only naturally occurring small animal model that can be infected with cell-free HIV or HIV-infected cells. Young rabbits can be infected by the peritoneal route after stimulation of peritoneal monocyte/macrophages with thioglycolate (Filice et al., 1988). The target cell for infection appears to be monocytes/macrophages, since these cells can be infected in tissue culture (Kulaga et al., 1988). Virus persists for up to 1 year and can be recovered from the peripheral blood as late as 8–10 months after infection. Additional work needs to be performed on the HIV-rabbit model to determine its suitability for drug testing.

TABLE 5 Criteria for Ideal Animal Model Systems of HIV-Like Infection

Animal is small, readily available, inexpensive, and amenable to experimental manipulation.
Pathogen is a lentivirus related to HIV with a similar genomic complexity, but does not infect humans or human cells.
Functional molecular clones are available to allow study of the molecular mechanisms of pathogenesis and level of drug or vaccine interaction.
Infections of the immune system are persistent with measurable pathologic lesions and recoverable virus.
Measurable immunosuppression is an endpoint in the infection and may be accompanied by an AIDS-like disease including opportunistic infections.
Diagnostic assays are available for measuring the presence of virus and accumulation of viral antigen.

Adapted from Gonda et al. (1990). In *Animal Models in AIDS*, pp. 233–255, with permission of the editors and Elsevier Science Publishers B.V., Amsterdam.

The rational design of animal models offers a novel approach to preclinical testing of antivirals. Probably one of the most promising biologically engineered small animal models for anti-HIV drug testing is the chimeric human immune system: severe combined immunodeficient mouse (Hu:SCID). Various immune tissues from humans have been used to reconstitute portions of the immune system in Hu:SCID mice. AZT treatment of HIV-infected Hu:SCID mice was effective in suppressing virus replication in infected animals (McCune et al., 1990). These data were the first demonstration that the efficacy of an antiviral compound against HIV can be tested directly in a small animal model. Genetically engineered transgenic mice harboring the HIV provirus may also have potential as useful animal models. HIV-transgenic mice have several advantages: they can be stably propagated through generations of offspring, are readily bred, and reproduce quickly. This will ensure a large pool of animals for testing. The transgenic animal has one drawback. It is probably less suited for studying compounds that block the initial stages of the virus life cycle (i.e., attachment, penetration, and reverse transcription), since all cells are predetermined to harbor provirus. However, in this regard, more about the life cycle and replicative capacity of HIV in latent infections remains to be determined. At the moment, HIV transgenics will probably best be suited to study therapeutic drugs that work at the level of viral transcription, translation, assembly, and release.

Of the nonhuman lentiviruses, the SIVs appear to be an important model of HIV-like infection and disease. They are the closest relatives to

HIV, share extensive nucleotide sequence similarity, correspond in genome organization, infect CD4+ cells, and induce an AIDS-like disease in a time frame suitable for laboratory investigation (Desrosiers and Ringler, 1989). One drawback to the use of SIV, and this is also applicable to HIV, is the possibility of an accidental infection of laboratory workers during experimentation, since both viruses replicate in human cells. In addition to SIV, several other lentivirus-animal model systems might have some application as safe models of HIV-like infection. These are the lentiviruses of ungulates and cats (Table 4). For the most part, the size of the ungulates excludes them from in vivo testing because of the large doses that may be needed. This is especially the case when only small quantities of compound are available. One of the ungulate lentiviruses, the bovine immunodeficiency-like virus (BIV) (Gonda et al., 1987), has been shown to infect rabbits readily and reliably (Pifat et al., submitted). BIV infections were induced by a single intraperitoneal inoculation of BIV-infected cells. The infection results in a rapid and sustained BIV-specific humoral response. BIV can be rescued from rabbits as early as 1 month and as late as 22 months after inoculation from spleen, lymph nodes, and peripheral blood leukocytes. The presence of BIV sequences was demonstrated by PCR in the same tissues, as well as in the bone marrow and brain. Macrophages in the spleen could also be stained immunohistochemically with BIV-specific antisera. These data suggest that BIV replicates in cells of the immune system. However, there was no clinical disease in animals evaluated for up to 2 years. Cats are naturally infected with a lentivirus, the feline immunodeficiency virus (FIV) (Pedersen et al., 1987). The FIV infection in the cat model appears to cause an AIDS-like syndrome including opportunistic infections (Pedersen, 1990). Recent data have also shown that FIV infection of cats is a suitable model in which to study the efficacy of antiviral compounds (Koolen and Egberink, 1990). None of the ungulate or cat lentiviruses are known to infect humans naturally or experimentally or to infect human cells in vitro. Thus, they are ideal for investigations in laboratories not equipped to handle infectious biohazardous agents such as HIV.

V. CONCLUDING REMARKS

Several classes of drugs have been discovered that have some inhibitory activity on HIV replication in vitro, thus indicating the immediate practicality of antiviral approaches to therapy. However, only a few of these drugs have proven useful in clinical trials at this writing (Mitsuya et al., 1990, 1991; Richman, 1990). Nevertheless, as information continues to accumulate about the structure and function of HIV proteins, the number of new antiretroviral agents will also grow.

The most pressing problems to be overcome in the development of new drugs are the selective targeting of virus-specific functions, avoiding side reactions with cellular systems involved directly or indirectly in virus replication, the lack of structural information about many of the potentially useful target proteins of HIV, and the derivation of the most effective and yet nontoxic form of useful drugs. Where the viral protein structure is known, target-oriented, rational drug design, as has been done for the HIV-1 protease, offers a promising approach. This makes the discovery of virus-specific inhibitors particularly challenging. Perhaps work on the structure of other viral proteins will eventually yield similar leads. The use of cell-based assays in the empirical or "blind assay" approach, as detailed here, offers a broad approach to screening large numbers of compounds for antiviral activities that may be directed to any portion of the virus life cycle, since the final outcome is the inhibition of virus replication. Regardless of the screening approach, once a compound is found effective in vitro, the use of animal models is appropriate to study in vivo toxicity, pharmacokinetics, and drug efficacy. The lentivirus–animal models described above appear to be the most relevant in this regard, and emerging data now indicate that animal-lentivirus models will be of enormous practical value in assessing strategies for the treatment of persistent HIV infections. The continual growth in the HIV pandemic and the potentially long time predicted before an effective vaccine for HIV will be available underscore the need for programs to identify and develop antiviral drugs to treat those infected with HIV.

ACKNOWLEDGMENTS

The authors thank G. Serig for excellent assistance in the preparation of the manuscript. This project has been funded in part with Federal funds from the Department of Health and Human Services under contract number NO1-CO-74102 with Program Resources, Inc. The content of this publication does not necessarily reflect the views or policies of the Department of Health and Human Services, nor does mention of trade names, commercial products, or organizations imply endorsement by the U.S. Government.

REFERENCES

Abrams, D. I., Kuno, S., Wong, R., Jeffords, J., Nash, M., Molaghan, J. B., Gorter, R., and Veno, R. (1989). *Ann. Intern. Med. 110*:183–188.

Achour, A., Picard, O., Zagury, D., Sarin, P. S., Gallo, R. C., Naylor, P. H., and Goldstein, A. L. (1990). *Proc. Natl. Acad. Sci. USA 87*:7045–7049.

Agrawal, S. (1991). In *Prospects for Antisense Nucleic Acid Therapy of Cancer and Viral Infections*, E. Wickstrom (Ed.). Wiley-Liss, Inc., New York, pp. 143–158.

Agrawal, S., Ikeuchi, T., Sun, D., Sarin, P. S., Konopka, A., Maizel, J., and Zamecnik, P. C. (1989). *Proc. Natl. Acad. Sci. USA 86*:7790–7794.

Ahluwalia, G., Cooney, D. A., Mitsuya, H., Fridland, A., Flora, K. P., Hao, Z., Dalal, M., Broder, S., and Johns, D. G. (1987). *Biochem. Pharmacol. 36*:3797–3800.

Alter, H. J., Eichberg, J. W., Masur, H., Saxinger, W. C., Gallo, R., Macher, A. M., Lane, H. C., and Fauci, A. S. (1984). *Science 226*:549–552.

Bader, J. P., McMahon, J. B., Schultz, R. J., Narayanan, V. L., Pierce, J. B., Harrison, W. A., Weislow, O. S., Midelfort, C. F., Stinson, S. F., and Boyd, M. R. (1991). *Proc. Natl. Acad. Sci. USA 88*:6740–6744.

Boyd, M. R. (1988). In *AIDS Etiology, Diagnosis, Treatment, and Prevention*, V. T. Devita, Jr., S. Hellman, and S. A. Rosenberg (Eds.). J. B. Lipincott, Philadelphia, pp. 305–317.

Callahan, L. N., Phelan, M., Mallinson, M., and Norcross, M. A. (1991). *J. Virol. 65*:1543–1550.

Capon, D. J., Chamow, S. M., Mordenti, J., Marsters, S. A., Gregory, T., Mitsuya, H., Byrn, R. A., Lucas, C., Wurm, F. M., Groopman, J. E., Broder, S., and Smith, D. H. (1989). *Nature* (London) *337*:525–531.

Clapham, P. R., Weber, J. N., Whitby, D., McIntosh, K., Dalgleish, A. G., Maddon, P. J., Deen, K. C., Sweet, R. W., and Weiss, R. A. (1989). *Nature* (London) *337*:368–370.

Cullen, B. R. (1991). *J. Virol. 65*:1053–1056.

Cullen, B. R., and Greene, W. C. (1990). *Virology 178*:1–5.

Daar, E. S., Li, X. L., Moudgil, T., and Ho, D. D. (1990). *Proc. Natl. Acad. Sci. USA 87*:6574–6578.

Dalgleish, A. G., Beverley, P. C. L., Clapham, P. R., Crawford, D. H., Greaves, M. F., and Weiss, R. A. (1984). *Nature* (London) *312*:763–767.

DesJarlais, R. L., Seibel, G. L., Kuntz, I. D., Furth, P. S., Alvarez, J. C., Ortiz de Montellano, P. R., DeCamp, D. L., Babe, L. M., and Craik, C. S. (1990). *Proc. Natl. Acad. Sci. USA 87*:6644–6648.

Desrosiers, R. C., and Ringler, D. J. (1989). *Intervirology 30*:301–312.

di Marzo Veronese, F., Sarngadharan, M. G., Rahman, R., Markham, P. D., Popovic, M., Bodner, A. J., and Gallo, R. C. (1985). *Proc. Natl. Acad. Sci. USA 82*: 5199–5202.

Dreyer, G. B., Metcalf, B. W., Tomaszek, T. A., Jr., Carr, T. J., Chandler, A. C., III, Hyland, L., Fakhoury, S. A., Magaard, V. W., Moore, M. L., Strickler, J. E., Debouck, C., and Meek, T. D. (1989). *Proc. Natl. Acad. Sci. USA 86*: 9752–9756.

Erikson, J., Neidhart, D. J., Van Drie, J., Kempf, D. J., Wang, X. C., Norbeck, D. W., Plattner, J. J., Rittenhouse, J. W., Turon, M., Wideburg, N., Kohlbrenner, W. E., Simmer, R., Helfrich, R., Paul, D. A., and Knigge, M. (1990). *Science 249*:527–533.

Esparza, J., and Osmanov, S. (1989). Global Programme on AIDS, World Health Organization, Geneva, Switzerland.
Filice, G., Cereda, P. M., and Varnier, O. E. (1988). *Nature* (London) *335*:366–369.
Fultz, P. N., McClure, H. M., Swensen, R. B., McGrath, C. R., Brodie, A., Getchell, J. P., Jensen, F. C., Anderson, D. C., Broderson, J. R., and Francis, D. P. (1986). *J. Virol. 58*:116–124.
Gardner, M. B., and Luciw, P. A. (1989). *FASEB J. 3*:2593–2606.
Gonda, M. A., Wong-Staal, F., Gallo, R. C., Clements, J. E., Narayan, O., and Gilden, R. V. (1985). *Proc. Natl. Acad. Sci. USA 83*:4007–4011.
Gonda, M. A., Braun, M. J., Clements, J. E., Pyper, J. M., Gallo, R. C., Wong-Staal, F., and Gilden, R. V. (1986). *Proc. Natl. Acad. Sci. USA 83*:4007–4011.
Gonda, M. A., Braun, M. J., Carter, S. G., Kost, T. A., Bess, J. W., Jr., Arthur, L. O., and Van Der Maaten, M. J. (1987). *Nature* (London) *330*:388–391.
Graham, G. J., and Maio, J. J. (1990). *Proc. Natl. Acad. Sci. USA 87*:5817–5821.
Groopman, J. E. (1991). *Am. J. Med. 90*(Suppl. 4A):275–305.
Gulakowski, R. J., McMahon, J. B., Staley, P. G., Moran, R. A., and Boyd, M. R. (1991). *J. Virol. Methods 33*:87–100.
Guyader, M., Emermann, M., Sonigo, P., Clavel, F., Montagnier, L., and Alizon, M. (1987). *Nature* (London) *326*:662–669.
Hamamoto, Y., Nakashima, H., Matsui, T., Matsuda, A., Ueda, T., and Yamamoto, N. (1987). *Antimicrob. Agents Chemother. 31*:907–910.
Harada, S., Koyanagi, Y., Yamamoto, N. (1985). *Science 229*:563–566.
Haseltine, W. A. (1990). In *AIDS and the New Viruses*, A. G. Dalgleish and R. A. Weiss (Eds.). Academic Press, San Diego, California, pp. 11–40.
Ito, M., Nakashima, H., and Baba, M. (1978). *Antiviral Res. 7*:127–137.
Jacks, T., Power, M. D., Masiarz, F. R., Luciw, P. A., Barr, P. J., and Varmus, H. E. (1988). *Nature* (London) *331*:280–283.
Javaherian, K., Langlois, A. J., McDanal, C., Ross, K. L., Eckler, L. I., Jellis, C. L., Profy, A. T., Rusche, J. R., Bolognesi, D. P., Putney, S. D., and Matthews, T. J. (1989). *Proc. Natl. Acad. Sci. USA 86*:6768–6772.
Kaneshima, H ., Shih, C.-C., Namikawa, R., Rabin, L., Outzen, H., Machado, S. G., and McCune, J. M. (1991). *Proc. Natl. Acad. Sci. USA 88*:4523–4527.
Karpas, A., Gillson, W., Bevan, P. C., and Oates, J. K. (1985). *Lancet* 2:695–697.
Kempf, D. J., Norbeck, D. W., Codacovi, L., Wang, X. C., Kohlbrenner, W. E., Wideburg, N. E., Paul, D. A., Knigge, M. F., Vasavanonda, S., Craig-Kennard, A., Saldivar, A., Rosenbrook, W., Jr., Clement, J. J., Plattner, J. J., and Erickson, J. (1990). *J. Med. Chem. 33*:2687–2689.
Kern, E. R. (1990). In *Antiviral Agents and Viral Diseases of Man*, 3rd ed., G. J. Galasso, R. J. Whitley, and T. C. Merigan (Eds.). Raven Press, New York, pp. 581–646.
Kohl, N. E., Emini, E. A., Schleif, W. A., Davis, L. J., Heimbach, J. C., Dixon, R. A. F., Scolnick, E. M., and Sigal, I. S. (1988). *Proc. Natl. Acad. Sci. USA 85*:4686–4690.
Koolen, M., and Egberink, H. (1990). In *Animal Models in AIDS*, H. Schellekens and M. C. Horzinek (Eds.). Elsevier, Amsterdam, pp. 165–183.
Kulaga, H., Folks, T. M., Rutledge, R., and Kindt, T. J. (1988). *Proc. Natl. Acad. Sci. USA 85*:4455–4459.

Kulaga, H., Folks, T., Rutledge, R., Truckenmiller, M. E., Gugel, E., and Kindt, T. J. (1989). *J. Exp. Med. 169*:321–326.

Larder, B. A., Darby, G., and Richman, D. D. (1989). *Science 243*:1731–1734.

Larder, B. A., and Kemp, S. D. (1989). *Science 246*:1155–1158.

Leonard, J. M., Abramczuk, J. W., Pezen, D. S., Rutledge, R., Belcher, J. H., Hakim, F., Shearer, G., Lamperth, L., Travis, W., Fredrickson, T., Notkins, A. L., and Martin, M. A. (1988). *Science 242*:1665–1670.

Letvin, N. L. (1990). *Immunol. Today 11*:322–326.

Lusso, P., Markham, P. D., Ranki, A., Earl, P., Moss, B., Dorner, F., Gallo, R. C., and Krohn, K. J. (1988). *J. Immunol. 141*:2467–2473.

Lyerly, H. K., Tyler, D. S., Nastala, C. L., and Weinhold, K. J. (1990). In *AIDS Vaccine Research and Clinical Trials*. S. D. Putney and D. P. Bolognesi (Eds.). Marcel Dekker, New York, pp. 157–177.

McCune, J. M. (1990). *Semin. Virol. 1*:229–235.

Meek, T. D., Dayton, B. D., Metcalf, B. W., Dreyer, G. B., Strickler, J. E., Gorniak, J. G., Rosenberg, M., and Moore, M. L. (1989). *Proc. Natl. Acad. Sci. USA 86*:1841–1845.

Mitsuya, H., Popovic, M., Yarchoan, R., Mitsushita, S., Gallo, R. C., and Broder, S. (1984). *Science 226*:172–174.

Mitsuya, H., Weinhold, K. J., Furman, F. A., St. Clair, M. H., Lehrman, S. N., Gallo, R. C., Bolognesi, D., Barry, D. W., and Broder, S. (1985). *Proc. Natl. Acad. Sci. USA 82*:7096–7100.

Mitsuya, H., and Broder, S. (1986). *Proc. Natl. Acad. Sci. USA 83*:1911–1915.

Mitsuya, H., Matsukura, M., and Broder, S. (1987). In *AIDS: Modern Concepts and Therapeutic Challenges*, S. Broder (Ed.). Marcel Dekker, New York, pp. 303–333.

Mitsuya, H., Yarchoan, R., and Broder, S. (1990). *Science 249*:1533–1544.

Mitsuya, H., Yarchoan, R., Kageyama, S., and Broder, S. (1991). *FASEB J. 5*(10):2369–2381.

Montefiori, D. C., Robinson, W. E., Jr., Schuffman, S. S., and Mitchell, W. M. (1988). *J. Clin. Microbiol. 26*:231–235.

Mosier, D. E., Gulizia, R. J., Baird, S. M., Wilson, D. B., Spector, D. H., and Spector, S. A. (1991). *Science 251*:791–794.

Nakashima, H., Matsui, T., Harada, S., Kobayashi, N., Matsuda, A., Ueda, T., and Yamamoto, N. (1986). *Antimicrob. Agents Chemother. 30*:933–937.

Nara, P. L., Hatch, W. C., Dunlop, N. M., Robey, W. G., Arthur, L. O., Gonda, M. A., and Fischinger, P. J. (1987a). *AIDS Res. Hum. Retroviruses 3*:283– 302.

Nara, P. L., Robey, W. G., Arthur, L. O., Asher, D. M., Wolff, A. V., Gibbs, C. J., Jr., Gajdusek, C., and Fischinger, P. J. (1987b). *J. Virol. 61*:3173–3180.

Nara, P. L., Robey, W. G., Gonda, M. A., Carter, S. G., and Fischinger, P. J. (1987c). *Proc. Natl. Acad. Sci. USA 84*:3797–3801.

Papsidero, L. D., Sheu, M., and Ruscetti, F. W. (1989). *J. Virol. 63*:267–272.

Pauwels, R., Balzarini, J. M., Baba, M., Snoeck, R., Schols, D., Herdewijn, P., Desmyter, J., and De Clerq, E. (1988). *J. Virol. Methods 20*:309–321.

Pauwels, R., Andries, K., Desmyters, J., Schols, D., Kukla, M. J., Breslin, H. J., Raeymaechers, A., Van Gelder, J., Woestenborghs, R., Heykants, J., Schellenhaus, K., Janssen, M. A. C., DeClerq, E., and Janssen, P. A. J. (1990). *Nature* (London) *343*:470–474.
Pedersen, N. C. (1990). In *Animal Models in AIDS*, H. Schellekens and M. C. Horzinek (Eds.). Elsevier, Amsterdam, pp. 165–183.
Pedersen, N. C., Ho, E., Brown, M. L., and Yamamoto, J. K. (1987). *Science* *235*:790–793.
Pifat, D. Y., Ennis, W. H., Ward, J. M., Oberste, M. S., and Gonda, M. A. (1991). *J. Virol.* (submitted).
Pincus, S. H., Wehrly, K., and Chesebro, B. (1991). *Biotechniques* *10*(3):336–342.
Popovic, M., Sarngadharan, M. G., Read, E., and Gallo, R. C. (1984). *Science* *224*:497–500.
Prusoff, W. H., Tia-Shun, L., August, M. E., and Marongiu, M. E. (1990). In *Advances in Chemotherapy of AIDS*, R. B. Diasio and J.-P. Sommadossi (Eds.). Pergamon Press, New York, pp. 1–9.
Rhodes, A., and James, W. (1990). *J. Gen. Virol.* *71*:1965–1974.
Richman, D. D. (1990). In *Antiviral Agents and Viral Diseases of Man*, 3rd edition, G. J. Galasso, R. J. Whitley, and T. C. Merigan (Eds.). Raven Press, New York, pp. 581–646.
Richman, D. D., Fischi, M. A., Grieco, M. H., Gottlieb, M. S., Volberding, P. A., Laskin, O. L., Leedom, J. M., Groopman, J. E., Mildvan, D., Hirsch, M. S., Jackson, G. G., Durack, D. T., Nusinoff-Lehrman, S., and the AZT Collaborative Working Group. (1987). *N. Engl. J. Med.* *317*:192–197.
Rink, T. J., Tsien, R. Y., and Pozzan, T. (1982). *J. Cell Biol.* *95*:189–196.
Roberts, J. D., Bebenek, K., and Kunkel, T. A. (1988). *Science* *242*:1171–1173.
Robey, W. G., Safai, B., Oroszlan, S., Arthur, L. O., Gonda, M. A., Gallo, R. C., and Fischinger, P. J. (1985). *Science* *228*:593–595.
Sarin, P. S., Sun, D.-K., Thornton, A. H., Naylor, P. H., and Goldstein, A. L. (1986). *Science* *232*:1135–1137.
Schinazi, R. F., Eriksson, B. F. H., and Hughes, S. H. (1989). *Antimicrob. Agents Chemother.* *33*:115–117.
Schwartz, O., Henin, Y., Marechal, V., and Montagnier, L. (1988). *AIDS Res. Hum. Retroviruses* *4*:441–448.
Sczakiel, G., and Pawlita, M. (1991). *J. Virol.* *65*:468–472.
Swanstrom, R., Kaplan, A. H., and Manchester, M. (1990). *Semin. Virol.* *1*:175–186.
Takeda, A., and Ennis, F. A. (1990). *AIDS Res. Hum. Retroviruses* *6*:999–1004.
Takeda, A., Sweet, R. W., and Ennis, F. A. (1990). *J. Virol.* *64*:5605–5610.
van Kuyk, R., Luciw, P. A., and Gardner, M. B. (1990). *AIDS Res. Hum. Retroviruses* *6*:831–834.
Varmus, H. (1988). *Science* *240*:1427–1435
Veno, R., and Kuno, S. (1987). *Lancet* *1*:1379–1380.
Vrang, L., Bazin, H., Remaud, G., Chattopadhyaya, J., and Oberg, B. (1987). *Antiviral Res.* *7*:139–149.
Walker, B. D. (1990). In *AIDS Vaccine Research and Clinical Trials*, S. D. Putney and D. P. Bolognesi (Eds.). Marcel Dekker, New York, pp. 179–194.

Weislow, O. S., Kiser, R., Fine, D. L., Bader, J., Shoemaker, R. H., and Boyd, M. R. (1989). *J. Natl. Cancer Inst. 81*:577–586.

Wlodawer, A., Miller, M., Jaskolski, M., Sathyanarayan, B. K., Baldwin, E., Weber, I. T., Selk, L. M., Clawson, L., Schneider, J., and Kent, S. B. H. (1989). *Science 245*:616–621.

Yarchoan, R., Klecker, R., Weinhold, K. J., Markham, P. D., Lyerly, H. K., Durack, D. T., Gelmann, E., Lehrman, S. N., Blum, R. M., Barry, D. W., Shearer, G. M., Fischl, M. A., Mitsuya, H., Gallo, R. C., Collins, J. M., Bolognesi, D. P., Myers, C. E., and Broder, S. (1986). *Lancet 1*:575–580.

Yarchoan, R., Perno, C. F., Thomas, R. V., Klecker, R. W., Allain, J. P ., Wills, R. J., McAtee, N., Fischl, M. A., Dubinsky, R., McNeely, M. C., Mitsuya, H., Pluda, J. M., Lawley, T. J., Leuther, M., Safai, B., Collins, J. M., Myers, C. E., and Broder, S. (1988). *Lancet 1*:76–81.

3

AIDS—VACCINES TO HUMAN IMMUNODEFICIENCY VIRUS

A Difficult Challenge

Edouard Kurstak, Christine Kurstak, A. Hossain, and A. Al Tuwaijri
Faculty of Medicine, University of Montreal, and International Comparative Virology Organization, Montreal, Quebec, Canada

I. INTRODUCTION

Substantial efforts have been made during the past few years to elucidate the structure, genetics, and biochemistry of the human immunodeficiency virus type 1 (HIV-1) as well as of its mechanisms of infectivity. The HIV-1 has been unequivocally identified as the primary cause of the acquired immunodeficiency syndromes (AIDS); Barre-Sinoussi et al., 1983; Gallo et al., 1984).

No other infectious disease in modern medical history has generated the concerns and unceasing efforts of physicians, scientists, and the community at large that AIDS has. The ever-increasing dimensions of the AIDS problem are indeed appealing. Since the first clinically diagnosed cases in 1981, over 200,000 cases of AIDS have been diagnosed in the United States and about 50% of these patients have already died (Epstein, 1991; AIDS Update, 1990, 1991). According to the World Health Organization's (WHO) estimates, 6–8 million people worldwide or perhaps as many as 1:400 adults are currently infected with HIV-1. By the year 2000, even conservative estimates of the WHO project a worldwide total of approximately 40 million HIV-1-infected persons. These statistics remind us that HIV continues its insidious spread despite the tremendous current prevention and control efforts.

The development of safe and effective HIV vaccines for the prevention and control of AIDS worldwide has thus emerged as an international public health priority. Significant scientific advances in the last 2 years in particular have prompted optimism that the development of safe and effective vaccine is indeed feasible, despite the genetic complexity and variability of HIV, and of retroviruses in general.

Several new approaches to development of AIDS vaccines have been noted, including possible alternative vaccine strategies, comprehensive insights into cell-mediated immune responses to HIV and related retroviruses, identification of new serologic epitopes, confirmatory vaccine-induced protection studies in experimental models, testing of novel vaccine adjuvants, and, above all, the problem of HIV variability and its impact on development of a vaccine against AIDS. The current status of potential problems and future prospects for an HIV-1 vaccine is covered in this chapter.

II. AIDS VACCINE CHALLENGE

At the present time it is by no means clear that an effective AIDS vaccine will be available in the near future. The fundamental issues confronting the development of a vaccine include those discussed below.

HIV infects cells of the immune system and, as such, the cells involved in the induction of an immune response and clearing the virus from the infected person may be susceptible to infection. This cells for a vaccine that would prevent infection rather than the development of the clinical disease.

Antigens inducing protective immunity have yet to be identified. Some virus-encoded proteins may prove to be toxic to uninfected cells (Barnes, 1987), elicit autoimmune reactions (Solinger et al., 1988), or even contribute to enhancement of the disease (Robinson et al., 1988).

Infected persons produce low concentrations of various neutralizing antibodies and some cell-mediated immune response occurs soon after primary infection (Spickett and Dalgleish, 1988) but whether these are protective remains unclear. The long and variable period between infection and the appearance of symptoms does suggest that stimulation of these immune responses may delay the onset of the disease. As such, postinfection immunization and re-stimulation of immune responses may be beneficial (Salk, 1987; Putney and Bolognesi, 1990; Williams, 1991).

Two major types of HIV, designated HIV-1 and HIV-2, have been identified (Barre-Sinoussi et al., 1983; Gallo et al., 1984; Clavel et al., 1986) and a similarity in genetic organization exists between them apart from an additional gene in HIV-2. They cross-react antigenically but nucleotide sequence analysis of different isolates reveals that these strains probably represent two ends of a very broad spectrum of virus variants. It is currently generally accepted that HIV is a rapidly evolving virus and that significant genetic heterogeneity exists between different isolates (Smith et al., 1988; Coffin, 1990). This heterogeneity has been associated with the generation of variants with diverse biological properties and includes those determining cell tropism and virulence (Cheng-Mayer et al., 1988a,b; Evans et al., 1988; Kong et al., 1988). It has been suggested that genetic variation among HIV isolates is probably attributable to the virus-encoded reverse transcriptase (Coffin, 1986). Reverse transcription is the key process in the replicative cycle and is known to be an error-prone event that may result in point deletion and insertion mutations. Variation, however, does not appear to be constant across the entire HIV genome since sequences within *gag* and *pol*, for example, are more highly conserved than those within *env*. This may reflect an inherent structural instability of certain regions of the genome or, as an alternative, the operation of mechanisms by which particular variants are selected based on their viability and, possibly, their ability to escape immune surveillance within the host (Huso and Narayan, 1990). As a result of this, many different HIV variants, each derived from a common progenitor and each with diverse biological properties, may be in circulating within an effected person at any one time (Hahn et al., 1986; Saag et al., 1988; Hossain et al., 1990). This has influence not only in the progression of the disease and the pathogenesis of AIDS but also for the design of control and preventive strategies.

Acquisition of HIV isolates from various regions worldwide followed by nucleotide sequencing of genetically variable regions has revealed the molecular epidemiology of HIV and identified more conserved regions of HIV proteins that could be potential targets for vaccine development. In addition, the recently developed pathogenetic lentivirus molecular clones now provide new tools for probing the immunologic consequences of genetic variation in HIV.

Making the correct challenge stock with carefully calibrated doses of HIV to test vaccine efficacy is undoubtedly a step of prime importance in the development of an AIDS vaccine. As an ideal, the strain in the vaccine and the challenge stock should be the same since this would facilitate carrying out an easier test for evaluation of the vaccine. Choosing the strains for the vaccine itself is also turning out to be a problem. After more than a decade of the AIDS epidemic, researchers remain baffled as to which strains are the most common.

The recent report (Dorozynski and Anderson, 1991) of two patients treated with an experimental vaccine who may have died from vaccine-related complications presents a note of caution. Behind the accusations against AIDS researcher Daniel Zagury was the evidence by Jean Claude Guillaume, a dermatologist, suggesting that two of Zagury's patients with AIDS developed a fatal vaccinia infection after being treated with a vaccinia virus preparation. The vaccinia virus had been genetically engineered to express HIV proteins. Zagury had hoped that these proteins would help to stimulating the immune system in fighting AIDS and contended that the herpes virus infection and not vaccinia caused the death. Zagury was exonerated of misconduct (Culliton, 1992).

The proximity of in vivo tests of an HIV vaccine brings with in intricate issues. Current problems include ways and criteria to guarantee developing countries access to potential HIV vaccines and the selection of sites for upcoming tests of vaccine efficacy.

The most sensitive of the issues, however, appears to be the so-called "distributive practice" (Cohen, 1991). One of the reasons for testing a vaccine in developing countries appears to be the greater chance of its being challenged by HIV infection. This, in turn, raises the question of whether a vaccine developed using HIV strains prevalent in the United States and Europe would prove effective in a Third World country where different strains are prevalent. In this respect the recent WHO decision to perform clinical trials with prototype HIV vaccines in Brazil, Rwanda, Thailand, and Uganda is certainly of interest and will generate new information on the immune response in local vaccinees.

III. APPROACHES TO HIV VACCINE DEVELOPMENT

In view of the lack of knowledge as to which of the immune mechanisms may confer protection against HIV infection, and the capability of HIV to be transmitted as a cell-free and cell-associated virus, an effective HIV vaccine must elicit long-term immunologic effects consisting of both humoral and cell-mediated responses (Koff, 1991). The suggestion that individuals may exhibit cell-mediated immune responses against HIV prior to or in the absence of seroconversion has prompted researchers to develop new vaccine strategies that involve the design of molecular combinations of antigens to be induced to a host immune system in diverse configurations so as to generate maximal responses.

The approaches currently being used include diverse strategies utilizing recombinant subunits, live recombinant viruses, synthetic peptides, inactivated viruses, live attenuated viruses, and recombinant viruslike particles (Berman et al., 1988). Given the fact that each of these strategies has a number of advantages and disadvantages, considerable effort may be required to determine which is the most appropriate for human use.

Most viral vaccines currently in use are essentially live attenuated viruses, which are highly effective due to their ability to initiate an infection of low grade with resultant long-lasting humoral and cell-mediated immunity. Two important characteristics of the AIDS virus, the high rate of mutagenic drift and insertion of genetic material into the chromosomes of infected cells, makes the development of a safe, live attenuated vaccine for AIDS a remote, and an unlikely, possibility. This, in conjunction with the recent reports of rhesus monkey and chimpanzees possibly being protected from HIV challenge after vaccination with inactive immunogen (Berman et al., 1990; Cranage et al., 1992; Gardner, 1990; Gibbs et al., 1991) emphasizes the need to work towards the development of safe, inactive candidate vaccines suitable for use in humans.

IV. CURRENT DEVELOPMENTS IN HIV VACCINE

Several research centers are actively engaged in producing an effective AIDS vaccine. Some proposed HIV vaccines are undergoing clinical trials.

The MicroGeneSys gp160 subunit vaccine produced by genetic engineering technology in insect cells was the first HIV vaccine, approved in 1987 for human trials. The first results indicated that this vaccine generated dose-related antibody responses and also some degree of cell-mediated immunity. Two other vaccines based on gp160 protein are the Bristol-Myers vaccinia virus-based gp160 vaccine and Immuno-AG recombinant form of gp160 vaccine. Both vaccines are being tested clinically.

Other HIV vaccines are based on gp120 protein components of the HIV envelope or on core protein of HIV, such as p17 and p24. For example, MicroGeneSys p24 vaccine was tested in healthy HIV-infected individuals to evaluate if the onset of disease symptoms could be delayed. A synthetic p17 subunit vaccine administered to uninfected volunteers elicited both cytotoxic T-cell and helper T-cell responses.

Genentech's recombinant gp120 vaccine produced in mammalian cells is effective in protecting chimpanzees from experimental infection with HIV. Biocine Corp. Env2-3 vaccine, based on the gp120 component of the HIV envelope protein gp160 genetically engineered in yeast cells, elicited strong antibody and cell-mediated immune responses in baboons and chimpanzees. Merk Sharp & Dohme's mouse–human chimeric monoclonal antibody directed against the gp120 principal neutralizing domain of HIV protects chimpanzees from HIV infection. Salk and collaborators' inactivated HIV envelope-depleted vaccine tested on HIV-infected individuals showed that the CD4 T-cell levels have remained stable in a patient they have monitored since 1987. There is no evidence of hastened clinical deterioration after killed-virus vaccine administration. However, the use of subunit vaccines over whole-virus vaccines is favored because of safety concerns.

Researchers are engaged in producing AIDS vaccines for different purposes, for example, to prevent maternal transmission of HIV to a fetus or to delay or prevent disease in infected individuals. At an AIDS Conference in Florence in June, 1991, it was claimed that when the HIV vaccine is given to persons already infected, their immune response is stimulated, with a stabilization of T cell decline over 2 years.

However, before any AIDS vaccine is used widely in human it will be appropriate to investigate more precisely all aspects of immunodeficiency in HIV-infected individuals and to know exactly what type of immune response the proposed vaccines will elicit in order to achieve adequate protection.

V. SOME INTERESTING ASPECTS OF VACCINE STRATEGIES

A. Pseudovirion Vaccine Strategy

Pseudovirions are whole virus particles, noninfectious due to the deletion of key elements of the viral genome required for infectivity and/or genome replication but with no known role in virion assembly. Pseudovirions used in AIDS vaccine development would be advantageous for several reasons:

1. They contain all of the virion antigens and should retain the ability to fuse with CD4+ cells, which should facilitate antigen presentation and make possible induction of cellular as well as humoral immunity.
2. The folded envelope glycoproteins of pseudovirions would permit the presentation of conformation and development of epitopes of importance.
3. Certain viral proteins within pseudovirions could be structurally modified to optimize their immunogenicity.

Despite the fact that only a limited number of reports have described the production of HIV *gag*, *pol*, and *gag–pol* plus *env* genes using vaccinia virus expression vectors (Haffar et al., 1990; Shioda and Shibuta, 1990), these preparations contain live recombinant vaccinia virus particles that are unsuitable for use in humans. In a recent communication Haynes et al. (1990) strongly suggested that HIV pseudovirions produced from stably engineered cell lines represent safe, inactive immunogens containing multiple antigens in their native conformations. Their strategy for the production of HIV-1 pseudovirions involved the deletion of LTR elements from the provirus of LAV-1 BRU and insertion of the remaining coding sequences into an expression vector containing a heterologous promoter and polyadenylation site. The inserted fragment retained the major 5′ splice donor to preserve the normal pattern of HIV RNA splicing and gene expression.

HIV-1 pseudovirions are known to be immunogenic in mice, leading to a strong humoral response to envelope and core proteins. Based on the notion that pseudovirions should contain correctly folded conformation-dependent epitopes and lead to antigen presentation on the surface of CD4+ cells, the authors emphasize the value of testing this pseudovirion-based AIDS vaccine in humans.

B. Recombinant BCG–HIV Vaccines

Primary immunization with live recombinant vectors in order to express HIV genes and generate cell-mediated immunity (CMI) memory is accompanied by booster immunizations with pseudovirions, HIV particles, or synthetic peptides. The recombinant vectors currently in development include vaccinia virus, *Mycobacterium bovis*–bacillus Calmette-Guérin (BCG), salmonella, and adenovirus. Apart from contributing to priming the T cell, salmonella and adenovirus could induce mucosal immune response, which is of important in the prevention of mucosal transmission of the virus.

The human tuberculosis vaccine, *Mycobacterium bovis*–BCG is a particularly attractive live recombinant vaccine vehicle. BCG and other mycobacteria are highly effective adjuvants and the immune response to mycobacteria has been studied extensively. BCG is a live bacterial vaccine that is safe for human use, being one of the few vaccines usually administered at birth, and elicits long-lasting immune responses with a single dose. With the availability of recently developed molecular genetic tools and methodology, it has bene possible to introduce foreign genes into BCG (Jacobs et al., 1987; Husson et al., 1990). More recently, Aldovini and Young (1991) have reported that a variety of HIV-1 polypeptides could be expressed in BCG recombinant under the control of the mycobacterial hsp 70 promoter and that the foreign polypeptides produced in BCG can induce antibody and T-cell responses. Investigations are centered on whether three different HIV-1 genes could be expressed in BCG. The results of these investigations give credence to the notion that BCG could be used as live recombinant vaccine vehicle to induce immune responses to pathogen proteins produced by the bacillus.

In a report by Gicquel et al. (1991) *nef* was chosen as a model to study the expression and immune response induced by recombinant BCG. Nef is an early expressed protein against which the majority of seropositive patients tested have developed a cytolytic T lymphocyte (CTL) response. A strong proliferation response of lymph node cells was observed in Balb/c mice immunized with BCG recombinants expressing *nef*. The fact that recombinant BCG vaccine vehicles can induce immune responses to foreign proteins produced by the bacillus indicates that BCG can act simultaneously as an adjuvant and as a vehicle to produce and deliver selected antigens to the immune system. Since the antigen continues to be produced by BCG replicating in vivo, a BCG recombinant may provide a more long-lasting immune response to the respective pathogen than that provided by the simple mixture of BCG and antigen. It may therefore be more cost-effective to obtain genetically engineered BCG recombinants than to produce mixture. Above all, the ease with which bacteria can be genetically manipulated offers the advantage that certain features of the BCG vaccine vehicle may be tailored to obtain maximal immune responses.

C. Cytolytic T Lymphocytes

Cytolytic T lymphocytes (CTL) have been suggested as possible critical components of the immune response to HIV-1, particularly at the early stage of the viral infection. In addition to neutralizing antibodies, CTL could be determined by eliminating the first infected macrophages. Thus, the induction of CTL might be a prerequisite for the success of a vaccine. Synthetic peptides and lipopeptides obtained by linking lipid moieties to synthetic peptides have been noted as candidate tools for such a vaccine and it has been shown recently that they are capable of inducing CTL (Koenig et al., 1990; Levy, 1990).

Incorporating the CTL approach in the design of vaccines assumes a careful delineation of the epitopes recognized by such CTL and a better understanding of their failure to protect infected individuals. In addition to the primary neutralizing epitopes and the significance of HIV gp120, other epitopes must be used in formulating vaccines to induce broad reactive humoral and cell-mediated immune (CMI) responses against HIV.

D. Subunit Vaccines

Subunit vaccines are generally made from antigen purified from virions or produced by genetic engineering. In relation to HIV proteins, many uncomplicated expression systems have been used in bacteria, yeast, and eukaryotic cell lines. A distinct advantage of subunit vaccines appears to be their safety. The main problem seems to be the choice of viral antigens to constitute a subunit vaccine. Envelope or core subunits have been used predominantly. Another disadvantage noted is their low immunogenicity. It has been suggested that the development of latent reservoirs could be blocked by an immune response directed against viral products for latency or even expressed at the surface of latently infected cells. Negative or differential regulatory genes such as *nef* (Guy et al., 1987) or *rev* (Pomerantz et al., 1990) could encode such products.

Phase I clinical trials in healthy human volunteers help to address the issues of safety and immunogenicity. Several trials of recombinant subunit gp160 vaccines (LAV-III B strain) have been conducted. Recent experiments suggest that the vaccinia-derived gp160 subunit vaccine in oil adjuvant may be more potent (Corey, 1991). It has recently been reported that immunizations (4 shots in 18 months) of human volunteers with a subunit vaccine made from the HIV-1 have induced immune responses that result in the killing of HIV-1-infected cells (Orentas et al., 1990). The vaccine contains the HIV-1 envelope precursor protein gp160 produced with recombinant DNA technology. The vaccines had gp160-specific CTLs that were shown by cloning to be CD4+. Although induced by exogenous antigens, most gp160-specific CTL clones also recognized gp160 synthesized endogenously in target cells. These clones lysed autologous CD4+ T lymphoblasts infected with HIV. Of particular interests was that certain vaccine-induced clones that lysed HIV-infected cells recognized gp160 from diverse HIV isolates, and did not participate in the killing of noninfected CD4+ cells that had bound gp120. The observations of Orentas et al. (1990) do suggest that recombinant gp160 preparation is capable of inducing specific, cross-reacting, and clinically relevant immune responses. Berman et al. (1990) have recently used recombinant DNA technology and developed a candidate AIDS vaccine. Their studies indicated that chimpanzees immunized with the gp120 variant showed no signs of infection after more than 6 months. It could be concluded from their studies that recombinant gp120, formulated in an adjuvant approved for human use, could elicit protective immunity against a homologous strain of HIV-1. Phase I clinical trials in healthy volunteers are also currently underway for a subunit gp160 vaccines produced in a baculovirus expression system (Smith and Volvovitz, 1990).

E. Immune-Stimulating Complexes and HIV Immunization

To reduce the risks of immunization with killed or live attenuated virus vaccines, it may be of advantage to use a purified and defined antigen containing determinants for both humoral and cellular immunity. However, although most nonliving intact protein preparations induce antibodies and CD4+ major histocompatibility complex (MHC) class II restricted helper and/or CTL, they do not elicits CD8+ MHC class I restricted CTL (Germain, 1986, 1988). With some exceptions (Wraith and Askonas, 1984; Staerz et al., 1987), it has not been possible to induce CD8+ CTL by immunizing with intact soluble proteins. Recently, however, Takahashi et al. (1990) showed that a single subcutaneous immunization in mice with immunostimulating complexes (stable molecular structures with protein or peptide antigens incorporated into a matrix of adjuvant glycoside) containing either purified intact gp160 envelope glycoprotein of HIV or influenza hemagglutinins resulted in reproducible, long-lasting priming of HIV-specific or influenza-specific CD8+ MHC class I restricted CTL. The precise mechanism by which these immune-stimulating complexes (ISCOMs) enter cells remain unclear. The lipid with which it is associated could be responsible not only for entry but also for the susceptibility to processing by the endogenous pathway (Bolognesi, 1990). The ISCOMs appear to be of particular interest to HIV vaccine developers because of the widely held belief that protective immune responses must be directed against both free virus and infected cells. Until now, only attenuated HIV preparations or replicating recombinant vectors were possible candidates, but the former were excluded due to safety considerations. From a practical point of view, ISCOM-based vaccines may achieve the long-desired goal of induction of both CTL and antibodies by a purified protein. Since killed HIV preparations for human vaccines carry considerable risk, and ISCOMs bear only selected viral components, the latter appears to be an attractive alternative.

F. Inactivated HIV Vaccines

Inactivated vaccines (killed viruses) are less immunogenic than live vaccines and generally require a significant increase in the antigenic load, potent adjuvants, and multiple injections. Distinct advantages are simplicity and safety.

Inactivated HIV is being tried as a vaccine but does not appear to be widely favored, particularly in view of the poor records of such types of vaccines against retroviruses. Apparent failure of this type of immunization to induce the production of CTLs that kill virus-infected cells as part of the normal immune responses and the impracticability of growing large amounts of HIV appear to be the main limitations. The most promising results to date have been obtained in protection against simian immunodeficiency virus (SIV) with inactivated vaccine preparations.

The SIV macaque (SIVmac) model is proving useful in research efforts to develop an HIV vaccine. SIVmac has extensive sequence similarity to

HIV-1 and HIV-2 (Chakrabarti et al., 1985) and, like human viruses, is tropic for CD4+ lymphocytes and macrophages (Kannagi et al., 1985; Watanabe et al., 1989). Following infection with SIVmac, rhesus monkeys develop lymphodenopathy and immunologic abnormalities that include a decline in circulating CD4+ lymphocytes. Infected monkeys eventually die from a spectrum of opportunistic infections and tumors similar to those seen in HIV-infected humans (Letvin et al., 1985). SIVmac-infected macaques would therefore serve as a model for the study of HIV infection in human. Success in preventing SIV infection in macaque monkeys with vaccine preparations made of inactivated virus has provided the impetus for developing an effective HIV vaccine (Desrosiers et al., 1989; Murphey-Corb et al., 1989). One basic question with regard to inactivated virus preparation that remains to be answered concerns the inactivation of HIV with a sufficiently wide margin of safety (Girard, 1989).

Recent observations demonstrated that macaque monkeys produced antibodies to SIV, despite the fact that they were inoculated only with inactivated human T cells that had not been infected. This raises the question of the mechanisms of immune response and of approaches to producing an effective AIDS vaccine (Anderson, 1991). In other experiments Kion and Hoffmann (1991) demonstrated that mice treated with T lymphocytes from another mouse strain but not exposed to HIV produced antibodies against two of the proteins characteristics of HIV known as gp120 and p24. It seems that the presence or absence of virus is not the sole determinant of the production of antibodies. The authors extend their suspicions to vaccines based on purified and then inactivated virus particles as well as another culture of T cells (Maddox, 1991).

G. Live Recombinant HIV Vaccines

Live recombinant vaccines are made by genetic recombination between different viral genomes. Recombinant vaccinia viruses expressing several virus and HIV genes have been constructed in many laboratories (Keny et al., 1981; Chakrabarti et al., 1987; Hu et al., 1989). The recombinant viruses have been injected into humans (Zagury et al., 1987) or animals (Hu et al., 1989), inducing a strong cellular immunity to themselves and to the inserted HIV epitopes, but they have been found to elicit a low anti-HIV humoral immunity even after several boosters. The cellular immunity against vaccinia that can pre-exist or be elicited by primo-vaccination limits, to a large extent, the efficacy of boosting. To counteract this problem Zagury and colleagues (1987) used an inactivated preparation: autologous cells infected in vitro with vaccinia-HIV-*env* recombinants and fixed with formalin. This approach, however, appears to be of limited practical application. Among the HIV vaccines used in phase I trials was a live vaccinia recombinant expressing gp160 (Zagury et al., 1988).

Shen et al. (1991) have recently used a live recombinant virus, SIVmac, to determine whether such a genetically restricted, T lymphocyte-mediated antiviral response could be generated in a primate. Vaccinia–SIVmac vaccination elicited on SIVmac *gag*-specific CD8+ CTL response in rhesus monkeys. These CTLs recognized a peptide fragment that spans residues 171–191 of the Gag protein. The rhesus monkey MHC class I gene product restricting this CTL response was defined. Both the vaccinated and SIVmac-infected monkeys showing this MHC class I gene product developed CTLs with the same *gag* epitope specificity. The results of this study demonstrate that a CD8+ CTL response to a conserved structural protein of SIVmac could be elicited in a higher primate with the use of a recombinant virus vector system. These findings support the feasibility of using recombinant viruses in vaccines for the eventual prevention of HIV infection in humans.

Recombinant virus vaccines that express a limited number of epitopes are currently being developed to prevent disease by changing the relative balance between viral spread and the immune response. Some circumstances, however, were noted in infections with a noncytopathic virus in which vaccination caused disease. Variables included the genetic background of the host, the time and dosage of injection, and the constituents of the vaccine. It is thus apparent that immunologic damage by T cells may be an unwanted consequence of vaccination with the new type of peptide or recombinant vaccines being investigated for the HIV and other pathogens. The recent report by Oehen et al. (1991), in which they evaluated the capacity of recombinant vaccinia viruses that express either lymphocytic choriomeningitis virus (LCMV)-glycoprotein or LCMV-nucleoprotein to protect high, low, and nonresponder mice from LCM disease, lends credence to this notion. Their results document that in noncytopathic virus infections an antiviral T-cell response may be induced by vaccination that may aggravate disease caused by a subsequent infection. It is thus imperative that vaccine strategies for HIV be reevaluated carefully because in some instances vaccination may cause rather than prevent T-cell-mediated immunopathologic disease.

VI. CONCLUSIONS

The following appear to be significant advances in AIDS vaccine research and important indicators of the potential effectiveness of HIV vaccines:

1. Neutralizing antibodies for different serotypes of the HIV-1.
2. Cytotoxic lymphocytes capable of destroying HIV-1-infected cells.
3. Resistance of vaccinated chimpanzees to experimental HIV-1 infection or with the SIV model and resistance of vaccinated monkeys to experimental HIV infection.
4. The V3 neutralizing antibody response may play a crucial role in chimpanzees challenged with HIV-1 and antibodies in HIV vaccine design.

Findings from three primate centers have shown that inactivated whole-virus-based SIV-1 can confer protective immunity on rhesus monkeys challenged with low dosages of SIV-1 (Gardner, 1990). Thus, under defined laboratory conditions it may be possible to prevent cell-free SIV-1 infection in some animals. Even though these results appear to be promising, questions remain as to whether these SIV-1 whole virus vaccines are capable of preventing cell-mediated viral transmission and if they evoke protective mucosal immunity. Nevertheless, the preliminary success with whole SIV-1 vaccine provides optimism that a whole-virus or subunit HIV-1 vaccine could be developed. The recent elegant experiments reported with the recombinant gp120 for immunization in an aluminium hydroxide adjuvant approved for human use (Berman et al., 1990) appear to important milestones in the development of an AIDS vaccine.

For any HIV vaccine, however, to be truly effective, it would be of prime importance to induce both humoral and cellular immune response and to take into account the HIV variability. The extraordinary antigenic variability of the AIDS viruses HIV-1 and HIV-2 and their remarkable capacity to escape the host immune system by remaining silent in the form of an integrated provirus or by seeking shelter in tissue (central nervous system) or cellular (macrophages) compartments where they cannot be reached by antibodies or cytotoxic T cells is one of the difficult challenges worthy of additional effort.

Developing a vaccine against AIDS viruses is proving particularly difficult because there is no naturally acquired immunity to the deadly HIV. No one who has become infected has been able to overcome the virus and become immune. The idea that the mechanism of AIDS may be that of an autoimmune disease should also be investigated more fully.

REFERENCES

AIDS Update (1990).
AIDS Update (1991).
Aldovini, A., and Young, R. A. (1991). *Nature 351*:479-482.
Anderson, C. (1991). *Nature 353*:287.

Barre-Sinoussi, F., Chermann, J. C., Rey, F., Nugeyre, M. T., Charmaret, S., Gruest, J., Danquet, C., Axler-Blin, C., Vezinet-Brun, F., Rouzioux, C., Rozenbaum, W., and Montagnier, L. (1983). *Science 220*:868-871.

Barnes, D. M. (1987). *Science 237*:971-973.

Berman, P. W., Gregory, T., Dowbenko, D., and Lasky, L. A. (1988). In *Applied Virology Research*, Vol. I, *New Vaccines and Chemotherapy*, E. Kurstak (Ed. in Chief). Plenum Medical, New York, pp. 17–24.

Berman, P. W., Gregory, T. J., Riddle, L., Nakamura, G. R., Champe, M. A., Porter, J. P., Wurm, F. M., Hershberg, R. D., Cobb, K. K., and Eichberg, J. W. (1990). *Nature 345*:622–625.

Bolognesi, D. P. (1990). *Nature 334*:818-819.

Chakrabarti, S., Robert-Guroff, M., and Wong-Staal, F. (1985). *Nature 320*:535–537.

Chakrabarti, L., Emerman, M., Trolos, P., and Sonigr, P. (1987). *Nature 328*:543–544.

Cheng-Mayer, C., Homsy, J., Evans, L. A., and Levy, J. A. (1988a). *Proc. Natl. Acad. Sci. USA 85*:2815–2819.

Cheng-Mayer, C., Seto, D., Tateno, M., and Levy, J. A. (1988b). *Science 240*:80–82.

Clavel, F., Guetard, D., and Brun-Vezinet, F. (1986). *Science 233*:343–346.

Coffin, J. M. (1986). *Cell 46*:1–4.

Coffin, J. M. (1990). In *Applied Virology Research*, Vol. 2, *Virus Variability, Epidemiology and Control*, E. Kurstak (Ed. in Chief). Plenum Medical, New York, pp. 11–33.

Cohen, J. (1991). *Science 251*:1312–1313.

Corey, L. (1991). In *Proc. Colloque des Cent Gardes*, 6th ed., M. Girard and L. Valette (Eds.). Marnes, Paris, pp. 3–4.

Cranage, M. P., Baskerville, A., Ashworth, L. A. E., Dennis, M., Cook, N., Sharpe, S., Farrar, Rose, J., Kitchin, P. A., and Greenaway, P. J. (1992). *Lancet 339*: 273–274.

Culliton, B. (1992). *Nature 335*:286.

Desrosiers, R., Wyand, M., Kodama, T., Ringler, D., Arthur, L., Schyal, P., Letvin, N., King, N., and Daniel, M. (1989). *Proc. Natl. Acad. Sci. USA 86*:6353–6357.

Dorozynski, A., and Anderson, A. (1991). *Science 252*:501–502.

Epstein, F. H. (1991). *N. Engl. J. Med. 324*:307–317.

Evans, L. A., Moreau, J., and Odehouri, K. (1988). *Science 240*:1522–1525.

Gallo, R. C., Salahuddin, S. Z., Popovic, M., Shearer, G. M., Kaplan, M., Hayes, B. F., Palker, T. J., Redfield, R., Olecke, J., Safai, B., White, G., Foster, P., and Markham, P. D. (1984). *Science 234*:500–503.

Gardner, M. B. (1990). *AIDS Res. Human Retrovirus 6*:835–846.

Germain, R. N. (1986). *Nature 332*:687–689.

Germain, R. N. (1988). *Cell 54*:441–444.

Gibbs, C. J., Peters, R., Gravell, M., Johnson, B. C., Jensen, F. C., Carlo, D. J., and Salk, J. (1991). *Proc. Natl. Acad. Sci. USA 88*:3348–3352.

Gicquel, B., Winter, N., Langranderie, M., Ranzier, J., and Gheorghin, M. (1991). In *Proc. Colloque des Cent Gardes*, 6th ed., M. Girard and L. Valette (Eds.). Marnes, Paris, pp. 56–57.

Girard, M. (1989). In *Proc. Colloque des Cent Gardes*, 4th ed., M. Girard, and L. Valette (Eds.). Marnes, Paris, pp. 265–269.

Guy, B., Kieny, M. P., and Riviere, Y. (1987). *Nature 330*:266–269.
Haffar, O., Garriques, J., Travis, B., Moran, P., Zarling, J., and Hu, S. L. (1990). *J. Virol. 64*:2653–2659.
Hahn, B. H., Shaw, G. M., and Taylor, M. E. (1986). *Science 232*:1543–1548.
Haynes, J. R., Rowinski, B., Sia, C., James, O., and Klein, M. H. (1990). In *Proc. Colloque des Cent Gardes*, 5th ed., M. Girard and L. Valette (Eds.). Marnes, Paris, pp. 193–197.
Hossain, A., Al Tuwaijri, A., Kurstak, C., and Kurstak, E. (1990). In *Applied Virology Research*, Vol. 2, *Virus Variability, Epidemiology and Control*, E. Kurstak (Ed. in Chief). Plenum Medical, New York, pp. 55–60.
Hu, W., Heyden, N. V., and Ratner, L. (1989). *J. Bacteriol. 172*:519–524.
Jacobs, W. R., Jr., Truckman, R., and Bloom, B. R. (1987). *Nature 327*:532–535.
Kannagi, M., Yetz, J. M., and Lervin, N. L. (1985). *Proc. Natl. Acad. Sci. USA 82*:7053.
Keny, M. P., Rautman, G., and Schmidt, D. (1981). *Biotechnology 4*:790–795.
Kion, T. A., and Hoffmann, G. W. (1991). *Science 253*:1138–1140.
Koenig, S., Fuerst, T. R., Wood, L. V., Woods, R. M., Suzick, J. A., Jones, Z. M., De la Cruz, V. F., Dovey, R. M., Venkaesson, S., Moss, B., Biddison, W. E., and Fauci, A. S. (1990). *J. Immunol. 145*:127–131.
Koff, W. C. (1991). *ASM News 57(2)*:73–76.
Kong, L. T., Lee, S. W., and Kappes, J. C. (1988). *Science 240*:1525–1529.
Letvin, N. L., Daniel, M. D., and Sehgal, D. K. (1985). *Science 230*:71–74.
Levy, J. P. (1990). In *Proc. Colloque des Cent Gardes*, 5th ed., M. Girard and L. Valette (Eds.). Marnes, Paris, pp. 147–151.
Maddox, J. (1991). *Nature 353*:297.
Murphey-Corb, M., Martin, L. N., and Dourdom-Fairbuan, B. (1989). *Science 246*:1293–1297.
Oehen, S., Hengartner, H., and Zinkernagel, R. M. (1991). *Science 251*:194–198.
Orentas, R. J., Hildreth, J. E. K., Obah, E., Polydefkis, M., Smith, G. E., Clements, M. L., and Siliciano, R. F. (1990). *Science 248*:1234–1236.
Pomerantz, R. J., Trono, D., Feinberg, M. B., and Baltimore, D. (1990). *Cell 61*:1271–1276.
Putney, S. D., and Bolognesi, D. P. (1990). *AIDS Vaccine Research and Clinical Trials*. Marcel Dekker, New York.
Robinson, W. E., Montefiori, D. C., and Mitchell, W. M. (1988). *Lancet 1*:790–795.
Saag, M. S., Hahn, B. H., and Gibbon, J. (1988). *Nature 334*:440–444.
Salk, J. (1987). *Nature 327*:473–476.
Shen, L., Zheng, W. C., Miller, M. D., Stollard, V., Mazzara, G. P., Panicali, D. L., and Letvin, N. L. (1991). *Science 252*:440–442.
Shioda, T., and Shibuta, H. (1990). *Virology 175*:139–148.
Smith, T. F., Srimvason, A., Schoehetman, G., Marcus, M., and Meyrs, G. (1988). *Nature 333*:343–346.
Smith, G., and Volvovitz, F. (1990). In *Proc. Intern. Conference on AIDS* (8th), San Francisco, p. 114.
Solinger, A. M., Adams, L. E., Friedman-Kien, A. E., and Hess, E. V. (1988). *J. Clin. Immunol. 8*:32–41.

Spickett, G. P., and Dalgleish, H. G. (1988). *Clin. Exp. Immunol. 71*:1–7.
Staerz, U. D., Karasuyama, H., and Gardner, A. (1987). *Nature 329*:449–451.
Takahashi, H., Germain, R. N., Moss, B., and Berzofsky, J. A. (1990). *J. Exp. Med. 171*:571–576.
Watanabe, M., Ringler, D., Nakamura, M., De Long, P. A., and Letvin, N. L. (1989). *J. Virol. 64*:656–660.
Williams, P. (1991). *ASM News 57(9)*:459–463.
Wraith, D. C., and Askonas, B. A. (1984). *Nature 308*:457–460.
Zagury, D., Lemond, R., and Famhard, M. (1987). *Nature 326*:249–250.
Zagury, D., Bernard, J., and Cheymer, R. (1988). *Nature 332*:728–731.

Part II

Viral Hepatitis

4

VIRAL HEPATITIS

Viruses, Clinical Aspects, Genetics, and Pathogenesis

A. Al Tuwaijri, Christine Kurstak, A. Hossain and Edouard Kurstak
Faculty of Medicine, University of Montreal, and International Comparative Virology Organization, Montreal, Quebec, Canada

I. INTRODUCTION

Viral hepatitis characterized as an inflammation of the liver is a recognized major public health problem in all parts of the world. Currently, at least four major types of hepatitis caused by different hepatitis viruses are known. The terms *hepatitis A* for infectious hepatitis spread through casual contact and *serum hepatitis* for hepatitis B have been known since the early 1970s following the identification and isolation of both these viral agents. Hepatitis A virus (HAV) is a single-stranded linear RNA enterovirus type 72, belonging to the Picornaviridae. Hepatitis B virus (HBV) is a double-stranded circular DNA associated with the Hepadnaviridae (Blumberg et al., 1970; Melnick, 1982).

Other virologically and immunologically distinct agents have been associated with viral hepatitis, including the delta agent or hepatitis D virus (HDV), a defective, single-stranded circular RNA virus, requiring the presence of hepatitis B virus for its replication and expression (Rizzetto et al., 1977). Clinical and epidemiologic findings suggest the presence of more than one infectious agent for non-A, non-B hepatitis (NANBH), so named because of the absence of serologic markers for hepatitis A or B in clinically diagnosed cases of hepatitis. A virus associated with the parenteral transmission of NANBH has been classified as hepatitis C virus (HCV) and a form of hepatitis transmitted enterically and previously known as epidemic or water-borne NANBH is now known as hepatitis E virus (HEV) (Bradley et al., 1987; Choo et al., 1989; Kurstak et al., 1990;

McLachlan, 1991). Hepatitis C virus remains to date the major causative agent of all NANBH in the United States (Alter et al., 1990). HCV infection, on the other hand, appears to play a relatively minor role in Taiwan, a hyperendemic area for hepatitis B and chronic liver disease, according to a recent study (Chen et al., 1990).

Acute viral hepatitis is a generalized infection with emphasis on inflammation of the liver. The clinical picture of the infection varies, and it can present as asymptomatic or subclinical infection, mild gastrointestinal symptoms and the anicteric form of the disease, acute illness with jaundice, severe prolonged jaundice, or acute fulminant hepatitis. Hepatitis B and coinfection with the hepatitis D virus, and infection with the parenterally transmitted NANBH, may be associated with persistent carrier state and may progress to chronic liver disease, which could be severe. Current evidence suggests a causative association between hepatitis B virus and hepatocellular carcinoma (HCC), a common malignant tumor worldwide (Szmuness, 1978; Bréchot et al., 1981; Hsu et at., 1989; Kurstak et al., 1990, Wang et al., 1990).

Together with cirrhosis, another important consequence of chronic infection, hepatocellular carcinoma appear to be a major source of morbidity and mortality in Southeast Asia and Africa and, to a much lesser extent, in North America and Europe. HCV may also be implicated in cases of HCC (Colombo et al., 1989; Kiyosawa et al., 1990, 1991), particularly in cases in which the tumor and/or underlying cirrhosis is related to autoimmune hepatitis or chronic alcoholism (Johnson and Williams, 1990). A recent study has also reported an association between HCV and cryoglobulinemia type II (Pascual et al., 1990).

II. VIROLOGY

A. Hepatitis A

Structural and Genomic Aspects

It is almost two decades since the causative agent of hepatitis A was identified by immune electron microscopic examination of the feces of infected patients (Feinstone et al., 1973). The subsequent purification of virus particles from such fecal samples and the demonstration of their similarities in a number of properties with the picornaviruses, which included well-characterized viral agents as poliovirus, encephalomyocarditis virus, rhinovirus, and foot-and-mouth disease virus, proved to be a step towards comprehensive understanding of the structure, replication, and pathogenicity of hepatitis A virus (HAV).

Based on its morphologic and structural features, HAV has been characterized as a typical enterovirus. The mature infectious virion is a naked spherical particle with a diameter of 27–28 nm, in close resemblance with other picornaviruses (Siegl, 1988). It bands at a density of between 1.33 and 1.34 g/ml in cesium chloride and sediments at 156–160 S.

Although several biophysical characteristics (sedimentation coefficient, buoyant density in CsCl, and stability at pH 3) of HAV enteroviruses and cardioviruses are similar, one of the outstanding properties of HAV appears to be its exceptional stability. Dissociation experiments as well as infectivity assays have indicated that in resistance to heating, HAV surpasses poliovirus by 20°C and, at physiological pH, retains its physical entirety and biological activity at 60°C for at least 30 min. In the presence of a stabilizing agent (Mg^{2+}) at a concentration of 1 M the virus resists even heating to 80°C for 10 min (Siegl et al., 1981). These characteristics place HAV among the most stable viral agents and favor its effective transmission via fecal material and contaminated water and food, both endemically and in epidemics.

Free chlorine (hypochlorous acid) at a concentration of 1 mg/L has been shown to be sufficient to inactivate HAV within 30 min (McCallum and Zuckerman, 1981). Complete inactivation of purified HAV during incubation with formalin at a final dilution of 1:4000 at 37°C/72 hr has also been reported (Provost et al., 1975). Frosner (1982) has observed a >4 $\log_{10}$ reduction of infectivity in viral harvests from cell cultures incubated with a comparable concentration of formalin at 37°C for 3 days. Under laboratory conditions, purified HAV in phosphate-buffered saline has been noted to be readily inactivated by irradiation with ultraviolet (UV) light at 1.1 W for approximately 1 min (Provost et al., 1975). Likewise, the inactivation kinetics of HAV during irradiation with cobalt 60 were reported to resemble closely the characteristics of polio virus (Frosner, 1982). It has been speculated (Siegl, 1988) that the prominent physical and biological stability of HAV may be linked to the amino acid composition, the size, and, in all probability, the arrangement of the capsid proteins.

The genome of HAV has been reported to be a linear, single-stranded RNA of positive polarity and infectious as such (Cohen et al., 1987). RNA extracted from two different strains has been cloned and sequenced and the molecule found to consist of around 7500 nucleotides in length. Like the genome of a typical picornavirus, it can be functionally divided into a 5′-terminal untranslated region composed of 733 nucleotides, a single open reading frame of 6,681 nucleotides, and a short, 64 nucleotide long untranslated segment at the 3′ end of the molecule (Cohen et al., 1987; Ticehurst, 1986).

The HAV virion consists of four major structural polypeptides with 60 copies of each VP1 to VP4 and molecular weights ranging characteristically from 8,000 to 33,000 (Couleps et al., 1980). In procapsids and empty capsids, the amino acid sequences representing VP2 and VP4 are present in the form of a precursor polypeptide, VP0. In the process of maturation of the virus, this precursor is cleaned to yield the final structural polypeptides. Protein analysis of HAV particles purified from human fecal samples or from infected cell cultures provides evidence that in composition and structural plan the HAV capsid resembles closely the capsid typical of picornaviruses (Siegl, 1988).

The HAV genome can be differential from the genomes of viruses classified within the established four genera of picornavirus family by an unusually low guanine-cytosine content of 38%. The pyrimidine nucleotides C and T appear to be clustered near the 5′ end of the genome between the nucleotides 31 and 249 (Cohen et al., 1987; Ticehurst, 1986).

Virion RNA itself is infectious (Siegl et al., 1981). Only a single major antigenic specificity has been identified with HAV, and is associated with the dominant surface polypeptide VP1 (Ostermayer, 1988).

Replication

It is now possible to propagate HAV in vitro in a variety of cell cultures of well-established susceptibility that includes primary cell cultures such as African green monkey kidney cells and human embryonic fibroblasts, frequently used cell lines as MRC-5 and Vero cells, and in barely known ones as fetal rhesus kidney (FRhK) (Provost and Hilleman, 1979; Frosner et al., 1979; Siegl et al., 1981). Despite the use of these cells to support replication of established strains of HAV, the recovery from clinical samples and in vitro growth adaptation of infectious virus appear to be still fraught with problems, and laborious.

Replication studies have elicited many differences between HAV and typical picornaviruses. All known HAV strains have been noted to have a highly protracted replication, culminating in persistent type of infection (Wheeler et al., 1986; deChastonay and Siegl, 1987) rather than a lytic type of infection effectively completed within hours, as in poliovirus (Koch and Koch, 1985). It has been possible to subpassage over a period of months and even years persistently infected HAV cultures with the concomitant production of hepatitis A virus antigen in the absence of mycoplasma or other adventitious cytolytic viruses (Wheeler et al., 1986). In contrast to the conditions under which picornaviruses like the poliovirus or coxsackieviruses have occasionally been found to establish persistent infection in cell, virtually all cells in a persistently infected HAV cell system appear to be infected with neither antiviral antibody nor interferon necessary to maintain the virus–cell equilibrium (Gauss-Muller and Dienhardt, 1984). Since isolation of HAV in cell cultures initially proved to be successful most frequently at temperatures of 32°C and 35°C as opposed to 37°C, it was assumed that the temperature sensitivity of HAV might contribute significantly to the establishment of persistent infection. In view of the increasing number of successful isolations of HAV at 37°C, this now seems likely.

The protracted course of replication, the failure of the HAV to shut off host cell macromolecular synthesis, and the low level of virus production have been posed as stumbling blocks in the direct analysis of HAV replication at the intracellular, molecular level. Evidence does, however, suggest that the partial block in HAV replication leading to low levels of virus production and ultimately to the establishment of persistent infection may be at the level of penetration and uncoating (Wheeler et al., 1986) or at the level of processing of viral precursor proteins (deChastonay and Siegl, 1987; Gauss-Muller and Dienhardt, 1984). According to these studies, the limiting factor in HAV replication seems to be in the synthesis of viral RNA. Anderson et al. (1988) studied the single-cycle growth kinetics of HM175; absorption and penetration into B-SC-1 cells did occur at similar rates for HM175 and poliovirus; however, uncoating of HM175 was found to be delayed for up to 12 hr after infection. After uncoating, infectious RNA accumulates at a logarithmic rate with concomitant accumulation of infectious virions, typically giving a yield of 20 plague-forming unit (PFU) per cell after 48 hr. Even though large amounts of double-stranded RNA could be detected in cells by indirect immunofluorescence within 2 hr of infection with poliovirus, little was detectable in HM175-infected cells before 24–48 hr, at which time the maximal yield of infectious virus was produced. On the basis of these results the authors suggest that uncoating of virus particles essentially delays the initiation of HAV replication for approximately 12 hr, after which the replication of viral RNA may possibly limit the growth rate and yield of infectious HAV.

Another feature that differentiates HAV in the cell systems from most other picornaviruses known thus far appears to be in the resistance of replication to all those antiviral substances known to reduce or to block synthesis of many picornaviruses. A total of 25 antivirals including guanidine, 2-(α-hydroxybenzyl) benzimidazale, rhodanine, amanitine, and methylquercitin (3-MQ) have been reportedly tested (Widell et al., 1986; deChastonay and Siegl, 1988; Siegl and Eggers, 1982). All were found to be ineffective when used in noncytotoxic concentrations and thus point to the uniqueness of HAV among the other well-known picornaviruses.

B. Hepatitis B

Structure and Genomic Aspects

Hepatitis B surface antigens (HBsAg) was discovered in 1965 by Blumberg and colleagues during their investigation of human serum protein polymorphism. The antigen was first found in the serum of an Australian aborigine when a precipitin line formed in agar gel diffusion between that serum and the serum of a patient with hemophilia who had received multiple blood transfusions. It was thus first named Australia antigen (Alter and Blumberg, 1966). Eventually it was associated with acute hepatitis B (Prince, 1968). HBsAg in blood remains to date the most useful marker of active HBV infection and the serum the principal source of viral material for the serologic characterization of hepatitis B virus (HBV).

A definitive characterization of the biophysical nature of HBV began with the subsequent identification of the infectious particle among the myriad of viral specific particles produced in the course of HBV infection. Dane and colleagues (1970) discovered the virus as a 42 nm particle consisting of an envelope surrounding a 27 nm core. These particles, although high in titer in infectious serum, were nevertheless a small minority of the total viral-specific particles that appear as empty envelopes with no internal core. The core of the Dane particle (core antigen, HBcAg) and the antibody (anti-HBc) directed against it were described by Almeida et al. (1971) and Magnius and Espmark (1972) highlighted a further antigen-antibody (anti-HBe). A flurry of interest at the time in viral-associated DNA and RNA polymerases prompted several groups to test Dane particles. In 1973 Kaplan et al. demonstrated conclusively that HBV contained a DNA polymerase activity that, in the presence of nonionic detergent to strip the virion of its outer envelope, used an endogenous but not exogenous template. Robinson et al. (1974) showed that the exogenous template appeared to be a small (approximately 3 kb pair) double-stranded circular DNA. Summers et al. (1975) further defined in their studies the structure of this DNA and the way in which the endogenous DNA polymerase used this molecule as a template for DNA synthesis. According to these authors, the viral DNA was not totally double-stranded but contained a large single-stranded gap of variable size. Thus one of the two strands was complete and the other was, on the average, only half complete and the endogenous DNA polymerase extended the incomplete strand using the complete strand as template.

Now, HBV is described as a 42-nm double-shelled particle. The center of the virion and present within the liver cell nucleus is a 27 nm nucleocapsid core containing HBcAg and HBeAg. Within the nucleocapsid are found the viral genome and DNA polymerase. The HBV genome (Tiollais, 1988) is a small, circular, double-stranded-DNA molecule (3.2 kb pairs long) with a single-stranded region of variable length.

It has also been established that the examination of serum containing HBsAg by electron microscopy reveals a remarkable pleomorphism of like particles, consisting of small, roughly spherical particles (22 nm in diameter), and tubular forms of varying length but 42 nm in diameter. The 42 nm particles consists of a core of about 28 nm in diameter with a 2 nm shell and an outer coat about 7 nm thick. The 42 nm particle is indeed the HBV whereas the small particles and tubular forms are noninfectious viral coat protein.

Subtypes

Serologic analysis of the HBsAg has shown that the HBsAg particles share a common group-specific antigen "a" and generally at least two mutually exclusive subdeterminants "d" or "y" and "w" or "r" (Bancroft et al., 1972; Courouce et al., 1976). Four principal phenotypes are recognized: *adw, adr, ayw, ayr*, but other complex permutations of these subdeterminants and new variants have been described, all apparently on the surface of the same physical particles (Courouce et al., 1976).

The major subtypes have differing geographical distribution. For example, in Northern Europe, the Americas, and Australia, subtype adw predominates; subtype ayw occurs in a broad zone that includes northern and western Africa, the eastern Mediterranean, eastern Europe, northern and central Asia, and the Indian subcontinent. Both adw and adr are found in Malaysia, Thailand, Indonesia, and Papua New Guinea while subtype adr predominates in other parts of southeast Asia including Japan, China, and Pacific islands (Zuckerman, 1988). Furthermore, an uneven geographic distribution of HBsAg subtypes in infected populations (Mazzur et al., 1974) is noticeable with subtypes adw, ayw, and adr found in extensive geographical regions of the world and ayr occurring much less frequently in most of the world. The geographical distributions of subtypes probably reflect the locations of their origins and migrations of infected human populations.

Replication

The replication cycle of hepatitis B viruses appears to be different from other DNA viruses and is in fact suggestive of a close relationship with the RNA viruses. The particular unusual feature is the use of an RNA copy of the genome as an intermediate in the replication of its DNA genome. Infecting DNA genomes are converted to a double-stranded form(s) that serves as a template for transcription of RNA. Multiple RNA transcripts are synthesized from each infecting genome with these transcripts characterized by either messenger function on DNA replicative function. Those with functions associated with DNA replication have been termed "pregenomes" or precursors of the progeny DNA genomes, in view of the fact that they are assembled into nucleocapsid cores and reverse-transcribed into DNA before being coated and leaving the cell. Each mature virion thus contains a DNA copy of the RNA pregenome and a DNA polymerase. This replication strategy for HBV DNA was proposed by Pekin ducks and ground squirrels and observations in humans. Obvious from this scheme is the fact that completion of the plus strand does not appear to be necessary for the release of the virus from the cell. This explains the finding that genomes in extracellular virions have incomplete plus strands of varying length (Scatto et al., 1985).

Budding of core particles into cisternae of endoplasmic-reticulum-related structures appears to be a possible mechanism for the formation of hepatitis B virus. Results of a recent study by Roingeard et al. (1990) seem to suggest that the exocytosis of cisternae to extracellular spaces may be a mechanism for release of hepatitis B virus particles.

Genetic Variation in Hepatitis B Virus

Use of conventional immunologic techniques had for some time indicated an association of HBsAg with a dominant epitope a. Two sets of mutually exclusive subtype epitopes d/y and w/r and generally a viral strain are known to express d or y, and w or r. All known antigenic subtypes of HBV are thus far known to contain the a determinant, antibody to which confers protection against all subtypes of HBV. The emergence of an escape mutant functionally locking the a determinant appears to be of concern. The study by Carman et al. (1990) indicates that the presence of anti-HBs apparently was unable to confer protection against infection with the mutant strain of HBV.

The application of molecular biology to the study of HBV has unmasked the interesting genetic sophistication of this compact DNA virus (Muller et al., 1988). The DNA amplification method using the polymerase chain reaction (PCR) has tremendously enhanced the detection and sequencing of the HBV gene (Sarki et al., 1988; Yokosuka et al., 1991). Earlier reports in the literature have indicated clinically important genetic variants of HBV (Carman et al., 1989). Individuals predominantly of Mediterranean origin have chronic HBV infection with continuing, often severe liver damage and high circulating levels of HBV DNA indicative of active viral replication in liver in the absence of HBeAg in serum. Absence or loss of HBeAg is generally believed to coincide with diminished intrahepatic viral replication. In such individuals with chronic HBeAg-negative, HBV, DNA-positive hepatitis B, HBeAg is not produced because of one or more point mutations in the precore region of the C gene of HBV.

A HBV variant has been recently described in which a novel core antigen resulting from a series of mutations in the precore and core regions of the genome is associated with failure of development of antibody to hepatitis B core antigen (anti-HBc) (Bhat et al., 1990). This occurred in a homosexual man infected with human immunodeficiency virus (HIV) who had received HBV vaccine before HBV infection was recognized. The patient may have been susceptible to HBV infection because of a lack of response to the vaccine due to immunosuppression not because HBV was a mutant form. The high levels of HBV DNA in the serum of this patient do, however, raise the possibility of a high rate of viral replication favoring spontaneous mutation (Martin and Friedman, 1991).

An extreme example of probable genetic variation in HBV is obvious in the transmission of hepatitis B to chimpanzees from patients with chronic hepatitis but no circulating markers of HBV (Thiers et al., 1988). Using a combination of a monoclonal antibody capture technique and the polymerase chain reaction, the viral genome has in one such case been cloned and sequenced and, furthermore, multiple nucleotide changes demonstrated compared to all known HBV subtypes (Liang et al., 1990). This study demonstrates that the viral DNA persists as a nonreplicating episomal form in the nucleus of hepatocytes. After a patient's clinical and serologic recovery from an acute hepatitis, low-level hepatitis B virus–related genome may persist in the liver despite the presence of antibodies to HBsAg. Such persistence of viral genome, according to the authors, may be a natural sequela of infection and may be a source of viral latency and possible reactivation. Further characterization of additional HBV isolates from patients without serologic markers would, however, help to define the extent and significance of genomic variations.

The studies by Carman et al. (1989, 1990) enhance the growing evidence for the genetic heterogeneity of HBV. They suggest that HBV infection by a variant that does not express the wild-type a determinant of HBsAg could possibly overcome immunity to HBV following vaccination. Whether natural immunity is also overcome by this variant has not yet been established, but according to Martin and Friedman (1991) this appears to be likely. A potential reason for concern that emerges from this study is whether universal vaccination against HBV could lead to an enhanced emergence of escape mutants.

The clinical importance of HBV mutants remains yet to be evaluated and the response to interferon therapy in chronic HBeAg-negative, HBV DNA-positive hepatitis B associated with the precore mutant remains unclear.

Attention has recently been focused on nonimmunogenicity of the HBV vaccine in persons lacking an immune-response gene. Immunogenicity of HBV vaccine has, to date, been largely equated with efficacy. The emergence of an escape mutant implies the possible occurrence of HBV infection after successful vaccination, not because of deficiencies in the host but primarily due to changes in the virus. Use of a monoclonal anti-HBs antibody in liver transplant recipients has apparently enhanced the emergence of a singular escape mutant (Carman et al., 1990). Yet another instance of viral multiplication in the presence of immunity to HBsAg is obvious from a recent report of an immunoselected HBV mutant (Moriyama et al., 1991). The possible development of escape mutants should thus be taken into active consideration in devising future vaccination strategies.

C. Hepatitis D

The discovery of the delta antigen by Rizzetto et al. (1977) has made the hepatitis D virus (HDV) the focus of worldwide research interest. The delta antigen, which was found as a poorly explained result of immunofluorescence staining in liver biopsy samples from chronic HBsAg carriers of Italian origin presently presents the nucleocapsid of a unique and important viral agent.

The HDV is an incomplete RNA virus dependent on the helper functions of HBV for its replication and survival. The requirements for the dual expression of these viruses are unknown and their relation is complex since HDV can replicate in cells without HBV sequences (European Association of the Liver Meeting Budapest, British Society Meeting, 1990). The HDV or delta agent is unique among human viruses and is basically a 35–37 nm, double-shelled particle. By electron microscopic examination it has been reported to be very similar to the "Dane particle" or HBV (Rizzetto, 1984). HDV has an external coat consisting of HBsAg encoded by HBV sequences (the helper virus) and an inner core consisting of the delta antigen (HDVAg provided by the genome of HDV) and the HDV viral genome. The genome of HDV is small circular molecule of RNA with a length of 1678 nucleotides; it is smaller than the genome of any known virus. The molecular weight is possibly around 500,000 daltons (Dernston,

1986; Kos, 1986; Wang et al., 1986). The virion RNA strand detected in serum is considered "genomic" and is single stranded with negative polarity. Both the genomic (–) strand and the antigenomic (+) strand of RNA have been detected in the liver of HDV-infected patients (Hoofnagle, 1989). Cloning and sequencing of HDV RNA has indicated a high cytosine–guanosine nucleotide base content (60%), also with many regions of internal complementary (Wang et al., 1986). Analysis of the nucleotide sequences of cloned HDV RNA has revealed sic "open-reading frames" that are considered possibly to represent the viral genes. Three of the open-reading frames are on the genomic and the remaining three on the antigenomic strand. Open-reading frame 5 on the antigenomic (+) strand has been suggested to be the gene for HDVAg, a 24 kb protein (Bergmann and Gerin, 1986).

HDV RNA isolated from infected liver is present in multiple forms, some linear, some circular, and others longer than genomic length, suggesting that HDV replicates its RNA by the "double-rolling circle model" (Branch and Robertson, 1984). The structure and replication cycle of HDV essentially places it outside of any known family of animal viruses (Hoofnagle, 1989).

HDV is currently assessed as a highly infectious pathogen with the potential to cause acute hepatitis, superimposed on acute or chronic hepatitis B infection and chronic hepatitis in HBsAg carriers. Since hepatitis B virus provides the means for hepatitis D virus secretion and release from infected cells, active HBV multiplication favoring the spread of HDV from cell to cell may increase the pathogenic potential of the defective agent (Smedile et al., 1981).

D. Non-A, Non-B Hepatitis

Virology

Non-A, non-B hepatitis is an important transmissible disease whose precise causative agents remain undetermined. Three epidemiologic types of NANBH have, however, been thus far recognized: enteric NANBH (ET-NANBH), posttransfusion or parenteral NANBH (PT-NANBH), and sporadically occurring, community-acquired NANBH (SPOR-NANBH).

The enterically transmitted epidemic non-A, non-B virus has been currently provisionally designated as the hepatitis E virus (HEV). It is a spherical, nonenveloped single-stranded RNA virus with a diameter of 27–34 nm and in all likelihood associated with the caliciviruses (Bradley, 1988). The viral agent responsible for the enterically transmitted form of NANBH has been recently (Reyes et al., 1990) serially transmitted in cynomolgus macaques (cynox) and resulted in typical elevation in liver enzyme levels and the detection of characteristic viruslike particles (VLPs) in both feces and bile. Infectious bile was used for the construction of recombinant complementary DNA libraries. One clone, ET 1.1, was found to be exogenous to uninfected human and cynogenomic liver DNA, as well as to genomic DNA from infected cyno liver. ET 1.1 did, however, hybridize to an approximately 7.6 kb RNA species present only in infected cyno liver. The translated nucleic acid sequence of a portion of ET 1.1 had a consensus amino acid motif consistent with an RNA-directed RNA polymerase, an enzyme common to all positive-strand RNA viruses ET 1.1 specifically identified similar sequences in complementary DNA from infected human fecal samples originating from five geographically distinct ET-NANBH outbreaks. This study thus suggests that ET 1.1 represents a portion of the genome of the principal viral agent, namely hepatitis E virus (HEV), responsible for epidemic outbreaks of ET-NANBH.

Parenterally transmitted NANB hepatitis is perhaps the most common form of posttransfusion hepatitis in most developed countries and may account for the majority of such cases. Recent work at the Centers for Disease Control and Chiron Corporation (Choo et al., 1989) has led to the isolation and characterization of the genome of the major causative virus of PT-NANBH, which is currently provisionally designated the hepatitis C virus (HCV). This is an enveloped single-stranded RNA virus with a genome of approximately 10,000 nucleotides, a diameter of 50–60 nm, and likely to belong to the flavivirus family. Filtration studies have further revealed that the virus is sensitive to such organic solvents as chloroform and has a relatively low buoyant density. Flavivirus, formally known as arboviruses, have been reclassified into five different groups. One of these groups, known as unclassified viruses, are bloodborne, cause chronic viremia, and include such viruses as the simian hemorrhagic fever virus of primates. Hepatitis C virus may belong to this class of viruses. The sporadic form of NANB hepatitis is most probably also caused by HCV.

Genetic Variation in Hepatitis C Virus

Although hepatitis C virus (HCV) has been identified as the predominant agent of chronic posttransfusion NANBH worldwide (Alter et al., 1989), the frequency of detectable anti-HCV in acute resolving NANBH infections reported appears to be much lower, ranging from 15 to 60% with a mean delay to seroconversion of almost 6 months after transfusion. hence, there is an urgent need for sensitive direct assays for viral markers. Considering the expected low titers of HCV antigens in infected individuals, antigen assays would very likely be limited by their inherent sensitivities. These considerations prompted Ulrich et al. (1990) to use reverse transcription (RT) in combination with the polymerase chain reaction amplification (RT-PCR) as a sensitive direct assay for the detection of HCV RNA in plasma. This RT-PCR amplification assay would be useful in differentiating infected from immune individuals. The polymerase chain reaction (PCR) has been recently used by Weiner et al. (1990) and, in a modified form as "nested PCR" assays, by Garson et al. (1990) towards the detection of hepatitis C viral sequences in blood donations. Nested PCR differs in using two successive rounds of amplification, with the second round using primers internal to or nested within the original two primers. Garson's use of nested primers achieved a level of sensitivity similar to that of the study by Weiner without resorting to a radioactive. This represents a significant amplification of the method and makes it potentially more amenable for use in clinical laboratories. Infectious HCV may be present in blood without detectable anti-HCV (Lucey and Traber, 1991). The application of PCR technology to the identification of HCV-RNA in potentially infected sera may provide a possible solution to this question of immense clinical importance.

Ulrich et al. (1990) reported in their recent study the prevalence of HCV RNA in plasma from symptomatic volunteers blood donors with elevated alanine aminotransferase (ALT) levels and its correlation with the presence of anti-HCV, HBsAg, and anti-HBc. The titers of HCV cDNA were determined to obtain quantitative information about the virus load in infected individuals. Amplified HCV cDNAs from plasma specimens with highest virus titer were directly sequenced and compared with chimpanzee-HCV (CH-HCV) cDNA sequence in an effort to determine the degree of genome heterogeneity among different HCV isolates. For a sensitive, specific RT-PCR assay it would be of importance to select primer binding sites that would presumably be conserved among different HCV isolates. The primer pair PKL 13-PKL 14 in the study of Ulrich et al. (1990) allowed efficient amplification of all HCV cDNA preparations thus far tested. The authors believe that they have managed to investigate the nucleotide sequence on that particular region of the HCV genome. The sequences of the CH-HCV and the three human HCV isolates are highly homologous, both at the nucleotide level and the predicted amino acid level, in the region between these two primers. The RT-PCR assay for the detection of HCV sequences in plasma could be a useful confirmatory test for the diagnosis of HCV infection and may provide concrete information on the frequency and duration of the symptomatic HCV carrier state.

III. CLINICAL ASPECTS

The symptoms of viral hepatitis are usually nonspecific. In individual cases the infecting viral agent remain indistinguishable by clinical features alone. Groups of serologically confirmed cases, however, show distinct clinical patterns.

A. Hepatitis A Infection

The development of specific serologic tests for the markers of the hepatitis A virus (HAV) has opened the possibility of differentiating with certainty the cases caused by HAV from attributable to either the hepatitis B virus (HBV) or the agents of NANBH. A practical result of these serologic tests has been the recognition of the asymptomatic cases of HAV infection and the characterization of the specific symptoms associated with hepatitis A.

The characteristic signs and symptoms of HAV infection are often indistinguishable from those of hepatitis B and NANBH. They include the malaise, fatigue, loss of appetite with which most cases of hepatitis A begin, and nausea and vomiting that may ensue within several days or simultaneous with the onset of other symptoms. Right upper quadrant abdominal pain may also occur. Jaundice, the recognition of which is dependent on its intensity and the patient's level of awareness may be present with the onset of fatigue and loss of appetite or it may develop 1–7 days later. Pale stool is yet another characteristic sign; other signs often present include hepatomegaly and splenomegaly.

Aspects of the presentation of a patient with hepatitis A that may, in certain cases, allow for a provisional diagnosis of HAV infection deserve consideration. In the environmental or epidemiologic context, a patient's infection may be most likely due to HAV if it occurs as part of a point-source outbreak following ingestion of water contaminated with sewage, or following close contact with a person identified with an HAV infection. Subsequent transmission of acute hepatitis to additional close contacts 1–6 weeks after onset is also suggestive of hepatitis A.

Findings most often associated with hepatitis A, but that may also be seen with hepatitis B, include fever (in those fulminant cases that rapidly evolve to coma) and extreme elevations of aminotransferase and bilirubin levels (Tabor, 1988). Fever appears to the one finding which occurs primarily in some acute HAV infections. No reports of fever in NANB hepatitis exist in the literature. In hepatitis A, fever rarely exceeds 39°C (102°F) and has been generally related to the intensity of the patients' illness. The fever in hepatitis A may be accompanied by chills. Diarrhea occasionally accompanies hepatitis A. Headache may also occur during infection with hepatitis A; this symptom has not been associated with other forms of hepatitis. In general, hepatitis A tends to have an abrupt onset whereas that of hepatitis B appears to be protracted and insidious. Acute illness is usually less severe in its clinical and biochemical findings in hepatitis A compared to hepatitis B.

Symptomatic cases of HAV may present in an atypical fashion. Severe diarrhea has been reported with HAV in stool during relapse (Benenson et al., 1980; Slubarczyk et al., 1984; Sjogren et al., 1987). Fever, diarrhea, cough, nausea, vomiting, abdominal pain, and anorexia may be the only symptoms recognizable in more than 50% of symptomatic children transmitting HAV (Storch et al., 1979). If one is uncertain whether these atypical symptoms are the result of HAV, ascribing them to other viral illness may lead one to underestimate the prevalence of asymptomatic HAV infections in children.

Asymptomatic cases of serologically documented HAV infections have been noted to be common. Asymptomatic infections appear to be predominant among children under 2 years of age (Hadler et al., 1980). The prevalence of asymptomatic infections is generally lowest among adults (Benenson et al., 1980; Jacobson et al., 1985).

It has been established that clinical or inapparent HAV infection gives rise to a specific antibody response conferring lifelong immunity, and that HAV is excreted in the feces shortly before for 1 or 2 weeks after onset. This is followed by the production of secretory coproantibodies, which eventually, would prevent reinfection at the intestinal level. The results of an epidemiologic study by Villarejos et al. (1976) carried out in Costa Rica, however, seem to be dissenting. These authors explain their results on persistence and reinfection with HAV as evidence of two separate infections with hepatitis A virus: the first without causing illness, presumably linked to the intestinal lumen, with neither systemic involvement nor consequently detectable antibody response; and the second occurring as a regular systemic infection with clinical signs and symptoms and a full-blown serologic immune response. As an explanation of this phenomenon, they further postulate the existence of strain variants that replicate in the intestinal lumen but do not have the potential to penetrate the gut and reach the bloodstream. This also could be the result of infection with very low doses of virus. The fact that immune persons can experience intestinal reinfection, together with the demonstration of prolonged viral excretion in the form of immune complexes from which HAV is liberated in the outer environment by proteolysis, may help to explain the mechanism of viral perpetuation in areas endemic for HAV.

Chronic hepatitis, a cause of long-term sequelae and death in some cases of hepatitis B and NANBH, has so far not been observed in patients with hepatitis A (Rakela et al., 1979). HAV infection has generally been noted to be self-limiting, with recovery occurring usually within 8–12 weeks. Fulminant hepatitis A is rare. Of the 11 reported cases of fulminant hepatitis A, 6 were reported by Rakela et al. (1979). The clinical presentation in fulminant HAV infection does not appear to be significantly different from other cases of symptomatic acute HAV infection (Rakela et al., 1977; Mathiesen et al., 1980). In the documented cases the incubation periods ranged from 3 to 4 weeks and symptoms at presentation included jaundice, dark urine, nausea, abdominal pain, and excessive thrust. At death, the duration of the disease from the time of onset of jaundice ranged from 10 to 48 days.

B. Hepatitis B Infection

Hepatitis B virus (HBV) infections can result in a variety of clinical manifestations of the disease. The commonly encountered ones are inapparent (subclinical) infection, acute infection of varying severity, or persistent infection with or without chronic liver disease. Persistent HBV infections have been found to occur at varying rates in different regions of the world, with the highest noted in certain regions of Asia and Africa. The difference in incidence of persistent infections is attributable to genetic factors and to age at infection. The trend is toward infection in very early life, leading to a chronic HBV carrier state, in contrast to infection occurring later in life. In the western world, approximately 45% of all HBV infections are known to result in acute disease, with a fatality rate of 1%, development of chronic infections in 5%, and 50% of the remaining cases being asymptomatic (Junge and Deinhardt, 1985).

Chronic infection can lead to progressive liver disease, cirrhosis, and primary hepatocellular carcinoma in 25–50% of cases (Hoofnagle and Alter, 1984; Seef and Koff, 1986). In a very recent study by Chang et al. (1991), the status of hepatitis B and nontumorous liver tissues of eight children with positive serum HBsAg and maternal HBsAg was investigated. Hepatocellular carcinoma from five of the eight children showed integration of HBV DNA into host cellular DNA sequences. A pattern of single-site integration in four children and multiple-site integration pattern in one child was demonstrated. HBV DNA could not be demonstrated in the remaining three children. With the use of subgenomic fragments of the HBV genome as probes, X gene fragments and the surface antigen gene fragment were found to be the most conserved sequences. The single-site integration of HBV DNA in childhood hepatocellular carcinoma may, as the authors speculate, have hit the critical region, resulting in insertional mutagenesis and early development of hepatocellular carcinoma. This emphasizes the idea that with a short incubation period and less exposure to environmental carcinogens during early life, childhood hepatocellular carcinoma may provide a useful model for the study of the carcinogenic potential of hepatitis B virus.

Clinical presentation varies with the nature and stage of the disease progression. Several factors predispose to the development of chronic carrier state, the most important being age, sex, and immunologic status. Some 95% of neonates born to mothers who are HBsAg/HBeAg carriers become chronically infected. Immunosuppressed or immunodeficient patients such as the cancer, those with Down's syndrome, lymphoma, leukemia, and those who have received dialysis or an organ transplant tend to have chronic disease. The intensity of viral replication appears to be unrelated to the clinical severity of hepatitis B infection.

The laboratory analysis of hepatitis B markers is of importance both in the diagnosis and management of infection.

Acute Hepatitis B Infection

The consequences of HBV infection may be grave. Rather than being associated with a typical clinical picture, HBV infection may produce a spectrum of different clinical and laboratory manifestations. The severity of acute HBV may range from inapparent infection to lethal fulminant hepatitis. The clinical course of acute HB is usually similar to that of hepatitis A or NANBH, with the onset of the disease perhaps being more insidious than that of hepatitis A. The first symptoms are usually noticeable 3–4 days before jaundice appears, but in atypical cases the symptoms may occur 2–3 weeks earlier. Malaise, lethargy, and anorexia are the most common prodromes. Food smells may cause nausea and there appears to be a loss of desire for cigarettes and alcohol. Vomiting could occur but is usually mild and lasts for a limited time. Constipation and mild diarrhea occur in some patients. Abdominal discomfort or right upper quadrant pain is commonly noted. All these symptoms result in weight loss averaging 2–4 kg (Junge and Dienhardt, 1985). Flulike symptoms with slightly elevated temperatures appear to be common: malaise, slight headache, and myalgia. Myalgia and arthralgia without clinical signs have been noted as the early symptoms in 10–30% of patients with acute hepatitis B (Gocke, 1975; Stewart et al., 1978).

With the development of the icterus phase, prodromal symptoms including arthralgia, myalgia, and fever subside; this is also referred to as "feeling better." Lethargy, weakness, anorexia, and right upper abdominal pain may persist or even increase. One to several days before the development of jaundice, the urine is brownish (dark urine). Jaundice is detectable in the conjuctivae or oral mucosa and may persist for a few days or weeks. Prolonged jaundice occurs particularly in patients with HB (Stewart et al., 1978) and notably among older women. Depending on the intensity of the icterus, patients have pale (light grey or yellow) stools. During the initial signs of icterus, mild and transient itching is common. Childhood infections appear to be mainly asymptomatic. The liver is usually palpable, slightly increased in size, with a smooth, tender edge but with almost normal consistency. Percussion of the right hypochondrium causes pain and there is evidence of a palpable spleen in about one-quarter of the patients. The posterior cervical lymph modes may show enlargement. Ascites have also been noted in severe cases of acute hepatitis B (Viola et al., 1983). In typical viral hepatitis, hepatic scintiscanning reveals a diffuse nonhomogeneous uptake pattern, mild hepatomegaly, and an enlarged spleen in about one-quarter of patients. Ultrasound findings could be nonspecific. Liver biopsy is only indicated in protracted disease when chronic hepatitis is suspected, serologic and laboratory values, especially serum aminotransferase levels, and clinical findings are extremely characteristic. The levels of liver enzymes serum aminotransferase (ALT) and aspartate aminotransferase (AST) are invaluable for the reliable diagnosis of acute viral hepatitis and monitoring of its course. Serum transaminase levels rise during the prodromal phase, usually preceding icterus by 8–10 days (Schmidt and Schmidt, 1983). In acute hepatitis, peak serum transaminase levels become characteristically high, than those varying between 500 and 3000 U/liter, with ALT levels recognizably higher than those of AST. The level of serum transaminases does not, however, always reflect the intensity of liver damage. According to the observations of Schmidt and Schmidt (1983), transaminase levels in patients with hepatitis B decrease more slowly than those in patients with hepatitis A, with a plateau more commonly observed. Very rarely is a second rise of transaminase activity of variable duration detected, as in cases of hepatitis A or NANBH. The relationship of serum transaminase activity to alkaline phosphatase activity appears to be of diagnostic significance primarily for patients with cholestatic icterus, with AST levels > 500 U/L (Schmidt and Schmidt, 1984). The more sensitive gamma glutamyl transpeptide (GGT) level is generally found to be elevated to 5–10 times the normal value and the GGT/AST or ALT ratio is less than 1 (Schmidt and Schmidt, 1983). Serum bilirubin elevations range widely and are indicative not only of hepatocellular damage but also the degree of cholestasis and hemolysis. In cases of uncomplicated viral hepatitis, peak values have been found noted to be 12 mg/100 ml and normal values are attained within 2–4 weeks (Koff and Galambos, 1982). Elevated levels of serum bilirubin would thus serve as an indicator of atypical hepatitis. Bilirubin is detectable in the urine several days before the development of jaundice. As with aminotransferase activity, serum bile acid levels are found to increase in patients with viral hepatitis, and elevated levels are maintained until recovery is complete. Bile acid levels, however, appear to be of no apparent diagnostic significance since no intricate differences in levels are detectable in acute and chronic hepatitis. Although elevated levels of IgM are detectable, with higher levels detected in hepatitis A than in hepatitis B, the large variations in IgM values limit its potential use in the unequivocal identification of the type of hepatitis. HBV infections could occur without any obvious signs and symptoms and even in the absence of any marked elevation in serum aminotransferase levels. Regular testing for HBsAg and/or anti-HBs provides the only evidence of the occurrence of these inapparent or subclinical infections. Anicteric hepatitis B has been noted to produce symptoms and laboratory-detected changes similar to the icteric form, but it more frequently becomes chronic. Inapparent or anicteric hepatitis B with a tendency towards chronicity appears to be the trend in patients receiving dialysis or those taking immunosuppressive drugs. Laboratory data indicative of mild cholestatis appear to be common in patients with acute hepatitis B. In patients with this rare, benign cholestatic-type B, itching and prolonged jaundice are frequently found. Serum transaminase levels are similar to those in typical cases of hepatitis, but levels of bilirubin and peak akaline phosphatase levels three times normal are found. Despite the severity and prolonged nature of cholestatic-type hepatitis, compared to icteric hepatitis, generally full recovery is the end result.

HBV infection could cause massive liver necrosis resulting in acute hepatic failure with a death rate more than 70%; however, fewer than 1% of all patients develop this fulminant hepatitis characterized by progressive jaundice, hepatic coma, shrinkage of the liver, and hemorrhagic diatheses. Prothrombin time appears to be low, serum ammonia levels elevated, and decreased levels of serum transaminase are detected. Functional renal failure, hypotension, acute pancreatitis, cerebral edema, gastrointestinal hemorrhage, and bacterial sepsis have been known to be the major complications (Horak, 1983). Symptoms of fulminant hepatitis may be initially present or develop during the course of what might appear to be a typical case of hepatitis B. Incidence of fulminant hepatitis B may perhaps be even more frequent than reported in the literature, particularly in view of the more rapid clearing rate of HBsAg than in regular hepatitis B (Trepo et al., 1976).

Chronic Hepatitis B Infection

This is conventionally defined as a state of hepatic inflammation associated with elevated alanine aminotransferase (SLT) levels lasting longer than 6 months. If HBsAg is detectable in the serum for 6 months or more, the patient is termed a chronic hepatitis B carrier. Most patients with chronic HBV infection have however, a history of symptomatic acute hepatitis B. Because the immune responses of such persons are inadequate, infectious viral particles persist, leading to continuous hepatocellular damage: chronic hepatitis, cirrhosis, and primary hepatocellular carcinoma (PHC) are often the result.

Three different clinical syndromes of chronic hepatitis are currently known:

1. chronic active hepatitis, a progressive and destructive liver disease
2. chronic persistent hepatitis, a benign form
3. chronic lobular hepatitis, recurrent bouts of "acute hepatitis" but asymptomatic between episodes; pathologically similar to acute and nonprogressive hepatitis.

Each of these forms of chronic hepatitis has a characteristic histologic appearance (Seef, 1975). Of these, chronic active hepatitis and chronic persistent hepatitis are the two clinically distinct forms generally recognized.

Most cases of chronic persistent hepatitis usually resolve over 1–2 years; in contrast to chronic active hepatitis, which often proceeds to terminal cirrhosis of PHC.

Chronic persistent hepatitis (CPH) may follow an acute attack of clinically recognized hepatitis B, but may also present insidiously (Iwarson, 1985). Approximately 50% of patients are symptomatic and the remainder tend to have vague, mild, and nonspecific symptoms such as fatigue and abnormal pain over the liver region. Jaundice and hepatomegaly may also be present. Transaminase enzymes (ALT, AST) are often elevated but are usually less than five times normal values. Serum gamma globulin levels as well as coagulation tests appear to be normal. The disease is most prevalent in young or middle-aged men. The histologic picture of CPH is not generally specific, clinical and laboratory data should be considered in achieving a reliable diagnosis. The majority of diagnosed cases of CPH appear to be attributable to HBV (Aldershivile et al., 1982). The main differences between chronic persistent hepatitis and acute viral hepatitis are the duration and severity of the symptoms, the degree of elevation of transaminase enzymes, and liver histologic findings. Chronic persistent hepatitis B is generally a benign disease that does not usually require specific treatment. The prognosis of chronic persistent hepatitis has been suggested to be generally good; the pathologic lesions may eventually resolve spontaneously.

Chronic active hepatitis (CAH) B is a severe and chronic inflammatory liver disease characterized by disarrangement of the architecture of the liver. A possible final development is liver cirrhosis. It may develop after an acute attack of hepatitis B but may also present silently. Rarely, chronic active hepatitis B or cirrhosis develops in children (Gershon et al., 1987). CAH may be due to varied causes. Judging by the trend in diagnosed cases, the role of HBV may be minimal (Koretz, 1989). The clinical picture of HBsAg-positive CAH may be variable but persistent changes in serum aminotransferase levels are common findings. Symptoms may include fatigue and anorexia but some patients are asymptomatic until late stages and may present with portal hypertension. A diagnosis of HBV-associated chronic active hepatitis is effectively achieved by evidence of chronic liver disease for at least 6 months, positive serum HBsAg and negative anti-HBc, 5–10-fold persistent elevation of transaminase enzymes, and piecemeal necrosis. The mainstay of treatment has been corticosteroids with or without azathioprine. There is no convincing evidence, however, that corticosteroids or other immunosuppressive agents could be of value in the treatment of HBV-associated CAH.

Patients receiving dialysis and renal transplants becoming chronically infected with HBV are at high risk for the development of chronic liver disease. They usually have no clinical symptoms and only mild elevations in serum aminotransferase levels. Liver biopsy specimens, are indicative of a severe chronic hepatitis. A recent study suggested that liver-membrane-specific activated T lymphocytes in peripheral blood may be important in the autoimmune attack of chronic active hepatitis in children (Wen et al., 1990). The indicated relative risk of contracting chronic hepatitis was 30 times greater for HBsAg-positive recipients or renal transplant recipients than for HBsAg-negative recipients. In another study (Quaglia et al., 1981), chronic liver disease was, however, found in only 35 of 405 renal transplant patients, with very few of these chronic cases attributable to HBV. It is thus obvious that HBV-associated chronic liver disease is not of major importance in renal transplant recipients, despite the chronic asymptomatic HBV infection in a certain number of patients, particularly when immunosuppressive therapy has been instituted. Furthermore, silent progression to chronicity seems to be common in patients receiving hemolysis (Miller et al., 1978). The prognosis of liver disease among HBsAg-positive dialysis or renal transplant patients with chronic persistent hepatitis documented histologically appears to be generally good and obviates any real need for treatment.

Although the majority of hemophiliacs have hepatitis B markers in serum, prospective studies indicate that less than 10% of patients with persistently elevated levels of aminotransferases are chronically infected with HBV and only 20% of those with chronic hepatitis have persistent HB infection (Hoofnagle and Seef, 1976; White et al., 1982). ALT elevations seemed to be higher in patients with CPH than in those with histologically milder forms of hepatic inflammation, but no correlation between liver histologic findings and hepatitis B serologic findings was obvious. Chronic HBV-associated liver disease could, however, pose a problem in hemophiliacs with persistent HBV replication (Kim et al., 1980). The high risk of hepatitis B exposure in male homosexuals, the apparent tendency to persistent HBV infection, and the development of chronic liver disease become obvious from studies conducted on HBsAg carriers. A bleak prognosis for HBV-associated chronic liver disease in male homosexuals compared wit nonhomosexuals is suggested by the studies of Aldershiville et al. (1982). Hepatitis B infection has been noted to be a major problem in drug addicts, and chronic liver disease due to HBV seems to occur more often than in nonaddicts.

C. Hepatitis D (Delta) Virus Infection

The hepatitis D virus (HDV) can cause either acute or chronic hepatitis (Rizzetto, 1984). Hepatitis D (delta hepatitis) resembles other forms of acute and chronic hepatitis in its clinical characteristics, it tends to be more severe than other forms (Caredda et al., 1987). The mortality rate of acute delta hepatitis (icteric) is reported to range form 2 to 20%, in comparison to less than 1% for acute hepatitis B. Chronic hepatitis D likewise appears to be more severe than other forms of viral hepatitis (Rizzetto et al., 1983; DeCock et al., 1986). Seventy to 80% of patients with chronic hepatitis D have been found to develop cirrhosis and complications of portal hypertension, in contrast to 15–30% of those with chronic hepatitis B. The rapid progressive course of chronic hepatitis D is also unusual in chronic hepatitis B or NANB hepatitis (Bonino et al., 1987).

Acute infection with HDV may occur simultaneously with HBV infection in a previously healthy individual (*coinfection*) or as a *superinfection*, signifying the appearance of acute HDV infection in a chronic HBV carrier. These two diseases have different clinical courses, outcome, and serologic markers (Rizzetto et al., 1984; Hoofnagle, 1989; Caredda et al., 1987).

In coinfection, the resultant illness is usually self-limiting and not more severe than an ordinary attack of HBV infection alone (Papaevangelou,

1983; Tabor, 1983), rarely leading to chronic hepatitis, even though morbidity may be significantly increased (Shattock et al., 1985). Prospective studies indicate less than 5% of patients with acute hepatitis develop chronic disease (Caredda et al., 1987). With a massive infecting dose, a more severe illness may occur either as fulminant hepatitis or as a prolonged biphasic illness: initial hepatitis followed by improvement and later by clinical and biochemical relapse (Govindarajan et al., 1988). In a recent study, Kosaka et al. (1991) suggest that precore-defective mutants of HBV have stronger activity to induce fulminant hepatitis B than do non-defective viruses. In a typical case of acute hepatitis D virus coinfection, hepatitis B surface antigen (HBsAg) followed by HDV RNA and HDVAg are first detectable during the incubation period of the disease. A rise in serum aminotransferase levels occur, often in a biphasic pattern, and clinical symptoms associated with jaundice appear. With clearance of HBsAg, HDV replication and acute liver disease resolve and shortly after the onset of clinical symptoms, antibody to HDV (anti-HDV) arises (Aragona et al., 1981).

In contrast to HDV coinfection, acute HDV superinfection of HBsAg carriers may produce severe hepatitis and lead to chronic acute hepatitis and cirrhosis, more often than with hepatitis B infection alone (Govindarajan, 1983; Hadler et al., 1984). Progression to chronic hepatitis D infection occurs in as many as 70–90% of all superinfections (Caredda et al., 1987). Most cases of chronic hepatitis D probably arise from superinfection (Hoofnagle, 1989). The factors contributing to chronicity remains as yet obscure. Clinical presentation of HDV infections has generally been noted to be similar to that of HBV. The HDV superinfection in a chronic HBsAg carrier is marked serologically by the appearance of serum aminotransferase level elevations and anti-HDV in the serum. Persistence of HDV replication is followed by persistence of abnormalities in liver biochemical test results and the rise of anti-HDV to high, sustained titers. Patients with delta superinfection develop HDV RNA in serum persisting in lower titer during the chronic infection (Smedile et al., 1981, 1987; Hoofnagle, 1989).

Possible modifications of chronic hepatitis B virus and HDV infections by human immunodeficiency virus (HIV) have been examined by Govindarajan et al. (1988) among household contacts of persons with hematologic disorders requiring hemotherapy, selected donors, recipients of blood component therapy, and persons with congenital clotting disorders requiring therapy with clotting factor concentrates. The replicative activities of HBV and HDV were assessed by analysis of detectability of serum HBV-DNA, IgM antibodies to hepatitis B core antigen (anti-HBc-IgM), and IgM antibodies to HDV antigen (anti-HDV-IgM). The hepatic necroinflammatory changes with HBV and coinfections are assayed by measurement of serum alanine aminotransferase (ALT) activities. No association between anti-HIV status and HBV-DNA, anti-HBcIgM, anti-HDV-IgM, or serum ALT activities was detectable.

D. NANBH Virus Infection

Enterically transmitted NANBH resembles hepatitis A infection clinically. The disease is self-limiting, with no report of long-term sequelae or chronic liver disease. One important feature of ET-NANBH/hepatitis E is its high mortality rate (20%) in infected pregnant women (Khuroo et al., 1981). Infection may lead to fatal fulminant hepatitis. In epidemics of ET-NANBH/hepatitis E, the overall mortality rate has been noted so far as 1–2% (Purcell and Ticehurst, 1988; Zuckerman, 1990; Lau et al., 1991).

Parenterally transmitted NANBH (PT-NANBH)/hepatitis C usually causes a milder disease clinically than hepatitis B, with a high proportion of symptomatic cases. In the United States and Europe, asymptomatic infections occur more often with PT-NANBH/HCV than with hepatitis B. The range of symptoms caused by parenteral HCV tend to be similar to those associated with acute hepatitis B. PT-NANBH is characterized by a high rate of chronicity, reportedly in 40–60% of cases noted in prospective studies (Purcell and Ticehurst, 1988). Ten to twenty-five percent of patients with chronic NANBH have developed cirrhosis, some of whom have since died (Alter and Hoofnagle, 1984). One report has indicated a limited number of cases of primary liver carcinoma in patients with PT-NANBH; the causal relationship, however, remains unproven (Kiyosawa, 1984). Very recently, Kiyosawa et al. (1987, 1990, 1991) have used anti-HCV testing of stored sera from patients with chronic hepatitis, cirrhosis, and hepatocellular carcinoma (HCC) and indicated additional evidence of a causal link between HCV and HCC. In Japan they found anti-HCV in 76% of patients with hepatocellular carcinoma. The casual link between HCV and HCC is also pointed out by Di Bisceglie et al. (1991), who found that the relative risk for hepatocellular carcinoma in HBsAg was 17.3 and for patients with anti-HCV was 7.3. Considering that the prevalence of HCV infection in the general population is higher than for HBV (14.4% vs. 6.7%), the authors concluded that in the United States HCV may play a more important role than HBV in the development of hepatocellular carcinoma.

IV. PATHOGENESIS

A. Hepatitis A

Despite the centuries-old recognition of viral hepatitis as a distinct clinical entity and the identification of the distinct nature of infectious hepatitis for several decades, a comprehensive understanding of the clinopathologic feature of acute hepatitis A and the hosts' immune response has been forthcoming only in the last few years. This has been possible subsequent to the development of methods for visualizing HAV and detecting virus antigen and antibody.

The morphologic lesions of acute hepatitis A are typical of the changes seen in all types of viral hepatitis. During the period of elevated serum aminotransferase activity, histologic features include activation of sinusoidal lining cells, focal hepatocellular nervous, portal, and periportal infiltration with mononuclear inflammatory cells, appearance of hepatocytes, and coagulative necrosis of hepatocytes resulting in the presence of acidophilic bodies (Friedman and Dienstag, 1984). The lesions in hepatitis A develop earlier and the duration of the morphologic changes is shorter, while the lesions in hepatitis B linger on, fluctuate, and regress slowly. While the distribution of lesions in hepatitis A is characterized by parenchymal changes being predominantly periportal, hepatitis B lesions tend to be accentuated around the hepatic vein tributaries. Streaks of focal necrosis may extend from the portal to hepatic vein tributaries (Popper et al., 1980; Abe et al., 1982).

The mechanisms underlying liver injury in hepatitis A remain obscure. The initial noncytopathic phase, during which the virus replicates and is released, is followed by decreased virus multiplication and inflammatory cell infiltration, suggesting that immune mechanisms may be involved in pathogenesis. Based on necrologic findings, the liver has been shown to be the first site in which the virus can be localized by immunofluorescence (Mathiesen et al., 1977). HAV can be detected by immunofluorescence staining as early as a week before, and sometimes coinciding with, the onset of fecal excretion. As shown by immunofluorescence staining, HAV first appears in a finely granular pattern, diffusely distributed throughout the hepatic parenchyma. As the course of infection continues, staining increases in intensity and becomes localized in fecal areas within hepatocytes and Kupffer's cells. Localization of HAV is restricted to the cytoplasm (Mathiesen et al., 1977; 1978).

Viremia is also an early event in hepatitis A, demonstrable as early as 12 days after inoculation (Giles et al., 1964). The brief duration of viremia and the extremely low concentration of HAV make the demonstration of

HAV in serum of patient with hepatitis A impractical clinically. Viremia is, however, most pronounced late in the incubation period, before symptoms or maximal elevations of serum aminotransferase activity occur.

Shedding of the virus in stools has been noted to be one of the earliest events detectable with in vitro techniques in clinical specimens. The onset of fecal excretion of HAV coincides with the appearance of nonspecific prodromal symptoms and peaks in intensity several days to more than a week before biochemical and histologic evidence of acute hepatitis is apparent (Dienstag et al., 1975). The bulk of fecal shedding of HAV precedes peak aminotransferase activity levels and onset of jaundice (Dienstag et al., 1975; Frosner et al., 1977). Thus by the time a patient with jaundice seeks medical attention, the level of fecal HAV may be inadequate for diagnosis. HAV has been detected in stools of both icteric and anicteric patients, but viral shedding appears to be more pronounced in icteric patients (Dienstag et al., 1975; Frosner et al., 1977). The apparent failure to detect HAV in feces of anicteric patients (Dienstag et al., 1975) and the demonstration of brief, low levels of fecal virus shedding in individuals with mild or inapparent illness suggest that the intensity of HAV fecal excretion is proportional to the severity of the disease.

The humoral immune response to HAV is intense, and anti-HAV is detectable during early acute illness, usually coincident with acute hepatocellular necrosis (Frosner et al., 1977; Rakela et al., 1977). Thus, anti-HAV is detectable in serum at a time during illness when viremia has been proven by immunologic testing and by infectivity in marmosets, suggesting that such early antibody may in fact be nonneutralizing. Titers of serum anti-HAV continue to rise after acute illness, reaching peak levels about 2–3 months later, and then falling gradually. Years after infection, relatively high anti-HAV titers are, however, easily detectable (Frosner et al., 1977) and anti-HAV can persist indefinitely. The pattern of anti-HAV development and the titers detected appear to be the same whether the infection is asymptomatic and accompanied by elevation of aminotransferase activity (Villarejos et al., 1976), asymptomatic in the absence of biochemical abnormalities (Krugman, 1976), mildly symptomatic, severe, or even fulminant (Friedman and Dienstag, 1984). Smooth muscle antibodies, antinuclear antibodies, liver cell membrane antibodies (Manns et al., 1980), antibodies to single-stranded DNA (Gust et al., 1980), antibodies to liver specific proteins (Meliconi et al., 1982), and liver-specific antigens (Dart and Kaldor, 1981) have been demonstrated in the sera of some patients with acute hepatitis A. This may be suggestive of the evidence that hepatic injury in general modifies the role of the liver in modulating immune responses. As is the case for many acute and chronic infectious diseases and diseases of the liver, evidence exists for the presence of circulating immune complexes in patients with HAV serum (Mathiesen et al., 1978). Unlike the humoral immune response to HAV, little attention has been focused on cellular immune responses to hepatitis A virus infection.

The pathophysiology of HAV-associated hepatocellular necrosis is currently obscure; a direct cytopathic role for the virus and for an immunologically mediated mechanism is possible. Despite the presence of anti-HAV in serum during early acute illness coinciding with acute hepatocellular necrosis, other observations lend support to the hypothesis that HAV, unlike HBV, behaves as a cytopathic agent and destroys hepatocytes without any significant contribution from the host's immune system (Friedman and Dienstag, 1984). The diagnosis appears to be dependent on the demonstration of anti-HAV IgM in serum during the acute phase of an HAV infection.

B. Hepatitis B

The pathogenesis of HBV-induced liver disease is not well understood but evidence suggests that immunologic events appear to be the primary pathogenic determinants. A basic point is that HBV is a noncytopathic virus, and that the mononuclear cells adjacent to dying hepatocytes in hepatic infiltrations are responsible for the death of these cells. Viral synthesis in patients without liver injury (the carrier state) does suggest that HBV is not directly cytopathic for hepatocytes. However, viral persistence is often associated with the development of chronic hepatitis, indicating that the virus is necessary, if not causative, in the disease process.

The precise role of the immune system in the disease process remains undefined. Several humoral and cellular immune responses to viral and host antigens have been described in HBV infection and HBsAg neutralized viral infectivity, and contributes to the formation of immune complexes that produce many extrahepatic disease manifestations, among them being notably arthritis. These immune complexes may be found in sera during the incubation period and acute phase of hepatitis B. Immune complexes have been found in the sera of patients with fulminant hepatitis B, but only infrequently in those with nonfulminant infection. Immune complexes are also important in the pathogenesis of syndromes characterized by damage of blood vessels: in polyarteritis nodosa and in the renal glomeruli in some forms of glomerulonephritis in children. HBsAg, anti-HBs, anti-HBc, and HBsAg-anti-HBs complexes have been found in variable proportions of patients with all the recognized chronic sequelae of acute hepatitis B.

Cellular immune responses are important determinants of the clinical features and course of HBV infection, as in some other viral diseases. Cell-mediated immunity to hepatitis B antigens has been demonstrated in most patients during the acute phase of hepatitis B and in a significant proportion of patients with HBsAg-positive chronic active hepatitis, but not in asymptomatic hepatitis B carriers (Prince and Trepo, 1971). These suggest that perhaps cell-mediated immunity may be important in terminating the infection and, under certain circumstances, in promoting liver damage. Altered suppressor and helper T-cell activity during infection may lead to immune-mediated liver injury (Dudley et al., 1972). It has also been suggested that the destruction of HBV DNA may be dependent on an immune response to HBsAg, and that failure of this process of elimination results in persistence of clones of cells with the potential for transformation.

C. Hepatitis D

The pathologic changes associated with HDV infection are indicative of a similarity of morphologic expressions induced by infection with NANB viruses and HDV. The predominant effect of HDV infection appears to be cytotoxic rather than lymphocytotoxic, which is the characteristic of hepatitis B (Popper, 1984). Histopathologic findings have also shown no significant differences in necroinflammatory features of patients with chronic liver disease (CLD) with or without HDV infection, suggesting that the presence of HDV does not result in an increase in necroinflammatory activity (Toukan et al., 1987).

A cytotoxic effect of HDV infection on hepatocytes, associated with specific histologic changes, characterizes a disease in young South American Indians. Initially, in an outbreak in remote valleys in Venezuela, epidemiologic investigations indicated a high HBsAg carrier rate and frequent HDV antibodies (Hadler et al., 1984). It was possible to reconstruct a sequence of pathologic events (Popper et al., 1983). In the early stage, a few days after onset of symptoms, the liver exhibited abundant microvesicular fat droplets in hepatocytes with focal necrosis, preceded by eosinophilic alterations and acidophilic bodies, unlike the findings of other forms of fulminant hepatitis. The cause of the unusual course of delta hepatitis remains unknown (Hoofnagle, 1989).

D. NANBH (Hepatitis C/E)

There is considerable evidence that PT-NANBH infection may be followed in many patients with prolonged viremia and the development of a persistent carrier state. Studies of the histopathologic sequelae of acute NANBH infection reveal chronic liver damage that may be severe and occur in 40–50% of patients. Hepatitis C is the major causative agent of all non-A, non-B hepatitis in the United States (Alter et al., 1990; Lau et al., 1991).

Histologic changes in the liver of patients with enterically transmitted non-A, non-B hepatitis (ET-NANBH; hepatitis E) are characteristic and differ from the histopathologic changes of parenterally transmitted NANB hepatitis (PT-NANBH). The typical changes observed in liver from patients with the disease include focal necrosis with little infiltration and no lobular predilection. The focal lesions appear to resemble those in some forms of drug-associated toxic hepatitis. At the cellular level there is a ballooning of hepatocytes, cytoplasmic cholestasis, and focal cytolytic necrosis with the formation of acidophilic bodies. At the lobular level, there is cholesterosis in canaliculi and pseudoglandular alteration of hepatocyte plates.

The resemblance of the histopathologic lesion of ET-NANBH to drug-induced cytotoxicity has raised questions as to the viral cause of the disease itself. The long incubation period and evidence of transmissibility in humans and primates, however, strongly suggest a viral cause. The high mortality rate of fulminant hepatitis in pregnant women appears to be particularly striking. The Shwartzman phenomenon has been proposed in this context (Popper et al., 1980, 1983; Purcell and Ticehurst, 1988). As noted in this article, viral damage to the sinusoidal cells, in particular the Kupffer cells, diminishes their ability to protect the hepatocytes against endotoxins of gram-negative bacterial origin in the intestinal tract. Direct injury of hepatocytes by endotoxin and secondary injury, mediated through release of eicosonoids, leads to prostaglandin-mediated chemotactic edema and cholestasis. This increased sensitivity of pregnant women to an endotoxin-mediated effect may explain the notable mortability of ET-NANBH in pregnancy.

Recently, the lack of association between circulating HCV-RNA and anti-HCV positivity in primary biliary cirrhosis (PBC) has been reported (Bertolini et al., 1991). In this study, serum samples from 106 consecutive patients with PBC were tested for anti-HCV by conventional ELISA (Ortho Diagnostics, Raritan, NJ). Positive samples (optical density ≥ 0.459) were retested in duplicate and further with the recombinant immunoblot assay (RIBA). To detect the HCV genome, RNA extracted from ELISA-positive samples was reverse-transcribed and amplified by the polymerase-chain reaction (PCR) with primers of the nonstructural region. Based on their results showing a 3% prevalence of anti-HCV positivity in the group of 88 patients who could be regularly evaluated and none with detectable HCV-RNA among those ELISA-positive with serum available for HCV determination, the authors conclude that the frequency of anti-HCV positivity in Italian patients with PBC appears to be somewhat higher than in the general population. Since none of the patients with PBC tested by PCR, unlike those with autoimmune chronic-active hepatitis, had detectable HCV-RNA in serum, it is unlikely that HCV plays a part in the pathogenesis of PBC.

REFERENCES

Abe, H., Beninger, P. R., Ikejini, N., Setoyama, H., Sata, M., and Tanikawa, K. (1982). *Gastroenterology 82*:938–947.

Aldershivile, J., Dietricksm, O., Skinkou, P., Kayger, P., Mathiesen, L. R., Christoffersen, P., and Nielsen, J. O. (1982). *Hepatology* 2:243–246.

Almeida, D., Rubenstein, D., and Statt, E. (1971). *Lancet* 2:1225–1227.

Alter, H. J., and Blumberg, G. S. (1966). *Blood 27*:297.

Alter, H. J., and Hoofnagle, J. H. (1984). In *Viral Hepatitis and Liver Disease.* G. N. Vyas, J. L. Dienstag, and J. H. Hoofnagle (Eds.). Grune & Stratton, New York, pp. 345–351.

Alter, H. J., Purcell, R. H., Shih, J. W., Melpolde, J. C., Houghton, M., Choo, Q. L., and Kuo, G. (1989). *N. Engl. J. Med. 321*:1494–1500.

Alter, M. J., Hadler, S. C., Judson, F. N., Manes, A., Alexander, J., Hu, P. Y., Miller, J. K., Moyer, L. A., Fields, H. A., Bradley, D. W., and Margolis, H. S. (1990). *JAMA 264*:2231–2235.

Anderson, D. A., Locarnini, S. A., and Gust, I. D. (1988). In *Viral Hepatitis and Liver Disease.* A. J. Zuckerman (Ed.). Alan R. Liss, New York, pp. 8–11.

Aragona, M., Macagno, S., and Caredda, F. (1987). In *Hepatitis Delta Virus and Its Infection.* M. Rizzetto, J. L. Gerin, and R. H. Purcell (Eds.). Alan R. Liss, New York, pp. 243–248.

Bancroft, W. H., Mundo, F. K., and Russell, P. K. (1972). *J. Immunol. 109*:842–848.

Benenson, M. W., Takafjui, E. T., Bancroft, W. H., and Lemon, S. M., Callogan, M. C., and Leach, D. A. (1980). *Am. J. Epidemiol. 112*:471–481.

Bergmann, K. F., and Gerin, J. L. (1986). *J. Infect. Dis. 514*:702–7005.

Bertolini, E., Zermiani, P., Battezzate, P. M., Bruno, S., Villa, E., Mannenti, F., Marelli, F., Moroni, G. A., Zuin, M., and Podda, M. (1991). *Lancet 337*:675–676.

Bhat, R. A., Ulnick, P. P., and Vyas, G.N. (1990). *Hepatology 11*:271–276.

Blumberg, B. S., Alter, H. J., and Visnish, S. (1965). *Bull. N.Y. Acad. Med. 40*:377–381.

Blumberg, B. S., Alter, H. J., and Visnish, S. (1970). *N. Engl. J. Med. 283*:349–354.

Bonino, F., Negro, F., Baidi, M., Brunetto, M., Chiaberge, E., Capalbo, M., Maron, E., Locarnini, C., Rocca, H., and Rocca, C. (1987). In *Hepatitis Delta Virus and its Infection*. M. Rizzetto, J. L. Gerin, and R. H. Purcell (Eds.). Alan R. Liss, New York, pp. 145–152.

Bradley, D. W. (1988). In *Viral Hepatitis and Liver Disease*. A. J. Zuckerman (Ed.). Alan R. Liss, New York, pp. 138–143.

Bradley, D. W., Krawczynski, W., and Cook, E. H. (1987). *Proc. Natl. Acad. Sci. 84*:6277–6281.

Branch, A. D., and Robertson, H. D. (1984). *Science 223*:450–458.

Bréchot, C., Nalpas, B., Courouce, A., Duhamel, G., Callard, P., Carnot, P., and Tiollais, P. (1981). *Proc. Nat'l. Acad. Sci. 78*:3906–3910.

Carman, W. F., Jacyna, M. R., Hadziyannis, S., Karayiannis, P., McGarvey, M. J., and Makris, A. (1989). *Lancet 2*:588–591.

Carman, W. F., Zanetti, A. R., and Harayiannis, P. (1990). *Lancet 2*:325–329.

Caredda, F., Antironri, S., Re, T., Pastecchia, C., and Moroni, M. (1987). In *Hepatitis Delta Virus and its Infection*. M. Rizzetto, J. L. Gerin, and R. H. Purcell (Eds.). Alan R. Liss, New York, pp. 267–276.

Chang, M. H., Chen, P. J., Chen, J. Y., Lai, M. Y., Hsu, H. C., Lian, D. R., Lui, Y. G., and Chen, D. S. (1991). *Hepatology 13*:316–320.

Chen, D. S., Kun, G. C., Sung, J. L., Lai, M. Y., Sheu, J. C., Chen, P. J., Yang, P. M., Hsu, H. M., Chang, M. H., Chen, C. J., Hahn, L. C., Choo, Q. L., Wang, T. H., and Houghton, M. (1990). *J. Infect. Dis. 162*:817–822.

Choo, Q. L., Kao, G., Winger, A. J., Overby, L. R., Bradley, D. W., and Houghton, M. (1989). *Science 244*:259–362.

Cohen, J. L., Ticehurst, J. R., Purcell, R. H., Buckler-White, A., and Baroudy, B. M. (1987). *J. Virol. 61*:50–59.

Colombo, M., Choo, Q. L., Dol-Ninno, E., Diogusodi, N., Kuo, G., Donato, M. F., Tommasini, M. A., and Houghton, M. (1989). *Lancet 2*:1006–1007.

Couleps, A. G., Locarnini, S. A., and Gust, I. D. (1980). *J. Virol. 35*:572–574.

Courouce, A. M., Holland, P. V., Muller, J. Y., and Saulier, J. P. (1976). *Bibl. Haematol.* (Basel) *42*:1–158.

Dane, D. S., Cameron, C. H., and Briggs, M. (1970). *Lancet 1*:685–698.

Dart, G. C., and Kaldor, J. (1981). *Pathology 13*:579–586.

de Chastonay, J., and Siegl, G. (1987). *Virology 157*:268–275.

de Chastonay, J., and Siegl, G. (1988). In *Viral Hepatitis and Liver Disease*. A. J. Zuckerman (Ed.). Alan R. Liss, New York, pp. 956–960.

DeCock, K. M., Govindarajan, S., Chin, K. P., and Redekar, A. G. (1986). *Ann. Intern. Med. 986*:108–114.

Dernston, K. (1986). *Science 232*:873.

Di Bisceglie, A. M., Order, S. E., Klein, J. L., Waggoner, S. G., Sjogren, M. H., Kuo, G., Houghton, M., Choo, Q. L., and Hoofnagle, J. H. (1991). *Am. J. Gastroenterol. 86*(3):335–338.

Dienstag, J. L., Feinstone, S. M., Kapikian, A. Z., Purcell, R. H., Boogs, J. D., and Conrad, M. E. (1975). *Lancet 1*:765–767.

Dudley, R. J., Fox, R. A., and Sherlock, S. (1972). *Lancet 1*:723–726.

Feinstone, S. M., Kapikian, A. Z., and Purcell, R. H. (1973). *Science 182*:1026–1028.

Friedman, L. S., and Dienstag, J. L. (1984). In *Hepatitis A*. R. J. Gerety (Ed.), Academic Press, New York, pp. 55–79.
Frosner, G. G. (1982). *Off. Gesundheitswes.* *44*:370–373.
Frosner, G. G., Overby, L. R., Flehmig, B., Gerth, H. J., Hans, H., Decker, R. H., Ling, C. M., Zuckerman, A. J., and Frosner, H. R. (1977). *Am. J. Mol. Biol.* *1*:163–173.
Frosner, G. G., Deinhardt, F., Scheid, R., Gauss-Muller, V., Holmes, N., Messenberger, V., Siegl, G., and Alexander, J. J. (1979). *Infection* *7*:303–306.
Garson, J. A., Tedder, R. S., Griggs, M., Tuke, P., Glazebrook, J. A., Trute, A., Parker, D., Barbara, J. A. J., Contreras, M., and Aloysiris, S. (1990). *Lancet* *335*:1419–1422.
Gauss-Muller, V., and Deinhardt, F. (1984). *Proc. Soc. Exp. Biol. Med.* *175*:10–15.
Gershon, A. A., Borkowsky, W., and Gerety, R. J. (1987). *Curr. Probl. Pediatr.* *17*(5):309–326.
Giles, J. P., Liebhaher, H., Krugman, S., and Latimer, C. (1964). *Virology* *24*:107–118.
Gocke, J. S. (1975). *Am. J. Med.* *270*:49–52.
Govindarajan, S. (1983). *Gastroenterology* *85*:162–165.
Govindarajan, S., DeCork, K. M., and Peters, R. L. (1986). *Gut* *27*:19–22.
Govindarajan, S., Edwards, V. M., Stuart, M. L., Operskalski, E. A., and Mosley, J. W. Transfusion Safety Study Group (1988). In *Viral Hepatitis and Liver Disease*. A. J. Zuckerman (Ed.). Alan R. Liss, New York, pp. 201–204.
Gust, I. D., Feinstone, S. M., Purcell, R. H., and Alter, H. J. (1980). *J. Med. Virol.* *6*:1–10.
Hadler, S. C., Webster, H. M., Erben, J. J., Swansin, J. E., and Maynard, J. E. (1980). *N. Engl. J. Med.* *302*:1222–1227.
Hadler, S. C., deMonzon, M., Panzetto, A., Anzola, E., Rivera, D., Mondolfi, A., Bracho, A., Francis, D. P., Gerber, M. A., Thung, S., Gevin, J. L., Maynard, J. E., Poppe, H., and Purcell, R. H. (1984). *Ann. Intern. Med.* *120*:339–344.
Hoofnagle, J. H. (1989). *JAMA* *261a*:1321–1325.
Hoofnagle, J. H., and Alter, H. (1984). In *Viral Hepatitis and Liver Disease*. G. N. Vyas, J. L. Dienstag, and J. H. Hoofnagle (Eds.). Grune & Stratton, New York, pp. 97–106.
Hoofnagle, J. H., and Seef, L. B. (1976). In *NIH Report*, 77–189. US Dept. of Health, Education & Welfare, Washington, DC, pp. 55–66.
Horak, W. (1983). In *Viral Hepatitis: Laboratory and Clinical Science*. F. Deinhardt and J. B. Deinhardt (Eds.). Marcel Dekker, New York, pp. 295–316.
Hsu, H. C., Wu, T. T., Sheu, J. C., Wu, C. Y., Chiou, T. J., Lee, C. S., and Chen, D. S. (1989). *Hepatology* *9*(5):747–750.
Iwarson, S. A. (1985). In *Hepatitis B*. R. J. Gerety (Ed.). Academic Press, New York, pp. 119–153.
Jacobson, I. M., Nath, B. J., and Dienstag, J. L. (1985). *J. Med. Virol.* *16*:163–169.
Johnson, P. J., and Williams, R. (1990). *J. Natl. Cancer Inst.* *82*:1784–1785.
Junge, U., and Deinhardt, F. (1985). In *Hepatitis B*. R. J. Gerety (Ed.). Academic Press, New York, pp. 93–118.
Kaplan, P. M., Greenman, R. I., Gerin, J. L., Purcell, R. H., and Robinson, W. S. (1973). *J. Virol.* *12*:995–1005.
Khuroo, M. S., Teli, M. R., Skidmone, S., Sofi, M. A., and Khuroo, M. I. (1981). *Am. J. Med.* *70*:252–256.

Kim, H., Saidi, P., Ackley, A., Bringelsen, K., and Goche, D. (1980). *Gastroenterology, 79*:1159.

Kiyosawa, K. (1984). *Gastroenterology 79*:777–779.

Kiyosawa, K., Akahoma, Y., Nogata, A., and Furuta, S. (1987). *Am. J. Gastroenterol. 78*:777–781.

Kiyosawa, K., Sodeyama, T., and Tanaka, E. (1990). *Hepatology 12*:671–675.

Kiyosawa, K., Sodeyama, T., and Tanaka, E. (1991). *Gastroenterology 100*(4):1145–1146.

Koch, F., and Koch, G. (1985). In *Molecular Biology of Poliovirus*. F. Koch and G. Koch (Eds.). Springer Verlag, New York. pp. 590.

Koff, R. S., and Galambos, J. In *Diseases of the Liver*, 5th ed. L. Schiff and E. R. Schiff (Eds.). J. B. Lippincott, Philadelphia, pp. 461–610.

Koretz, R. L. (1989). *Am. Fam. Physician 39*:197–202.

Kos, A. (1986). *Nature 323*:558.

Kosaka, Y., Takase, K., Kojima, M., Shimizu, M., Inoue, K. (1991). *Gastroenterology 100*(4):1087–1094.

Kurstak, E., Al Tuwaijri, A., and Kurstak, C. (1990). Second International Symposium on Viral Diseases, Beijing, pp. 28–33.

Krugman, S. (1976). *J. Infect. Dis. 134*:70–74.

Lau, J. Y. N., Alexander, G. J. M., and Alberti A. (1991). *Gut (Suppl.)*S47–362.

Liang, T. J., Blum, H., and Wands, J. R. (1990). *Hepatology 12*:204–212.

Lucey, M., and Traber, P. G. (1991). *Hepatology 13*:193–195.

Magnius, L. O., and Espmark, J. A. (1972). *Immunology 109*:1017–1021.

Manns, M., Meyer Zun Buschenfelde, K. H., Hutternoth, T. H., and Hess, G. (1980). *Clin. Exp. Immunol. 42*:263–272.

Martin, P., and Friedman, L. S. (1991). *Gastroenterology 100*:578–579.

Mathiesen, L. R., Feinstone, S. M., Purcell, R. H., and Wagner, J. (1977). *Infect. Immun. 18*:524–530.

Mathiesen, L. R., Drucker, J., Lorenz, D., Wagner, J., Gerety, R. J., and Purcell, R. H. (1978). *J. Infect. Dis. 138*P:369–377.

Mathiesen, L. R., Skenhof, P., Nielsen, J. O., Purcell, R. H., Wong, D., and Ranek, L. (1980). *Gut 21*:72–77.

Mazzur, S., Burget, S., and Blumberg, B. S. (1974). *Nature 247*:38.

McCallum, R. W., and Zuckerman, A. J. (1981). *J. Med. Virol. 8*:1–29.

McLachlan, A. (1991). *Molecular Biology of the Hepatitis B Virus*. CRC Press, Boca Raton, Fla.

Meliconi, R., Perperas, A., Jensen, D., Alberti, A., McFarland, I. G., Eddleston, A. L. W. F., and Williams, R. (1982). *Gut 23*:603–607.

Melnick, J. L. (1982). *Intervirology 18*:105–106.

Miller, D. J., Williams, A. E., Le Bouvier, G., Dwyer, J. M., Grant, and Klatskin, G. (1978). *Gastroenterology 74*:1208–1213.

Miller, R. H., Kaneko, S., Chung, C. T., Girones, R., and Purcell, R. H. (1989). *Hepatology 9*:322–327.

Moriyama, K., Nakajima, E., Hohjoh, Asayama, R., and Okochi, K. (1991). *Lancet 337*:125.

Muller, R., Lauchart, W., Farle, M., Klein, H., Niehoff, G., and Pichlmayr, R. (1988). In *Viral Hepatitis and Liver Disease*, A. N. Zuckerman (Ed.). Alan R. Liss, New York, pp. 810–812.

Ostermayer, R. (1988). In *Viral Hepatitis and Liver Disease*. A. J. Zuckerman (Ed.). Alan R. Liss, New York, pp. 59–64.

Papaevenagelou, G. (1983). *Lancet 1*:917–920.

Pascual, M., Perrin, L., Giostra, E., and Schifferli, J. A. (1990). *J. Infect. Dis. 162*:569–570.

Popper, H. (1984). In *Viral Hepatitis and Liver Disease*. G. N. Vyas, J. L. Dienstag, and J. H. Hoofnagle (Eds.). Grune & Stratton, New York, pp. 381–384.

Popper, H., Dienstag, J. L., Feinstone, S. M., Alter, J. J., and Purcell, R. H. (1980). *Virchow Arch.* [A] *387*:91–106.

Popper, H., Thung, S. N., and Gerber, M. A. (1983). *Hepatology 3*:906–912.

Prince, A. M. (1968). *Proc. Nat'l. Acad. Sci. 60*:814–821.

Prince, A. M., and Trepo, C. (1971). *Lancet 1*:1309–1312.

Provost, P. J., and Hilleman, M. R. (1979). *Proc. Soc. Exp. Biol. Med. 160*:213–2221.

Provost, P. J., Ittensohn, Villarejos, V. M., and Hilleman, M. R. (1975). *Proc. Soc. Exp. Biol. Med. 148*:962–969.

Purcell, R. H., and Ticehurst, J. R. (1988). In *Viral Hepatitis and Liver Disease*. A. J. Zuckerman (Ed.). Alan R. Liss, New York, pp. 131–138.

Quaglia, M. P., Tolkoff-Rubin, N. E., and Dienstag, J. L. (1981). *Transplantation 32*:504–506.

Rakela, J., Redeker, A. G., Edwards, V. M., Decker, R., Overby, L. R., and Mosley, J. W. (1977). *J. Clin. Microbiol. 5*:110–111.

Rakela, J., Redeker, A. G., Edwards, V. M., Decker, R., Overby, L. R., and Mosley, J. M. (1979). *Gastroenterology 74*:879–882.

Reyes, G. R., Purdy, M. A., Kim, J. P., Luk, K. A., Young, L. V., Fry, K. E., and Bradley, D. W. (1990). *Science 247*:1335–1339.

Rizzetto, M. (1984). *Hepatology 3*:729–737.

Rizzetto, D. W., Canese, M. G., Arico, S., Crivelli, O., Trepo, C., Bonino, E., and Verme, G. (1977). *Gut 18*:997–1003.

Rizzetto, M., Verme, G., and Recchia, S. (1983). *Ann. Intern. Med. 98*:437–441.

Rizzetto, M., Verme, G., and Gerin, J. L. (1984). In *Progress in Liver Disease* Vol. VIII. H. Popper and F. Schaffner (Eds.). Grune & Stratton, Orlando, pp. 417–431.

Robinson, W., Clayton, D., and Greenman, R. (1974). *J. Virol. 14*:384–391.

Roingeard, P., Lu, S., Siereau, C., Freschlin, M., Arbeille, B., Essex, M., and Romet-Lemonne, J. L. (1990). *Hepatology 11*:277–285.

Sarki, R. K., Gelfand, D. H., Stoffel, S., Scharf, S. J., Higuchi, R., Horn, G. T., Mulles, K. B., and Erlich, H. A. (1988). *Science 239*:487–491.

Scatto, J., Hadchouel, M., and Wain-Hobson, S. (1985). *J. Infect. Dis. 151*:610–617.

Schmidt, E., and Schmidt, F. W. (1983). In *Viral Hepatitis: Laboratory and Clinical Science*. F. Deinhardt and T. Deinhardt (Eds.). Marcel Dekker, New York, pp. 411–487.

Schmidt, E., and Schmidt, F. W. (1984). *Dtsch Med Wochenschr. 109*:139–144.

Seef, L. B., Zimmerman, H. J., and Wright, E. C. (1975). *Am. J. Med. Sci. 270*:41–47.

Seef, L. B., and Koff, R. S. (1986). *Semin. Liver Dis. 6*:11–17.
Shattock, A. G., Irwin, F. M., Morgan, E. M., Hillary, I. B., Kelly, M. G., Fielding, D. F., Kelly, D. A., and Weir, D. G. (1985). *Br. Med. J. 290*:1377–1380.
Siegl, G. (1988). In *Viral Hepatitis and Liver Disease.* A. J. Zuckerman (Ed.). Alan R. Liss, New York, pp. 3–7.
Siegl, G., and Eggers, H. J. (1982). *J. Gen. Virol. 61*:111–114.
Siegl, G., Frosner, G. G., Gausa-Miller, V., Tratschin, J. D., and Dienhardt, F. (1981). *J. Gen. Virol. 57*:331–341.
Smedile, A., Dentico, P., and Zanetti, A. (1981). *Gastroenterology 81*:992–997.
Smedile, A., Baroudy, B. M., Bergmann, K. F., Rizzetto, M., Purcell, R. H., and Gerin, J. L. (1987). In *Hepatitis Delta Virus and Its Infection.* M. Rizzetto, J. L. Gerin, and R. H. Purcell (Eds.). Alan R. Liss, New York, pp. 231–234.
Stewart, J. S., Farrow, L. J., Clifford, R. E., Lamb, S. G. S., Coghill, N. F., Lincoln, R. L., Sanderson, J. M., Dodd, P. A., Smith, H. G., Preece, J. W., and Zuckerman, A. J. (1978). *Q. J. Med. 187*:365–384.
Storch, G., McFarlande, L. M., Kelso, K., Heilman, C. J., and Caraway, C. T. (1979). *JAMA 242*:1514–1518.
Summers, J., and Mason, W. S. (1982a). *Cell 29*:403–415.
Summers, J., and Mason, W. S. (1982b). *Hepatology 2*:61–66.
Summers, J., O'Connell, A., and Millman, I. (1975). *Proc. Natl. Acad. Sci. USA 72*:4597–4601.
Szmuness, W. (1978). *Progr. Med. Virol. 26*:40–69.
Tabor, E. (1983). *Lancet 1*:765–769.
Tabor, E. (1988). *Adv. Pediatr. Infect. Dis.* 3:19–23.
Thiers, V., Nakajima, E., Kresmsdorf, D., Macke, D., Schellekers, H., Driss, P., and Gorideam, A. (1988). *Lancet* 2:1273–1276.
Ticehurst, J. R. (1986). *Semin. Liver Dis. 6*:46–55.
Tiollais, P. (1988). In *Viral Hepatitis and Liver Disease.* A. J. Zuckerman (Ed.). Alan R. Liss, New York, pp. 295–301.
Toukan, Au, Omayma, A., El-Rub, A., Abu-Laban, Sa, Tarawneh, Ms, Kamal, M. F., Hadler, S. C., Krawizynski, K., Marcolis, H. S., and Maynard, J. E. (1987). *Hepatology* 7:1340–1346.
Trepo, C. G., Robert, D., Mutin, J., Trepo, D., Sepetjern, M., and Prince, A. M. (1976). *Gut 17*:10–13.
Ulrich, P. P., Romeo, J. M., Lane, P. K., Kelly, I., Daniel, L. J., and Vyas, G. N. (1990). *J. Clin. Invest. 86*:1609–1614.
Villarejos, V. M., Gutiermez-Diermessen, A., Anderson-Visona, K., Rodriguez-Aragonas, A., Provost, P. J., and Hilleman, M. R. (1976). *Proc. Soc. Exp. Biol. Med. 153*:205–208.
Villarejos, V. M., Hu, R., and Visona, K. A. (1988). In *Viral Hepatitis and Liver Disease.* A. J. Zuckerman (Ed.). Alan R. Liss, New York, pp. 111–112.
Viola, C., Vinetta, L., Bosch, J., and Rhodes, J. (1983). *Hepatology* 3:1013–1015.
Wang, K. S., Choo, Q. L., and Weiner, A. J. (1986). *Nature 323*:508–514.
Wang, J., Chenivesse, X., Henglesn, B. and Bréchot, C. (1990). *Nature 343*:555–557.

Weiner, A. J., Juo, G., Bradley, D. W., Bonino, F., Soracco, G., Lee, C., Rosenblatt, J., Choo, Q. L., and Houghton, M. (1990). *Lancet 335*:1–3.
Wen, Li, Peakman, M., Lobo-Yeo, A., McFarlane, B. M., Mowat, A. P., Mieli-Vergani, G., and Vergani, D. (1990). *Lancet 336*:1527–1530.
Wheeler, C. M., Fields, H. A., Schable, C. A., Meinke, W. J., and Maynard, J. E. (1986). *J. Clin. Microbiol. 23*:513–517.
White, G. C., Zeitler, K. D., Lesesne, H. R., McMillan, C. W., Wareren, M. S., Roberts, H. R., and Blatt, P. M. (1982). *Blood 60*:1259–1262.
Widell, A., Hansson, B. G., Oberg, B., Nordenfelt. (1986). *Antiviral Res. 6*:103–112.
Yokosuka, O., Omata, M., Hosoda, K., Toda, M., Ehata, T., and Ohto, M. (1991). *Gastroenterology 100*:175–181.
Zuckerman, A. J. (1988). Monograph, Schering Corp. USA.
Zuckerman, A. J. (1990). *Br. Med. J. 300*:1475–1476.

5

VIRAL HEPATITIS

Current Trends in Prevention, Control, and Treatment

Edouard Kurstak, A. Hossain, A. Al Tuwaijri, and Christine Kurstak
Faculty of Medicine, University of Montreal, and International Comparative Virology Organization, Montreal, Quebec, Canada

I. INTRODUCTION

Hepatitis (inflammation of the liver) has been attributed to a variety of causes: drugs, toxins, bacteria, excessive alcohol intake, and, most commonly, several different viruses.

Viral hepatitis remains to date a global health problem. The most common causative viruses are the hepatitis A (infectious hepatitis) and hepatitis B (serum hepatitis) viruses (HAV and HBV, respectively), identified and isolated in the 1970s (Feinstone et al., 1973; Miller et al., 1975; Dane et al., 1970; Almeida et al., 1971). Others include the delta agent, or hepatitis D virus (HDV), identified in 1977 (Rizzetto et al., 1977), which requires the presence of HBV to express itself clinically as hepatitis D and the non-A, non-B hepatitis (NANBH). NANBH is presently known to include a primary form caused by hepatitis C virus (HCV), which includes most transfusion-associated hepatitis; a sporadic form most probably attributable to HCV; an epidemic form observed primarily on the Asian continent, identified as enteric hepatitis and caused by hepatitis E virus (HEV); and other unidentified variants (Bradley et al., 1987; Chao et al., 1989). All forms of viral hepatitis do, however, pose a serious public health problem worldwide. In the United States, viral hepatitis ranks third among reportable communicable diseases (Hollinger et al., 1991).

The three approaches towards the prevention and control of viral hepatitis currently in use are general measures (education, screening, and improved standards of hygiene), passive immunization (prophylactic immunoglobulin), and active immunization. These are discussed in depth in this chapter in the context of hepatitis A, hepatitis B, non-A, non-B hepatitis (hepatitis C, hepatitis E), and hepatitis D.

Few drugs for the treatment of the hepatitis viruses have been studied; however, the development and marketing of antiviral drugs in recent years appear to be heading toward new and extensive research in antiviral therapy for many viruses including the hepatitis viruses. None of the antiviral drugs marketed thus far have been found effective for the treatment of viral hepatitis. The current status of the therapy of viral hepatitis is also discussed.

II. HEPATITIS A

Hepatitis A is a common viral infection in most parts of the world and the disease continues to pose a significant problem even in the most highly industrialized nations. It is more prevalent, however, in areas with a high population density and poor hygiene or sanitation standards. Infections acquired early in life tend to be subclinical, while in adults there is more likelihood of them being symptomatic.

The most important and long-lasting control measures have been the implementation of standard public health approaches that include provision of clean water, proper sewage disposal, and improved personal hygiene (Gust, 1988).

A. Passive Immunization

Human normal immunoglobulin (HNIG, ISG, gamma globulin) is of value for both pre-exposure and postexposure prophylaxis. The value of these preparations was first demonstrated some time ago (Gellis et al., 1945; Neefe and Stokes, 1945) and many field studies have since substantiated that HNIG administered before exposure or during the incubation period protects against symptomatic infection.

For postexposure prophylaxis (e.g., controlling outbreaks in households or institutions), HNIG is most effective (80–90%) when given early in the incubation period (Mosley et al., 1968). Administering immunoglobulin more than 2 weeks after exposure is unlikely to be effective (Centers for Disease Control, 1981). Usually, Ig containing at least 100 IU/ml anti-HAV with a dosage of at least 2 IU anti-HAV/kg body weight will prevent or attenuate a clinical illness.In special cases, such as pregnant patients or in patients with liver disease the dosage may be doubled. Serologic confirmation of HAV in the index case before treatment of contact is recommended but screening of contacts for HAV IgG is not.

Pre-exposure prophylaxis is recommended mainly for nonimmune persons traveling from nonendemic to endemic areas where exposure to HAV is likely to occur. This generally includes travelers from developed countries to underdeveloped areas with the risk of exposure to HAV varying with the prevalence of hepatitis A in areas visited, the general living conditions, sanitation, and length of stay. The duration of stay has been reported to be most directly related to the risk of exposure to hepatitis A (Maynard, 1978). Parry et al. (1988) have assessed a salivary anti-HAV assay in travelers and conclude that screening is worthwhile in those over 40 years old, in frequent or long-stay travelers, in those traveling to areas endemic for HAV, and in those with a history of jaundice. Travelers are particularly advised to take general precautions against HAV and other enteric diseases by avoiding potentially contaminated food (such as uncooked shellfish) and untreated water.

B. Active Immunization

HAV has a number of features that suggest that control through vaccination is possible. The virus can be grown in cell culture and suitable animal models exist for testing candidate vaccines. A single serotype is involved and infections are associated with lifelong immunity.

A safe and efficient vaccine for hepatitis A would be of particular benefit to certain high-risk groups including children attending day care centers, certain overseas travelers, homosexuals, persons in military service, and selected institutional persons. General childhood immunization might even deserve consideration, depending on the characteristics of the vaccine and the duration of the expected immunity (Lemon, 1985).

Several types of HAV vaccines are feasible, including conventional attenuated and inactivated vaccines as well as recombinant or synthetic peptide-subunit vaccines based on new biotechnological developments.

It is now possible to produce both inactivated and live attenuated hepatitis A vaccines from virus grown in cell culture. Initial studies indicated potential difficulties due to the long replicative cycle of the virus, the virus for the most part being cell associated, and the relatively low titers generated. These problems have been largely overcome by rapid passage of the virus and selection of mutants that release substantial quantities of the virus into the supernatant fluid.

A vaccine-induced escape mutant of hepatitis B has recently been reported (Carmen et al., 1990). Infection by the escape HBV mutant in a successfully vaccinated and presumably protected individual, should it be confirmed, would be cause for concern. With widespread HBV vaccination, it is hoped that herd immunity will develop. The appearance of an escape mutant raises the specter of "antigenic drift," as is observed with influenza A viruses (Martin and Friedman, 1991). Until now, host-related factors have been identified as the principal impediments to universal protection against HBV infection by vaccination.

Inactivated Vaccines

In early studies HAV antigen prepared from the livers of infected marmosets and inactivated with formalin-elicited antibodies in susceptible marmosets, albeit after multiple doses, provided protection against live-virus challenge (Provost and Hillemant, 1978). This study established the possibility of producing hepatitis A vaccine. However, since marmoset liver was an unsatisfactory substrate for a human vaccine, efforts intensified to adapt strains to cell cultures and to produce a conventional cell-culture-derived vaccine. The Merck group has reported (Provost et al., 1986) results with CR326 adapted to LLC-MK2, a continuous line of monkey kidney cells. The antigenicity of the vaccine was evaluated in mice and marmosets. Doses as low as 0.01 μg produced seroconversion in 50% of marmosets. The vaccine appears to be very promising but the substrate LLC-MK2 may pose a potential problem in licensing. To obviate this, CR326 has recently been adapted to diploid fibroblasts.

Reports from research groups in Europe and China have also indicated progress toward production of inactivated HA vaccines (Binn et al., 1986; Flehmig et al., 1986). HAV produced in cell culture and inactivated with formalin was shown to be immunogenic in owl monkeys (Binn et al., 1986).

Evaluation of the inactivated HA vaccines by the various groups is proceeding. These vaccines have been demonstrated to be safe, antigenic, and protective in animals. Phase I clinical studies are underway. Desmyter et al. (1990) vaccinated volunteer medical students in a randomized, double-blind comparison of killed hepatitis A vaccines, prepared on MRC-5 cells and formaline-inactivated. Injections of 1 ml of vaccine were given in the deltoid muscle every 3 months. Since seroconversion by enzyme-linked immunosorbent assay (ELISA) was 100% in several vaccinees after one injection, Desmyter and his colleagues suggested that three injections within 60 days may not be necessary. Recently Sjogren et al. (1991) have shown that the FI-1/HM175 vaccine was immunogenic in 86% of the subjects and that three doses were as immunogenic as four. The vaccine was found to be safe and acceptable for use in healthy adults.

Live Attenuated Vaccines

Live attenuated hepatitis A vaccines have also been developed by serial passage of selected HAV strains in cell cultures. Attentuation was demonstrated in marmosets and chimpanzees (Provost et al., 1983, 1984). Several cell-culture-adapted strains of the CR-326 strain of HAV that were shown to be attenuated in nonhuman primates have been tested in human beings as candidate vaccines (Provost et al., 1984). The most attenuated of these variants failed to show evidence of infectivity for human beings and did not elicit antibody.

In 1989, Mao et al. carried out a primary study of attenuated live hepatitis A vaccine (H2 strain) in 12 healthy human volunteers. They found that the H2 strain vaccine gave a much better immune response than the F-strain studied by Provost et al. (1986), with seroconversion found in all subjects using the same tests. Based on the results of a follow-up study on 127 children (age 4–12 years) with H2 strains of the live attenuated hepatitis A vaccine, Mao et al. (1989) suggest that the H2 strain has a good immunogenicity without side effects in humans.

Other Strategies for Hepatitis A Vaccines

Other possible approaches to vaccine development include the in vitro expression of viral antigens from recombinant DNA in prokaryotic or eukaryotic vectors or the chemical synthesis of oligopeptides corresponding to immunoreactive epitopes on the virus (Kleid et al., 1981; Jameson et al., 1985). Based on studies with HAV and poliovirus, a critical neutralization epitope involves the major surface polypeptide VP1 (Hughes et al., 1985; Emini et al., 1985). A recombinant plasmid producing in bacteria (*Escherichia coli*) a hepatitis A virus (HAV) capsid protein that may be useful as a subunit vaccine has been reported (Johnston et al., 1988).

C. Treatment

No specific therapy has yet been developed that is effective for hepatitis A. Despite the availability of methods for propagation of the hepatitis A virus (HAV), reports in the literature of studies leading to screening of proposed drugs appears to be rather limited. The fact that HAV infection is a self-limited infection for most patients, and the easy availability of immune globulin for effective prophylaxis in outbreaks, may perhaps have undermined the motivation for study of HAV antiviral drugs. HAV infection has not been known to become chronic and progress to a carrier state. Fulminant hepatic failure, however, develops in 1–4% of hospitalized patients who may then die. No therapy is yet available to prevent this.

A feature that differentiates HAV in the cell systems from most other picornaviruses thus far known appears to be in the resistance of replication to all antiviral substances known to reduce or block synthesis of many picornaviruses. A total of 25 antiviral compounds including guanidine, 2-(α-hydroxybenzyl) benzimidazole rhodarine, amanitine, and methylquersitin (3-MQ) have been tested (Widell et al., 1986; Siegl and Eggers, 1982; deChastonay and Siegl, 1988). All were found to have no effect on HAV replication when used in noncytotoxic concentrations. However, reduction of HAV antigen titer and, to a lesser extent, reduction of HAV infectivity were reported to occur in vitro in response to arabinosylcytosine (ara-C) (Widell et al., 1986). The recent development by deChastonay and Siegl (1988) of assay systems that may be of general use for evaluating with rapidity the cytotoxicity of potential chemotherapeutic compounds, particularly against HAV, appears to be interesting.

Recently, the immunogenicity of a purified inactivated HAV vaccine in cynomolgus macaques has been described (Chaudhury and Mao, 1990). HAV was isolated from the stool of a patient from the People's Republic of China in fetal rhesus monkey kidney (FRhk-4). The virus HAV LCDC-1 was adapted to produce a chronic infection in FRhk-4 cells. The vaccine was developed from HAV grown from chronically infected FRhk-4 cells. The cynomolgus macaques selected for vaccine trial were all negative for anti-HAV according to results of HAVAB radioimmunoassay (RIA). Three groups of monkeys were inoculated intramuscularly with 0.1 ml of vaccine containing 3, 1.5, and 0.75 μg/ml HAV. The control monkey was inoculated with phosphate-buffered saline (PBS) containing 1 mg/ml aluminium hydroxide. Postvaccination blood samples were also tested for anti-HAV. The anti-HAV titers varied from 1.5 to 1.30 by RIA. The HAV titers obtained were indicative of immune response being related to dose of vaccine. The anti-HAV titers produced in the cynomolgus macaques were similar to those reported in owl monkeys with a formalin-inactivated HAV vaccine (Binn et al., 1986) and also to the antibody titers of chimpanzees inoculated with an attenuated HAV vaccine (Karron et al., 1988). A higher yield of HAV was obtainable from chronically infected cells and hence the production of an inactivated, purified, immunogenic vaccine was shown to be feasible.

III. HEPATITIS B

Hepatitis B is a viral disease of global importance with an estimated 300 million persistent carriers worldwide. As the single most important cause of persistent viral carriage on a global basis, it is responsible for a high proportion of the world's cases of cirrhosis and is involved in the causes of up to 80% of hepatocellular carcinoma. It is second only to tobacco smoking as a cause of cancer mortality (WHO, 1983). The serious consequences are a result of development of persistent viral carrier state, which is estimated to occur in 70–90% of acute infections in infancy and to decline to between 6% and 10% of infections occurring after the 6th year of life (Maynard et al., 1988). Geographic patterns of HBV prevalence have been noted to vary from areas of low endemicity (fewer than 1% of adults as chronic HBV carriers and less than 10% of the adult population who would probably experience infection) to areas of intermediate and high endemicity (chronic carrier rates of 2–15% in adults and 30–100% of the population experiencing infection) (Al Tuwaijri et al., 1990). Currently, nearly 4 billion persons reside in areas of the world where hepatitis B virus is of intermediate or high endemicity (Maynard et al., 1988).

In areas of low endemicity, HBV infection occurs predominantly in adults and due to sexual contact for the most part, while maternal–infant transmission or close contact in early life attributes to infection in areas of intermediate and high endemicity. In hyperendemic areas, however, the relative contribution of perinatal transmission to the prevalence of persistent viral carrier state has been found to be variable, accounting for about up to 50% of chronic carriers in China and Southeast Asia and approximately 20% in other hyperendemic areas. For all hyperendemic areas, HBV horizontal transmission resulting from close contact of susceptible children with persistent carriers appears to be the predominant contributor to the pool of persistent carriers (Howard and Zuckerman, 1984; Kurstak et al., 1990).

Several effective measures of importance to control and prevent HBV infection would include:

1. Education of high-risk groups and health care personnel as to how to avoid infection and infecting others; infection control measures and vaccination.
2. Screening of blood and blood products, donor organs/tissues.
3. Passive immunization with hepatitis B immunoglobulin (HBIG) for postexposure prophylaxis.
4. Active immunization. The availability of highly safe and effective hepatitis B vaccines now makes possible the establishment of immunization programs aimed at eventually eliminating HBV infection. Strategies for immunization are based on endemicity of HB. In areas of low endemicity, vaccine prophylaxis has generally been recommended for particular high-risk groups, the majority being adults, whereas mass immunization of infants appears to be the priority in areas of high endemicity.

The passive prophylaxis and the active immunization vaccines available to date or tested are discussed in detail in this chapter.

A. Passive Immunization

Hepatitis B immunoglobulin (HBIG) prepared from pooled plasma with a high titer of anti-HBs may confer temporary immunity against certain defined conditions. The major indication for the administration of HBIG is a single acute exposure to HBV, such as that occurring in health-care personnel when blood containing HBsAg is inoculated, ingested, or splashed onto mucous membranes or conjunctiva. Other indications would be for sexual partners of HBsAg-positive individuals and babies born to carrier mothers. Although an optimal dose has not been established, doses in the range of 250–500 IU have been used effectively.

HBIG is most effective when given within 24 hr of exposure, after which its efficacy declines rapidly. In adults, 3 ml containing 200 IU anti-HBs/ml is usually given and it is generally recommended that two doses of HBIG be given 30 days apart. Results with the use of HBIG for prophylaxis in babies at risk of infection with HBV are encouraging if the immunoglobulin is given as soon as possible after birth (within 12 hr). The chance of the baby developing the persistent carrier state is reduced to about 70%. It has been recently suggested that long-term passive–active immunization with high intravenous doses of HBIG may be effective in preventing HBV reinfection for more than 8 months in at least some liver transplant recipients (Muller et al., 1988). Recent studies using combined passive and active immunization indicate an efficacy approaching 90% with the dosage of HBIG recommended as 1–2 ml (200 IU of anti-HBs/ml) (Stevens et al., 1988; Chen et al., 1987). The HBIG is simultaneously administered at a site different from the vaccine.

B. Active Immunization

Indications

Immunization against hepatitis B is required particularly for groups at increased risk of acquiring this viral infection. These include persons requiring repeated transfusions of blood or blood products, prolonged inpatient treatment, frequent tissue penetration for repeated access to circulation, natural or acquired immune deficiency, or with malignant diseases. Viral hepatitis appears to be an occupational hazard among health-care workers as well as in semiclosed institutions. High rates of infection with HBV have been reported in drug addicts, drug abusers, homosexuals, and prostitutes. Those working in high endemic areas are also at an increased risk of infection. Women in areas of the world with a high carrier rate are another segment of the population requiring immunization, because of the increased risk of transmission of the infection to their offspring. Young infants, children, and susceptible persons living in certain tropical and subtropical areas with poor living conditions and high prevalence of HBV could also be candidates for HBV immunization (Kurstak et al., 1989, 1990; Lau et al., 1991).

Safety of the Vaccines

Inability to grow HBV in tissue culture has directed efforts to the use of other preparations for active immunization. Since HBsAg leads to production of protective surface antibody, purified 22 nm spherical surface antigen particles have been developed as vaccines. These have been prepared from the plasma of symptomless carriers. The first HBV vaccines were licensed in France and the United States in 1981 and may be regarded as the first anticancer vaccines to become available for human use. There are currently 13 hepatitis B vaccines available worldwide, which include the yeast-derived recombinant HBV vaccines licensed in 1986. There is no risk known yet of transmission of the acquired immune deficiency syndrome (AIDS) or other infection by plasma-derived vaccines meeting the WHO requirements.

Dosage, Administration Route, and Vaccination Schedules

The usual course in an adult given as prophylaxis before or after exposure consists of three doses at 0, 1, and 2 months and a booster dose at 12 months.

In a recent study by Jilg et al. (1989), three different schedules for vaccination against hepatitis B were compared. The schedule used injections at months 0, 1, 2, and 12, at months 0, 1, and 6, or at months 0, 1, and 12 in healthy young adults. Concentration of antibodies to hepatitis B surface antigen (anti-HBs) after the third injection was found to be dependent on the interval between the second and the third dose, with geometric mean titers (GMTs) in the three groups being 53 IU/L 5,846 IU/L and 19,912 IU/L, when the third dose was given at month 2, 6, or 12, respectively. Whereas the HBs responses to the third dose at month 6 or 12 were typical booster reactions, the kinetics after a third dose given at month 2 resembled those after only two doses but at a significantly higher level. A fourth dose given at month 12 to the individuals vaccinated at months 0, 1, and 2 led to a prompt anti-HBs response similar to the response in those vaccinated at months 0, 1, and 12 months may be preferable to vaccination at months 0, 1, and 6. For individuals at high risk of hepatitis B infection, vaccination at months 0, 1, 2, and 12 might be considered for achieving an optimal early seroconversion as well as long-term protection. The vaccine is given intramuscularly (or subcutaneously) into the deltoid in adults and the anterolateral thigh in infants. Adverse reactions reported after immunization have been minimal and basically confined to soreness and reddening at the inoculation site.

Antibody Persistence and Booster Doses

Seroconversion rates following HB vaccination have been reported to vary between 80 and 100% in healthy adults; a good response is defined as an anti-HBs level 100 m IU/ml. It has been noted that the elderly, the immunodeficient (including those with AIDS), patients receiving hemolysis, and obese individuals tend not to respond well and may require larger or even additional doses. Few reports of long-term follow up of HB vaccines exist. Stevens et al. (1988) and Hadler et al. (1986) have addressed this question in homosexual men. Data derived from such observations may be influenced by the level of immunologic suppression in homosexuals and from frequent natural exposure to hepatitis B in this population. Gibas et al. (1988) studied the 5 year persistence of anti-HBs in male and female health workers and found that even at 5 years 53% retained moderate or high levels of anti-HBs. In the absence of sufficient long-term follow-up studies, the duration of immunity following HB vaccination remains unclear and the timing of and need for booster doses controversial. It was initially thought that booster doses would probably be required at 3–5 years. Many laboratories have since advised monitoring anti-HBs levels and administering booster doses when levels fall below 10 m IU/ml. To obviate repeated dosing of vaccines, some advise booster doses at 5 years in all who respond well, since the majority will have maintained protective anti-HBs levels for this period.

C. Hepatitis B Vaccines

Although safe and effective vaccines manufactured from the plasma of chronic carriers of HBV have been available since the early 1980s, only a small proportion of candidates for vaccination have been immunized. The reasons include high cost and limited capacity for production of plasma-derived vaccines and reluctance of individuals to be vaccinated with products originating from human blood. The development in recent years of vaccines produced from genetically engineered yeast cells (Petre et al., 1987) has considerably improved the prospects for control of hepatitis B, since they can be produced in unlimited quantities at reasonable cost without the need for human blood. An overview of HB vaccines currently available or tested is presented below.

Polypeptide Vaccines

Hepatitis B polypeptide vaccines containing specific hepatitis B virus determinants of the major nonglycosylated peptide I of the surface antigen with a molecular weight (mol wt) in the range of 28,000–30,000 daltons have been prepared. The induced polypeptides of the surface antigen are immunogenic and the purified 25,000 (p25) and 30,000 (p30) mol wt polypeptides are effective antigens.

Hepatitis B Vaccines by Recombinant DNA Techniques

Recombinant DNA techniques have been used for expressing HBsAg and HBcAg in prokaryotic cells (*E. coli* and *B. subtilis*) and in eukaryotic cells as mutant mouse LM cells, HeLa, and yeast cells (*Saccharomyces cerevisae*). Recombinant yeast–derived hepatitis B vaccines (YDV) have undergone extensive evaluation by clinical trials. The safety, reactogenicity, immunogenicity, and protective efficacy of an rDNA YDV have been demonstrated in 27 countries involving over 8,500 healthy, immunodeficient, and high-risk subjects. Reactions attributable to the vaccine have been reportedly mild and transient and similar in type, incidence, and severity to those induced by the plasma-derived vaccine (PDV). No antiyeast antibody production was detected. Recently André and Safary (1988) in double-blind, comparative trials have found that the YDV and PDV elicit similar immune responses, with seroconversion rates approaching 100% in healthy subjects. Furthermore, the YDV was also shown to be capable of boosting anti-HBs levels initially induced by PDV. The decay rates of antibodies elicited by PDV and YDV were similar, with a 20 mg YDV dose selected as optimal to ensure long-term protection in the majority of vaccines.

Hybrid Vaccinia Virus Vaccines

Potential hybrid vaccines using recombinant vaccinia virus have been constructed for hepatitis B and also for herpes simplex, rabies, and other viruses. Foreign viral DNA is introduced into the vaccinia DNA by construction of chimeric genes accomplished by homologous recombination in cells, since the large size of the genome of vaccinia virus precludes in vitro gene insertion. A chimeric gene consisting of vaccinia virus promoter sequences ligated to the coding sequence for the designed foreign protein is flanked by vaccinia virus DNA in a plasmid vector. The recloned vaccinia virus containing HBsAg sequences has been used successfully for priming experimental animals. Currently, however, there is no acceptable laboratory marker of attenuation or of virulence of vaccinia virus for humans, either on the host directly inoculated with the virus on after several passages in the same species. The advantages of recombinant vaccinia virus as a vaccine include cost-effectiveness, ease of administration by multiple pressure or scratch technique, vaccine stability, long shelf-life, and the possible use of polyvalent antigens (Maynard et al., 1988; Zuckerman, 1988).

Hepatitis B Vaccines Using Hybrid Particles

Recent developments in hepatitis B vaccine research include the use of envelope proteins of HBV (HBsAg) in a particulate form by expressing the proteins in mammalian cells. In phase insertions of variable length and sequence of another virus (poliomyelitis virus type 1) were made in different regions of the S gene of HBV. The envelope proteins carrying the surface antigen and the insert were assembled with cellular lipids in the cultured mammalian cells after transfection. The inserted polio neutralization peptide was found to be exposed on the surface of the hybrid envelope particles and induced neutralizing antibodies against poliovirus in experimentally immunized mice. The expression and secretion of hybrid envelope particles by established cells would thus provide an efficient system for the production of new vaccines. Another potentially excellent carrier vehicle for human and veterinary vaccines in addition to hepatitis B would be core particles of HBV. The advantage of the core structure as a particle includes its ability to augment helper T cell function. The feasibility of this approach has been recently demonstrated with synthetic and biosynthetic peptides of foot and mouth disease virus (FMDV) after fusion to hepatitis B virus core (Clarke et al., 1987).

Reported recently (Adamowicz et al., 1988) was the production of a new hepatitis B vaccine (Gen Hevac B) that may open a new era both in hepatitis B vaccination (since it contains S and pre-S2 products) and in vaccine production since recombinant HBsAg particles were synthesized in mammalian cells. The substrate Chinese hamster ovary (CHO) cells were transfected with a plasmid containing the nucleotide sequence encoding the HBV S and pre-S antigens. These cells continuously synthesize HBsAg proteins and excrete into the culture medium particles resembling the HBsAg proteins found in the plasma of human chronic HBsAg carriers. To achieve this, a CHO cell line lacking the dihydrofolate reductase (DHFR) gene, and thus sensitive to aminopterine, was transfected with a plasmid containing two transcriptional units, the mouse DHFR gene, and the HBV S and pre-S antigen genes. The utilization of CHO continuous mammalian cells for the production of HBsAg particles has several potential advantages: fidelity of the recombinant protein to the natural product, the glycosylation and appropriate folding of the protein, and excretion into the medium. The protective efficacy of the vaccine was evaluated in chimpanzees and all animals were found to develop strong anti-HBs and anti-pre–S2 responses. No local or general clinical side effects of the vaccine were reported and no biological abnormalities observed in trials in 17 humans, demonstrating an excellent tolerance of the vaccine.

Similar results are obtained using baculovirus expression vector system with a much higher yield of HBV-immunizing antigens in insect larvae (Kang et al., 1988).

Potential Chemically Synthesized Hepatitis B Vaccines

Chemical synthesis of small oligopeptides representing specific regions of HBsAg-S and pre-S is currently advancing. Antisera to these peptides cross-react with the native surface antigen particles, and protective immunity has been demonstrated in limited experimental studies. Enhancement of the immunogenicity of the pre-S region of HBsAg has been demonstrated in mice with chemically synthetic amino acid residues. The immune response to the pre-S2 region was shown to be regulated by H-2-linked genes, distinct from those regulating the response to S region. It was also shown that immunization of a nonresponder murine strain with particles containing both S and pre-S2 can circumvent nonresponsiveness. Recently also, a protein sequence mediating the attachment of HBV to human hepatoma cells was identified. A synthetic peptide analog, recognized by both cell receptors and viral antibodies elicited antibodies reacting with the virus. Such a preparation may elicit protective antibodies by blocking attachment of the virus to the cells. Successful mimicking of determinants of HBsAg using chemically synthesized peptides in linear and cyclical forms has been reported. Studies have also confirmed that selected overlapping peptides corresponding to relevant epitopes of HBsAg may be useful as synthetic vaccines when combined with adjuvants (Zuckerman, 1988; Maynard et al., 1988). Chemically synthesized peptides would thus undoubtedly be an alternative approach to the development of a safe and effective hepatitis B vaccine at low cost.

Anti-idiotype Antibody as a Prospective HB Vaccine

Jerne's theory (1974) has opened the possibilities of regulating the immune response at the level of idiotype recognition via an idiotype reaction. The possibility of manipulating immune response by injecting anti-idiotype antibodies has been evaluated (Rodkey, 1980). Anti-idiotype antibodies have also been successfully used together with the HBsAg (Kennedy et al., 1983) or HBsAg synthetic peptides (Kennedy et al., 1984) to enhance the immune response to HBsAg.

Recently (Korec et al., 1988) a test was developed for anti-idiotype antibodies prepared against polyclonal and monoclonal animal antibodies. The anti-idiotype antibodies provoked the production of anti-HBs antibodies when injected into BALBc mice. Sera of humans repeatedly immunized with human anti-HBs antibody gave positive results in an RIA for anti-idiotype antibody. These antibodies were found to elicit an anti-HBs response in BALBc mice and Syrian hamsters. This therefore represents the basis for a potential human anti-idiotpye vaccine against hepatitis B.

D. Simultaneous Vaccination for Hepatitis A and B

Since the prevalence of antibodies against HAV is declining in industrialized countries, large populations of adults appear to be susceptible to infection with HAV. Therefore, vaccination for HAV is recommended and perhaps could be combined with vaccination for HBV, especially for people in high-risk groups.

Flehmig et al. (1990) have recently shown that a combined vaccine containing a genetically engineered hepatitis B surface antigen and HAV vaccine produced from HAV propagated in diploid human fibroblast cell culture successfully induced high levels of neutralizing antibodies against HAV and good antibody against HBV. Because HAV could be grown in human embryo fibroblasts, production of large amounts of antigen for vaccine production poses merely a technical problem.

Combined HAV and HBV vaccines rather that separate vaccines may be more convenient in vaccinating homosexually active men, those attending day care centers, patients living in centers for the mentally retarded, and travellers to endemic areas.

E. Treatment

Acute Hepatitis B

Recovery from hepatitis B (HBV) infection is dependent on the integrated activities of the patient's interferon and immune systems. Chronic HBV infection arises because of defects in these defenses. Therapeutic measures available thus far are unable to suppress inflammatory activity, stimulate liver regeneration, or enhance virus elimination and hence the natural course of acute hepatitis B cannot be influenced. In the early stages of acute HBV infection, however, following the production of alpha-interferon, major histocompatibility antigen (MHC) expression on hepatocytes has been found to increase and coincidentally transaminase levels rise. Interferon also activates a series of enzymes including the 2-5A synthetase system, leading to the inhibition of viral protein syntheses. It is believed that these changes will produce an antiviral state of uninfected regenerating liver cells, preventing reinfection. Together with the virus-neutralizing antibodies developed, this would prevent short and long-term relapse or reinfection (Thomas, 1988).

Since hepatitis B is normally a self-limited disease, the treatment of acute hepatitis B generally centers on preventing clinical deterioration. Glucocorticoids, even though they may cause an initial rapid decline in both serum bilirubin and serum aminotransferase activities, do not appear to be of any benefit in acute hepatitis and may even be harmful due to their side effects (Stutz et al., 1969). In fulminant viral hepatitis, a serious complication that only 10–20% of patients with hepatitis B survive when coma grade IV is reached (DeCoch et al., 1986), an improvement of liver function and disappearance of coma have been recently closely correlated with the institution of foscarnet (trisodium phosphonofromate) treatment (Hedin et al., 1987).

In the early phase of acute hepatitis, metoclopramide has been found to increase the rate of gastric emptying and seems to be the drug of choice for antiemetic treatment. Immunoglobulin as well as high titers of anti-HBs have been reported to be of no value in the treatment of either ordinary acute hepatitis B or fulminant hepatitis B (Eisenburg et al., 1975).

Chronic Hepatitis B

The development of the chronic carrier state is believed to be attributable to many different causes. The two predominant situations are chronic HBV infection following infection in neonatal life and exposure after the neonatal period. Large quantities of naturally derived anti-HBc may predispose to prolonged infection but other factors, such as the immunity of the neonatal immune system, the presence of immunosuppressive factors such as alpha-fetoprotein, and the large inoculum of the virus, may also contribute to the high incidence of chronic infection resulting from exposure at or before birth (Thomas, 1988). In marked contrast to the situation at birth, with 90% of babies born to HBV "e" antigen-positive mothers becoming infected and over 90% of them developing chronic carrier state (Beasly et al., 1981), only 5–10% of the subjects infected after the neonatal period develop chronic infection. There are probably several different causes for the development of chronic infection at this stage of life. One recently documented defect, is the production of subnormal quantities of alpha interferon by peripheral blood mononuclear cells (Ikeda et al., 1986). There is evidence of abnormal activation of hepatocytes by interferon and significant elevations of hepatic 2-5A synthetase.

There is no established place in the treatment of chronic HBV infection for regimens involving solely anti-inflammatory or immunosuppressive drugs (Scullard et al., 1981). A variety of synthetic and natural antiviral compounds have been developed and currently evaluated in clinical trials.

Chronic HBV carrier state is now a condition for which patients need assessment for possible therapy rather than simple conservative management. Treatment of carriers has provided a model with which to approach other chronic viral infections with the aim of harnessing the immune system and readjusting the host/parasite relationship in favor of the host (Lever, 1988).

The indications for therapy have not yet been definitely been identified but the general guidelines appear to be infectivity (HBeAg and HBV DNA positivity) and evidence of progressive liver disease (histologic signs of chronic active hepatitis). The primary objectives include inhibition of HBV replication directly or by stimulation of the host antiviral response long-term control of inflammatory necrosis of hepatocytes and prevention of malignant transformation of hepatocytes.

According to Thomas (1988), three levels of responses to therapy may be achieved. A transient response is characterized by inhibition of HBV replication, loss of HBV-DNA and polymerase but not HBeAg or HBsAg during therapy, but return of these markers when therapy is ended. Incomplete response is characterized by sustained inhibition of HBV replication, loss of HBV-DNA and DNA polymerase even after therapy is ended, conversion from HBeAg to anti-HBe, but continued HBs antigenemia. Complete response involves inhibition of HBV replication: loss of HBV DNA and DNA polymerase continuing after ending of therapy with permanent seroconversion from HBsAg and HBeAg to anti-HBs and anti-HBe.

The principal antiviral drugs tested thus far for treatment of chronic hepatitis B include suramin, acyclovir, adenine arabinose, zidovudine, ribavarin, phosphonoformate, and alpha, beta, and gamma interferons..

Suramin To date, only one antiretroviral agent has been reported to have been tried against hepadnavirus infection. Suramin with antiretroviral properties in vitro against a variety of retroviruses including HIV was shown to inhibit the DNA-polymerase activity of the hepadnavirus duck hepatitis B virus in vitro (Kessler et al., 1986). A subsequent study showed that suramin had no effect in vivo on the hepatitis B virus DNA-polymerase activity in the serum of three humans with severe hepatitis (Loke et al., 1987).

Acyclovir (Acycloguanosine) At low concentrations in herpes simplex virus infection, this drug is active due to phosphorylation to active metabolites by virus-encoded thymidine kinase. This enzyme has, however, not been detected in HBV-infected cells. Higher concentrations partially inhibit HBV replication but the clinical usefulness remains unknown. Preliminary results with acyclovir for the treatment of hepatitis B have been reported with small numbers of patients.

Intravenous acyclovir over a period of 5–7 days resulted in reduction in levels of DNA-polymerase and HBV DNA in the serum of four of six patients with chronic HBV infection. HBeAg remained positive in all and there was no report of follow-up (Weller et al., 1983). A randomized controlled trial of intravenous acyclovir for 28 days compared with no therapy in chronic HBV infection resulted in some reduction in DNA-polymerase levels in 10 of 15 treated patients, with loss of DNA-polymerase in 5 (Alexander et al., 1987). In a study with the combined use of alpha-interferon (8 weeks) and intravenous acyclovir (the first 2 weeks), Schalm et al. (1985) detected a profound decrease in levels of DNA-polymerase and HBeAg in all of five treated patients, a change far greater than that seen earlier with either treatment alone in these patients.

Adenine Arabinoside Adenosine arabinoside (ara-A) and adenosine arabinoside nomophosphate (ara-AMP) have been studied in chronic HBV infection in humans. Recent work in vitro has demonstrated that, when it is within a cell, the virus may also be able to inhibit IFN-induced antiviral system and thereby reduce the ability of that cell to produce antiviral proteins and enzymes. Inhibiting replication of the virus may impair its own defenses sufficiently for the host immune system to eliminate the virus. This happens to be the basis for antiviral treatment with viral inhibitions such as ara-A and ara-AMP (Lever, 1988). Ara-A is a potent inhibitor of HBV replication but its clinical use is limited by its poor aqueous solubility. Bessendine et al. (1981) have reported sustained HBe antigen/antibody seroconversion after a 10 day course in 40% of cases in a small, randomized controlled study. A course of 10 mg/kg/24 hr for 3 days followed by 5 mg/kg/24 hr for a further 23 days of ara-AMP has been evaluated in small controlled studies in humans with chronic HBV (Hoofnagle et al., 1984; Trepo et al., 1984). In the controlled study reported by Trepo et al. (1984), DNA-polymerase and/or HBeAg disappeared in 12 of 18 (67%) patients with chronic hepatitis B of undefined duration treated with one or more courses of ara-AMP compared to 5 of 19 (26%) placebo recipients. In another controlled study however, with 20 patients with chronic hepatitis B of at least 1 year's duration given either 4 weeks of ara-AMP or no treatment, no benefit was obvious. Equal numbers of patients in each group became and remained negative for HBV DNA-polymerase and HBV DNA in serum, accompanied by biochemical improvement (Hoofnagle et al., 1984).

Interferons With the availability of recombinant DNA technology and advanced culture systems able to produce large quantities of interferons, the prospects for treating patients with chronic HBV infections have changed completely. In the United Kingdom carriers not infected at birth are reportedly being treated, with an approximate 50% chance of treatment permanently inhibiting viral replication (Lever, 1988).

Based upon theoretical considerations, interferons are some of the most promising antiviral agents since they have direct antireplicative and immunomodulatory effects (Blackman and Morris, 1985; Weil, 1983). Both natural and recombinant DNA-produced preparations of type I interferon (alpha and beta) and type II (gamma) have been examined. A number of studies have suggested that interferons may augment the rate of seroconversion to anti-HBe, which is associated with clinical, biochemical, and histologic remission. Although natural seroconversion is often associated with a reduction in the titer of HBsAg, clearance of HBsAg and the development of anti-HBs occur infrequently (Sampliner et al., 1979). In an effort to investigate the therapeutic potential of lymphoblastoid alpha interferon in hepatitis B virus infection, 59 consecutive previously untreated male carriers seropositive for HBeAg for at least 12 months were assessed by Alexander et al. (1988). During interferon therapy at an initial daily dosage of $10 \times 10^6\ \mu m^{-2}$ and adjusted according to toxicity, the serum aspartate aminotransferase (AST) level rose to more than twice the baseline value in 11 of 23 patients. In six patients in whom this was marked, there was permanent loss of HBeAg. Each of them developed anti-HBe and five lost HBsAg. The results of this study illustrate that interferon induces seroconversion in a proportion of patients, characterized by loss of HBsAg. Furthermore, patients with a marked elevation of serum AST levels stand an increased chance of losing HBeAg. Nevertheless, the proportion of patients responding to interferon appears to be small.

Caselman et al. (1988) carried out a controlled and randomized trial in 20 patients using a combination of antiviral human fibroblast (IFN-beta) and immunomodulating immune interferon (IFN-gamma) for the treatment of chronic active hepatitis. The effects of therapy on viral DNA were evaluated by nucleic acid hybridization. After therapy, virus replication was no longer detectable in 4 of 10 patients, 2 of whom eliminated the virus completely from the serum and liver and recovered from chronic infection. In the other two responders, hepatitis B surface antigenemia persisted in the absence of virus multiplication. The authors suggest that this was presumably due to hepatitis B viral sequence integrated into the hepatocyte genome in one case and to nonreplicating episomal virus DNA in the other. The results of this preliminary study thus indicate the potential of combined human fibroblast and immune interferons in the therapy of chronic active hepatitis B.

Monoclonal Antibody to HBsAg Murine monoclonal antibody to HBsAg has been evaluated recently in an attempt to clear chronic infection (Lever et al., 1988). Two patients with primary hypogammaglobulinemia who were chronic HBeAg-positive HBV carriers were treated with the murine monoclonal antibody to HBsAg. Both patients lost HBeAg after treatment, and one who has HBV DNA-positive prior to treatment became HBV DNA-negative. Transaminase levels normalized in both patients after treatment and neither reported relapse.

Interleukin-2 In HBV-induced liver disease, cytotoxic T cells are probably responsible for destruction of liver cells (Lau et al., 1991; Thomas et al., 1982). Interleukin-2 (IL-2), a lymphokine that amplifies immune function, causes cytotoxic T cells to increase in number and maturity (Gillis et al., 1978). T cells in the peripheral blood from patients during an exacerbation of chronic hepatitis have been found to produce more IL-2 than in remission (Onya et al., 1987). A possibility exists that exogenous IL-2 may make cytotoxic T cells proliferate and eliminate infected liver cells. Ohta et al. (1988) evaluated the therapeutic use of recombinant IL-2 (rIL-2) against viral antigens and antibodies, various immunologic parameters, and liver function tests. Their data indicate that rIL-2 acts as an immunomodulating agent to enhance host immune activity in HBeAg-positive patients, but the effectiveness of their regimen in producing long-term inhibition of HBV replication remains to be evaluated.

IV. HEPATITIS D

Because hepatitis D (delta hepatitis) is intricately linked to hepatitis B, it seems realistic to envision that any prevention of delta hepatitis should in fact be initiated with prevention of hepatitis B. Likewise, patients susceptible to hepatitis B and seronegative for antibodies to HBV, could be considered susceptible to hepatitis D virus (HDV) infection as well. Given the possibility of large epidemics and the severity of hepatitis D, immunization with HBV vaccine should be a definite recommendation.

No specific prophylaxis against HDV exists and the kinetics of its inactivation by physical and chemical agents remains obscure. Prevention of superinfection in an HBV carrier appears to be limited to environmental and barrier measures. The risk of acquiring HDV infection from screened HBsAg appears to be very low, but infection of hemophiliacs treated with factor VIII prepared from pooled plasma from donors has been reported.

Protection against transmission of both HBV and HDV could be achieved by administration of HBIG of HB vaccine to babies and children. Noncarriers of HBV in high-risk groups or in areas in which HDV is endemic are likewise protected against HDV infection by HBV vaccine.

At present there is no established therapy for hepatitis D. Retrospective studies have suggested that corticosteroids are ineffective in amelioriating the course or preventing progression of this disease (Rizzetto et al., 1983). Limited results reported to date do, however, suggest that patients with HDV respond to interferon. Interferon appears to inhibit HDV replication, and a prolonged course of therapy has been associated with improvement (Hoofnagle and Di Bisceglie, 1988; Rosina et al., 1987; Hoofnagle et al., 1987). Although antiviral therapy appears to be promising for some patients with chronic hepatitis D, it has little hope of efficacy in patients with fulminant hepatitis or with advanced disease.

Reports by Hedin et al. (1987) and by Price et al. (1986) indicate that fulminant HBV/HDV hepatitis may respond to treatment with foscarnet (trisodium phosphonoformate), an inhibitor of some viral DNA polymerases, including HBV. In those with terminal HDV disease, liver transplantation has been considered a feasible option; however, recurrence of HBV and HDV after transplantation poses a potential problem (Rizzetto et al., 1987).

V. NON-A, NON-B HEPATITIS (HEPATITIS E AND HEPATITIS C)

A. Prevention and Control

Control measures for enterically transmitted non-A, non-B hepatitis (ET-NANBH) would presumably be similar to those for HAV and include the provision of clean water, sanitary disposal of human excreta, and improved personal and food hygiene. It has also been reported that passive immunization with immunoglobulin prepared from healthy donors in endemic areas may protect pregnant women who are particularly vulnerable. Active immunization could only be achieved with the unequivocal identification and characterization of the causative virus (hepatitis E virus) (Zuckerman, 1990).

Posttransfusion non-A, non-B hepatitis (PT-NANBH), or hepatitis C may result in chronic liver disease and possibly hepatocellular carcinoma. In the absence of serologic markers, preventive measures have been based on the use of "surrogate" markers to screen blood and blood products and viral inactivation. Two surrogate tests used in the routine screening of blood in the United States include alanine aminotransferase (ALT) and HBV core antibody (anti-HBc). The PT-NANBH virus (hepatitis C virus) has been reported to be inactivable with the use of heat, lipid solvents, and photochemical inactivation (Study Group, 1988). This report indicates that severe dry heating at 80°C is highly effective in inactivating NANBH viruses (HCV and HEV) in coagulation factor concentrates. Several measurements of serum aminotransferase levels for 4 months revealed no patterns of rises attributable to NANBH in 32 patients (coagulation-factor-deficient) investigated. According to the authors, this severe dry heating method appears to have reduced the risk of NANBH transmission from about 90% in untreated concentrates to a statistically determined rate of 0–9%. No evidence of infection with hepatitis B or HIV was obvious in these recipients. A combination of specific assays for HBV, HIV, HCV, and viral inactivation would thus help to increase and further ensure the safety of the blood supply.

There have been reports of certain batches of human normal immunoglobulin (HNIG) reducing icteric cases of NANBH after transfusion. In the absence of serologic markers for diagnosis of infection, the efficacy of such prophylaxis remains to be fully assessed.

A recent study found immune serum globulin (ISG) effective in preventing HCV infection; however, more investigations are required (Sanchez-Quiyano et al., 1988). In this 5 year study Spanish patients undergoing heart surgery were assigned to either a control group or to a group that received Ig. The Ig was a commercially available 16% solution obtained from donors and given at a dosage of 10 ml/day before and a week after surgery. Transfusion-associated hepatitis was significantly more common in the control than in the Ig-treated group. Although more cases of hepatitis B virus infection occurred in the control than in the Ig-treated group, the difference was not statistically significant. In contrast, transfusion-associated NANBH (hepatitis C) appeared to be statistically less significant in the Ig-treated group and the incubation periods were noted to be shorter and the peak aminotransferase levels lower in the few recipients of Ig with hepatitis than in the controls with hepatitis. The authors do suggest that Ig could serve as an inexpensive form of immunoprophylaxis against transfusion-associated hepatitis C. It appears, however, that the efficacy of such passive prophylaxis cannot be properly assessed until serologic markers are available for diagnosing infection and the antibody in the immunoglobulin measured.

The availability of a vaccine remains dependent on the isolation and characterization of the virus(es) (HCV) causing PT-NANBH. The isolation of one of the agents of PT-NANBH, the hepatitis C virus, reported recently (Chao et al., 1989) appears to be a step towards development of a possible vaccine. In this study, a random-primed complementary DNA library was constructed from plasma containing the uncharacterized NANBH agent and screened with serum from a patient diagnosed with NANBH. A complementary DNA clone was isolated that was shown to encode an antigen associated specifically with NANBH infections. The clone was not derived from host DNA but from an RNA molecule present in NANB hepatitis infections consisting of at least 10,000 nucleotides and positive-stranded with respect to the encoded NANB hepatitis antigen. Their data appeared to be consistent with the clone being derived from the genome of NANB hepatitis agent.

B. Treatment

Non-A, non-B hepatitis has a marked propensity to progress to chronic liver disease. In 60–70% of cases of posttransfusion NANBH patients have been noted to have elevations in serum aminotransferase levels for more than a year (Aach et al., 1981). Despite the fact many cases of chronic NANBH turn out to be symptomatic and mild, 15–25% lead to pronounced liver injury, with an insidious progression to cirrhosis, portal hypertension, and hepatic failure (Berman et al., 1979). There is currently no established therapy for chronic NANBH. Assessment of treatment protocols for chronic NANBH has been hampered by lack of viral markers, the fluctuating nature of the transaminase levels, the risk attached to serial biopsies in certain patients (coagulation problems in those undergoing chronic renal dialysis and in hemophiliac patients), and the uncertain natural history in some patient populations (Ellis, 1990).

Prophylactic administration of immune serum globulin to patients receiving blood transfusions has been shown to reduce the incidence of icteric hepatitis (DeVoss et al., 1983) and chronic hepatitis (Prior et al., 1987), but these results remain refuted by some (Brown et al., 1986). However, it does seem logical to administer immunoglobulin after exposure to needle-stick injuries (Ellis, 1990).

Corticosteroids have yielded disappointing results and do not appear to be beneficial (Alter and Hoofnagle, 1984). Acyclovir has likewise produced no apparent short-term or long-term benefits (Pappas et al., 1985).

As with hepatitis D, interferons appear to be the only successful drugs used against NANBH (Hoofnagle and Di Bisceglie, 1988). The availability of highly purified and potent preparations of recombinant human alpha interferon has allowed trials of this antiviral and immunomodulating agent in the treatment of chronic NANBH. In fact, both recombinant alpha and human lymphoblastoid interferons have been shown to be effective in the treatment of chronic hepatitis B (Thomas and Scully, 1985) and hepatitis D (Hoofnagle et al., 1985).

In one of the pilot studies for the evaluation of recombinant human alpha interferon as a potential antiviral agent for NANBH, Hoofnagle et al. (1986) reported eight patients responding with a fall of serum ALT activities to normal or near normal. In two patients the disease relapsed after therapy was stopped but responded after its resumption. Liver biopsy specimens obtained after 1 year of the therapy demonstrated marked improvement in hepatic histologic appearance, even with the use of low doses of alpha interferon. Although this study was not adequately controlled, the overall response was regarded as very encouraging.

Recently, a prospective, randomized, controlled parallel group study of active treatment with low dose interferon alpha (human lymphoblastoid interferon) to determine its effect on ALT activities in chronic NANBH vs. no treatment has been reported (Jacyna et al., 1989). Though all 14 treated patients showed a reduction in aspartate aminotransferase activities, in two patients these did not return to normal. Whether the failure of treatment in these two was related to the type of NANBH or to misdiagnosis of chronic NANBH, or was a reflection of an individual difference in response to interferon was not obvious. This is the first controlled study that has shown that alpha interferon could rapidly return ALT activity to normal in most patients with chronic NANBH.

REFERENCES

Aach, R. D., Szmuness, w., and Mosley, J. W. (1981). *N. Engl. J. Med. 304*:989–994.

Adamowicz, F. T., Vinas, R., Mevelec, M. N., Diaz, I., Courouce, A. M., Mazert, M. C., Lagarde, D., and Girard, M. (1988). In *Viral Hepatitis and Liver Disease*. A. J. Zuckerman (Ed.). Alan R. Liss, New York, pp. 1087–1090.

Alexander, G. J. M., Fagan, E. A., Hegarty, J. E., Yeo, J., Eddleston, A. L. W. F., and Williams, R. (1987). *J. Med. Virol. 21*:81–87.

Alexander, G. J. M., Brahm, J., Fagan, E. A., Smith, H. M., Daniels, H. M., Eddleston, L. W. F., and Williams, R. (1988). In *Viral Hepatitis and Liver Disease*. A. J. Zuckerman (Ed.). Alan R. Liss, New York, pp. 862–863.

Almeida, J. D., Rubenstein, D., and Stott, E. (1971). Lancet 2:1225–1227.

Alter, H. J., and Hoofnagle, J. H. (1984). In *Viral Hepatitis and Liver Disease*. G. N. Vyas, J. L. Dienstag, and J. H. Hoofnagle (Eds.). Grune & Stratton, Orlando, FL, pp. 345–354.

Al Tuwaijri, A., Desmyter, J., Hossain, A., Kurstak, C., and Kurstak, E. (1990). *Inst. Pasteur Res. Virol. 141*:473–477.

Andre, F. E., and Safary, A. (1988). In *Viral Hepatitis and Liver Disease*. A. J. Zuckerman (Ed.). Alan R. Liss, New York, pp. 1025–1030.

Beasly, R. P., Hwang, L. Y., and Lin, C. C. (1981). *Lancet*: 388–398.

Berman, M., Alter, H. J., Ishak, H. E. G., Purcell, R. H., and Jones, E. A. (1979). *Ann. Intern. Med. 91*:1–6.

Bessendine, M. F., Chadwik, R. G., Sabenon, J., Thoman, H. C., and Sherlock, S. (1981). *Gastroenterology 80*:1016–1022.

Binn, L. N., Bancroft, W. H., Lemon, S. M., Marchwicki, R. H., LeDuc, J. W., Trahan, C. J., Staley, E. C., and Keenan, C. M. (1986). *J. Infect. Dis. 153*:749–758.

Blackman, M. J., and Morris, A. G. (1985). *Immunology 56*: 451–458.

Bradley, D. W., Krawczynski, W., Cook, E. H., Jr. (1987). *Proc. Natl. Acad. Sci. USA 84*:6277–6281.

Brown, C., Peterson, J., Underwood, J. R., Gust, I., and Tob, B. A. (1986). *J. Clin. Lab. Immunol. 19*:1–4.

Carmen, W. F., Zanetti, A., Karayiannis, P., Walters, J., Manzillo, G., Fanzi, E., Zuckerman, A. J., and Thomas, H. C. (1990). *Lancet 336*:325–329.

Caselman, I. W. H., Elsenburg, J., Hofschneide, P. H., and Koshy, R. (1988). In *Viral Hepatitis and Liver Disease*. A. J. Zuckerman (Ed.). Alan R. Liss, New York, pp. 875–878.

Centers for Disease Control. (1981). *MMWR 30*:423–428.

Chao, Q. L., Koo, G., Weinger, A. J., Overby, L. R., Bradley, D. W., and Houghton, M. (1989). *Science 244*:359–362.

Chaudhury, R. K., and Mao, J. S. (1990). *J. Infect. Dis. 161*:586–587.

Chen, D. S., Hus, HN-M., Sung, J. L., Hsu, T. C., Hsu, S. T., Kuo, Y. T., Lo, K. J., and Schich, Y. T. (1987). *JAMA 257*:2597–2603.

Clarke, B. E., Newton, S. E., and Carrol, A. B. (1987). *Nature 330*:381–384.

Dane, D. S., Cameron, C. H., and Briggs, M. (1970). *Lancet 1*:695–698.

deChastonay, J., and Siegl, G. (1988). In *Viral Hepatitis and Liver Disease*. A. J. Zuckerman (Ed.). Alan R. Liss, New York, pp. 956–960.

DeCoch, K. M., Goubau, P., D'Hondt, E., Delem, A., Safary, A., and André, F. (1990). First International Symposium In Immunization and Immunotherapy. Riyadh, ICVO, 40.

Desmyter, J., Goubau, P., D'Hondt, E., Delem, A., Safary, A., and André, F. (1990). First International Symposium in Immunization and Immunotherapy. Riyadh, ICVO, 49.

DeVoss, R., Vanstapel, M. J., and Desmyter, J. (1983). *Hepatology 3*:532–544.

Eisenburg, J., Mersher, P., Holl, J., and Grunst, J. (1975). *Fortsch. Med. J. 93*:1085–1092.

Ellis, E. S. (1990). *J. Infect. 21*:235–240.

Emini, E. A., Hughes, J. V., Perlow, D. S., and Boger, J. (1985). *J. Virol. 55*:836–839.

Feinstone, S. M., Kapikian, A. Z., and Purcell, R. H. (1973). *Science 182*:1026–1028.

Flehmig, B., Haage, A., and Pfistener, M. (1986). *J. Med. Virol. 22*:7–16.

Flehmig, B., Heinricy, U., and Phisterer, M. (1990). *J. Infect. Dis. 161*:865–868.

Galambos, J. F. *Gastroenterology 44*:267–274.

Gellis, S. S., Stokes, J., Jr., Broker, G. M., Hall, W. M., Gilvert, H. R., Beyer, E., and Murrisey, R. A. (1945). *JAMA 128*:1062.

Gibas, A., Watkins, E., Hinkle, C., and Dienstag, J. L. (1988). In *Viral Hepatitis and Liver Disease*. A. J. Zuckerman (Ed.). Alan R. Liss, New York, pp. 998–1001.

Gillis, S., Ferm, M. M., Ouw, and Smith, K. A. (1978). *J. Immunol. 120*:2027–2033.

Gust, I. D. (1988). In *Viral Hepatitis and Liver Disease*. A. J. Zuckerman (Ed.). Alan R. Liss, New York, pp. 77–80.

Hadler, S. C., Frances, D. P., Maynard, J. E., Thompson, S. E., Judson, F. N., Echenverg, D. F., Ostrow, D. G., O'Malley, P. M., Penley, D. A., Altman, N. L., Braff, E., Shipman, G. F., Coleman, P. J., and Mandel, E. J. (1986). *N. Engl. J. Med. 315*:209–214.

Hedin, G., Weiland, O., Ljunngren, K., Trombury, A., Nordenfelt, E., Hannson, B. G., and Oberg, B. (1987). In *Progress in Clinical and Biological Research*, vol. 234. M. Rizzetto, J. L. Gerin, and R. H. Purcell (Eds.). Alan R. Liss, New York, pp. 309–320.

Hollinger, F. B., Lemon, S. M., and Margolis, H. (1991). *Viral Hepatitis and Liver Disease*. Williams & Wilkins, Baltimore.

Hoofnagle, J. H., Hanson, R. G., and Minuk, G. Y. (1984). *Gastroenterology 86*: 150–157.

Hoofnagle, J. H., Smedile, A., and Mullen, K. D. (1985). *Gastroenterology 88*:1665.

Hoofnagle, J. H ., Midlen, K. D., Jones, B. D., Rustgi, V., Di Bisceglie, A. D., Peters, M., Waggoner, J. E. G., Yoon Park, R. N., and Jones, E. A. (1986). *N. Engl. J. Med. 315*:1575–1578.

Hoofnagle, J. H., Mullen, K., and Peters, K. (1987). In *Hepatitis Delta Virus and its Infection*. M. Rizzetto, J. L. Gerin, and R. H. Purcell (Eds.). Alan R. Liss, New York, pp. 291–298.

Hoofnagle, J. H., and Di Bisceglie, A. D. (1988). In *Viral Hepatitis and Liver Disease*. A. J. Zuckerman (Ed.). Alan R. Liss, New York, pp. 823–830.

Howard, C. R., and Zuckerman, A. J. (1984). In *Control of Virus Diseases*. E. Kurstack (Ed.). Marcel Dekker, New York, pp. 33–55.

Hughes, J. V., Bennett, C., Stanton, L., Linemwyer, D. L., and Mitra, S. W. (1985). In *Vaccines*. R. A. Lerner, Chanock, R. M., and F. Brown (Eds.). *Cold Spring Harbor Laboratories, Cold Spring Harbor, NY.*

Ikeda, T., Lever, A. M. L., and Thomas, H. C. (1986). *Hepatology 6*:962–965.

Jacyna, M. R., Brooks, M. G., Loke, R. H. T., Main, J., Murray-Lyn, E. M., and Thomas, H. C. (1989). *Br. Med. J. 298*:80–82.

Jameson, B. A., Bonin, J., Murray, M. G., Wimmer, E., Kew, O.. (1985). In *Vaccines*. R. A. Lerner, R. M. Chanock, and F. Brown (Eds.). Cold Spring Harbor Laboratories, Cold Spring Harbor, NY.

Jeren, N. N. (1974). *Ann. Immunol. Inst. Pasteur 125c*:373–389.

Jilg, W., Schmidt, M., and Deinhardt, F. (1989). *J. Infect. Dis. 160*:766–769.

Johnston, J. M., Harmon, S. A., Binn, L. N., Richards, O. C., Ehrenfeld, E., and Summers, D. F. (1988). *J. Infect. Dis. 157*:1203–1211.

Kang, C. Y., Vernet, T., and Thomas, D. Y. (1988). In *Applied Virology Research*, Vol. 1, New Vaccines and Chemotherapy. E. Kurstack (Ed. in Chief). Marcel Dekker, New York, pp. 31–42.

Karon, R. A., Duener, R., Ticehurst, J., d'Hindt, E., Popper, H., Melnick, R., Phillips, J., Feinstone, S., and Purcell, R. H. (1988). *J. Infect. Dis. 157*:338–345.

Kennedy, R. C., Adler-Storthz, A., Henkel, R. D., Sanchez, Y., Melnick, J. L., and Dressman, G. R. (1983). *Science* 853–855.

Kennedy, R. C., Parrow, J. T., Sanchez, I., Melnick, J. L., and Dressman, G. R. (1984). *Virology 136*:247–252.
Kessler, H. A., Pottage, J. C., Trenholme, G. M., Benson, C. A., and Levin, S. (1986). *AIDS Res. 6*:962–965.
Kleid, D. G., Yansuva, D., and Small, B. (1981). *Science 214*:1125–1129.
Korec, E., Hlozanek, I., Stara, J., and Nemecek, V. (1988). In *Viral Hepatitis and Liver Disease*, A. J. Zucklerman (Ed.). Alan R. Liss, New York, pp. 1102–1103.
Kurstak, E., Jabbar, F. A., Gezairy, H. A., and Pavilliard, R. (1989). *Bull. Inst. Pasteur 87*:289–295.
Kurstak, E., Al Tuwaijri, A., and Kurstak, C. (1990). Second International Symposium on Viral Diseases, Beijing, ICVO, 28.
Lau, J. Y. N., Alexander, G. J. M., and Alberti, A. (1991). *Gut. Suppl.* S47–S62.
Lemon, S. M. (1985). *N. Engl. J. Med. 313*:1059–1067.
Lever, A. M. L. (1988). *J. Infect. 16*:221–229.
Lever, A. M. L., Waters, J., Brook, M. G., Karayiannis, P., and Thomas, H. C. C. (1988). In *Viral Hepatitis and Liver Disease*. A. J. Zuckerman (Ed.). Alan R. Liss, New York, pp. 961–962.
Loke, R. H. T., Anderson, M. G., Coleman, J. C., Tsequaye, K. N., Zuckerman, A. J., and Murray-Lyn, D. M. (1987). *J. Med. Virol. 21*:97–99.
Mao, J. S., Dong, D. X., Zhang, H. Y., Chen, N. I., Zhang, X. Y., Huang, H. Y., Xu, R. I. Y., Zhow, T. J., Wan, Z. J., Wang, Y. Z., Hu, Z. H., Cao, Y. Y., Li, H. M., and Chu, C. M. (1989). *J. Infect. Dis. 159*:621–624.
Martin, P., and Friedman, L. S. (1991). *Gastroenterology 100*:578–579.
Maynard, J. E. (1978). *Am. J. Epidemiol. 107*:77–86.
Maynard, J. E., Kane, M. A., Alter, M. J., and Hadler, S. C. (1988). In *Viral Hepatitis and Liver Disease*. A. J. Zuckerman (Ed.). Alan R. Liss, New York, pp. 967–969.
Miller, W. J., Provost, P. J., McAleer, W. J., Itensohn, O. L., Villarejos, V. M., and Hilleman, M. R. (1975). *Proc. Soc. Exp. Biol. Med. 149*:254–261.
Mosley, J. W., Reisler, D. M., Brachott, D., Roth, D., and Weiser, J. (1968). *Am. J. Epidemiol. 87*:539–550.
Muller, R., Lauchert, W., Farle, M., Klein, H., Niehoff, G., and Pichlmayr, R. (1988). In *Viral Hepatitis and Liver Disease*. A. J. Zuckerman (Ed.). Alan R. Liss, New York, pp. 810–812.
Neefe, J. R., and Stokes, J. Jr. (1945). *JAMA 128*:1063.
Ohta, Y., Onji, M., Kondoh, H., Yamaguchi, S., Horiike, N., and Ogawa, Y. (1988). In *Viral Hepatitis and Liver Disease*. A. J. Zuckerman (Ed.). Alan R. Liss, New York, pp. 884–886.
Onya, M., Kondoh, H., Horiike, N., Yamacuchi, S., Ogawea, Y., Juman, L., and Ohta, Y. (1987). *Hepato-gastroenterology 34*:141–144.
Pappas, S. G., Hoofnagle, J. H., Young, N., Stevens, S. E., and Jones, E. A. (1985). *J. Med. Virol. 15*:1–9.
Parry, A., and Barrington, C. P. (1988). *Lancet 1*:1447.
Petre, J., Van Wynendeele, F., DeNeys, B., Conrath, K., Van Opstal, O., Hauser, P., Rutgers, T., Cabenon, T., Capiou, C., Hartford, N., DeWilde, M., Stephenne,

J., Carr, S., Hemling, H., and Swadesh, J. (1987). *Postgrad. Med. J. 63* (suppl 2):73–81.

Price, J. S., France, A. J., Maonen, L. D., and Welsby, P. D. (1986). *Lancet 1*:1273.

Prior, C., Fuchs, D., and Hansen, A. (1987). *Lancet* 2:1235–1237.

Provost, P. J., Conti, P. A., and Gresa, P. A. (1983). *Proc. Soc. Biol. Med. 172*:357–363.

Provost, P. J., Burynak, E. B., McLean, A. A., Hilleman, M. R., and Scolnick, E. M. (1984). In *Viral Hepatitis and Liver Disease*. G. N. Vyas, J. L. Dienstag, and J. A. Hoofnagle (Eds.). Grune & Stratton, Orlando, FL, pp. 467–475.

Provost, P. J., Hughes, J. V., Miller, W. J., Gresa, P. A., Banken, P. S., and Emini, E. A. (1986a). *J. Med. Virol. 19*:23–31.

Provost, P. J., Bishop, R. F., Gerety, R. J., Hilleman, M. R., McAleur, W. J ., Skilnich, E. M., and Stevens, C. E. (1986b). *J. Med. Virol. 20*:165–175.

Rizzetto, M., Ganese, M. G., Arico, S., Crivelli, O., Trepo, C., Bonino, E., and Verme, G. (1977). *Gut 18*:997–1003.

Rizzetto, M., Verme, G., Recchia, S., Bonino, F., Farci, P., Arico, S., Calzia, R., Picciotto, A., Colombo, M., and Popper, H. (1983). *Ann. Intern. Med. 98*: 437–441.

Rizzetto, M., Macagno, S., Chiaberge, E., Verme, G., Negro, P., Marinucci, G., DiGiacommo, G., Alfani, D., Contesini, R., Milazzo, F., Dogina, M., Fassati, R., and Galmarini, D. (1987). *Lancet* 2:469–471.

Rodkey, L. S. (1980). *Microbiol. Rev. 44*:631–659.

Rosina, F., Sararco, G., Actis, G. C., Brunetto, M. R., Maran, E., Pindtus, C., Dianzani, F., Verme, G., and Rizzetto, M. (1987). In *Hepatitis Delta Virus and its Infection*. M. Rizzetto, J. L. Gerin, and R. H. Purcell (Eds.). Alan R. Liss, New York, pp. 299–303.

Sampliner, R. E., Hamilton, F. A., Iser, O. A., Taor, E., and Bortnott, J. (1979). *Am. J. Med. Sci. 277*:17–22.

Sanchez-Quiyano, A., Pinedo, J. A., and Lissen, E. (1988). *Lancet 1*:1245–1249.

Schalm, S. W., Heytink, R. A., Van Buuren, H. R., and deMan, R. A. (1985). *Lancet* 2:358–360.

Scullard, G. H., Smith, C. I., Morigan, T. C., Robinson, W. S., and Gregory, P. G. (1981). *Gastroenterology 81*:987–991.

Siegl, G., and Eggers, H. J. (1982). *J. Gen. Virol. 61*:111–114.

Sjogren, M. H., Hoke, C. H., Binn, L. N., Eckels, K. H., Dubois, D. R., Lyde, L., Tsuchida, A., Oaks, S., Marchwicki, R., Lednar, W., Chloupek, R., Ticehurst, J., and Bancroft, W. H. (1991). *Ann. Intern. Med. 114*:470–471.

Stevens, C. E., Taylor, P. E., Tong, M. J., Toy, P. T., Vyas, G. N., Zang, E. A., and Krugman, S. (1988). In *Viral Hepatitis and Liver Disease*. A. J. Zuckerman (Ed.). Alan R. Liss, New York, pp. 982–988.

Study Group UK Hemophilia Centre. (1988). *Lancet 1*:814–816.

Stutz, R., Blum, A. L., Haemmenli, U. P., Schmed, P., and Schmid, M. (1969). *Am. J. Med. 47*:93–100.

Thomas, H. C., Montano, L., Goodall, A., Oladapo, J., and Wiecleman, K. H. (1982). *Hepatology* 2:1165–1215.

Thomas, H. C., and Scully, L. J . (1985). *Br. Med. Bull. 41*:374–386.

Thomas, H. C. (1988). In *Viral Hepatitis and Liver Disease*. A. J. Zuckerman (Ed.). Alan R. Liss, New York, pp. 817–822.

Trepo, C., Hantz, O., Ouzan, D., Chossegros, P., Chevallier, P., Berthellon, P., and Brette, P. (1984). *Hepatology* 4:1055.

Weil, J., Epstein, C. J., Epstein, L. B., Sedmak, J., Sabran, J. L., and Grossberg, S. E. (1983). *Nature 301*:437–439.

Weller, I. V. D., Careno, V., Fowler, M. J. F., Monjardino, J., Mankinen, D., Varghese, Z., Sweny, P., Thomas, H. C., and Sherlock, S. (1983). *J. Natimicrobial Chemother. 11*:223–231.

Widdel, A., Hansson, B. G., Oberg, B., and Nordenfelt, E. (1986). *Antiviral Res. 6*:103–112.

World Health Organization Meeting on Prevention of Liver Cancer. (1983). *WHO Tech. Rep. 691*:1–29.

Zuckerman, A. J. (1988). Monograph, Schering Corp., USA.

Zuckerman, A. J. (1990). *Br. Med. J. 300*:1475–1476.

6

World Health Organization Strategy for Control of Hepatitis B

Yuri Ghendon *World Health Organization, Geneva, Switzerland*

I. INTRODUCTION

Viral hepatitis is a major public health problem in all parts of the world. At least four forms of the disease that differ as to their causes are recognized. These are referred to as hepatitis A, hepatitis B (HB), hepatitis C (parenterally transmitted non-A, non-B hepatitis), and hepatitis E (enterically transmitted non-A, non-B hepatitis). Recently, the delta virus was discovered, a defective virus that is only capable of replication with hepadnavirus.

All hepatitis viruses cause a systemic infection with pathologic changes in the liver. However, HB is the most important of all the viral hepatitides.

Hepatitis B infection and its sequelae, which include chronic persistent hepatitis B, chronic active hepatitis B, cirrhosis, and primary hepatocellular carcinoma (PHC), remain major public health problems. Every year, more than 50 million people are infected with the hepatitis B virus (HBV). More than 2 billion individuals have already been infected by HBV. It accounts for half of all clinical hepatitis seen in some countries and is responsible for much of the mortality, with an acute case fatality rate of about 1%. Even more important is that 5–10% of patients infected with HBV become chronic carriers (Ghendon, 1990a; Kane et al., 1991). Persistent infection (the carrier state) constitutes the reservoir of infection, with 0.1% to as many as 15% or more of the general population affected in different regions. It is currently estimated that there are nearly 300 million carriers of the hepatitis B virus worldwide. The importance of hepatitis B is shown by the fact that 30% of persistently infected persons who reach adulthood will die of the chronic sequelae of their infection (i.e., cirrhosis of primary liver cancer) (Maynard et al., 1989).

HBV is responsible for up to 80% of all cases of primary hepatocellular carcinoma (Deinhardt et al., 1983). In countries where the HBV carrier rates reached or exceed 10%, HBV infection may account for as much as 3% of total mortality (Beasley and Hwang, 1984). More than 1 million persons die annually due to serious sequelae of hepatitis B (Progress in control of viral hepatitis, 1988). This number is expected to increase substantially in the next decades due to rapid population increases and reduced infant mortality.

Fortunately, HB is now preventable with safe and effective vaccines. HB vaccines can prevent disease and the carrier state in almost all vaccinees. These vaccines have been used in more than 50 million persons, and have proved themselves to be among the safest, most immunogenic, and most effective viral vaccines yet developed.

II. GEOGRAPHIC DISTRIBUTION

The prevalence of HB is not the same in different countries and regions.

Hepatitis researchers have classified the world into area of high, intermediate, and low endemicity, basing this division on the prevalence of HBV markers and on the primary modes of HBV transmission (Progress in the control of viral hepatitis, 1988; Integration of hepatitis B vaccines into EPI, 1990).

Areas of high endemicity include those where most of the population becomes infected with the virus, usually during the perinatal period or childhood. The low limit of the prevalence of HBV carriers for this category is from 5% to 10%, with 50% to 95% of the population having serologic evidence of HBV infection. The upper limit of the prevalence of the carrier state is about 20%. Africa, Asia east of the Indian subcontinent, the Pacific basin, the Amazon basin, the Arctic rim, and portions of the Middle East, Asia Minor, and the Caribbean are areas of high endemicity.

Areas of intermediate endemicity generally have an HBV carrier prevalence of 2–5%, with 30–50% of the population having serologic evidence of HBV infection. Some parts of southern Europe, most of eastern Europe, the Middle East, western Asia through the Indian subcontinent, and parts of Central and South America are included in this category. In these areas both child to child and adult transmission occur, and perinatal transmission is not common because only about 10–15% of carrier mothers are HBeAg-positive. Acute viral hepatitis with jaundice is a major cause of morbidity because a substantial proportion of infection occurs in older adolescents and adults, and infection at this age is much more likely to present with acute clinical disease.

North America, western Europe, Australia, and parts of South America are considered to be areas of low endemicity. In these areas perinatal and child to child transmission is relatively uncommon, and most infections occur in adults through sexual activity, needle sharing during drug abuse, or during occupational exposure to blood. Acute hepatitis B is a major cause of morbidity in many countries in this category (see also Sung, 1990; Fay, 1990; Kiire, 1990; Goudeau, 1990; Hollinger, 1990; Toukan, 1990).

Of the global population of 5 billion individuals, 3.5 billion live in areas where HBV endemicity is moderate or high (HBV chronic carrier rate >2%), and more than 122 million babies are born each year who are at substantial risk of becoming chronic carriers. The geographic burden of chronic carriage is predominantly in Asia, where >75% of the HBV chronic carriers live (Maynard et al., 1988). The next highest proportion of chronic carriers reside in sub-Saharan Africa. A crucial geopolitical fact concerning the global distribution of HBV carriers is that >90% of these individuals reside in the developing world, where access to adequate health care delivery services and financial resources to provide them are extremely limited. Of the some 122 million infants born in 1985, 1.3 million will be expected to die an HBV-induced death due to liver disease. The high proportion of these deaths (76%) will occur in Asia, with the next highest proportion (18%) occurring in Africa (Maynard, 1990).

III. EPIDEMIOLOGIC FACTORS AND MODES OF TRANSMISSION

The most important epidemiologic feature of HB that directly affects endemicity and must be recognized in the planning and implementation of prevention strategies is age at infection. At <1 year 70–90% of infections result in persistent HBV carriage; at age 2–3 years, from 40 to 70%; at the age of 4–6 years, from 10 to 40%; and at the age of 7 years and older only 6–10% of infections result in persistent HBV carriage (Stevens et al., 1975; Maynard, 1990).

Age at infection is also the primary correlate for route of infection. In areas of low HBV endemicity, infection occurs primarily in adult life and by sexual transmission. In areas of intermediate and high endemicity, infection occurs primarily among infants and children through mother–child transmission and through close personal contact among children. Since the probability of chronic HBV carriage, given an acute HBV infection, increases dramatically in infancy and early childhood an early age of infection substantially increases the overall burden of chronic carriage in endemic regions. Early age of induction of chronic carriage also increases HBV-induced mortality because of the longer survival of chronic carriers. Thus, HB prevention efforts for the majority of the world's population must be directed at entire populations reachable in infancy or at a very early age.

HBV infection is transmitted to susceptible persons through close contact with the blood and other body fluids of chronic infectious carriers or persons suffering acute infection. In low-incidence countries, the risk of HB infection is still high among certain groups of health-care workers, patients receiving treatment by maintenance hemodialysis or blood products, residents of institutions for the mentally handicapped, prisoners, drug addicts, male homosexuals, and the sexually promiscuous. In high-incidence areas, such as southeast Asia, perinatal transmission of HBV from carrier mothers to children is a major mode of infection. In other high-incidence areas, such as Africa, the main mode of transmission is horizontal (see Ghendon, 1987).

Perinatal (mother to child) transmission is one of the most efficient and serious modes of HBV transmission. The first demonstrations of possible transmission of HBV from mother to child were reported in 1972 by Obayashi et al. (1972), and then by Okada et al. (1975) and Stevens et al. (1975). In 1976 the WHO Expert Committee on Viral Hepatitis noted that "transmission of infection from carrier mothers to their babies can occur during the perinatal period and appears to be an important factor in determining the prevalence of HBV infection in some regions" (Advances in viral hepatitis, 1977). In 1982 the WHO Meeting on Viral Hepatitis postulated that "transmission from HBV carrier mothers to their babies appears to be the single most important factor for the high prevalence of HBV infection in some areas" (Deinhardt and Gust, 1982).

Perinatal transmission occurs from mothers who are positive for both the hepatitis B surface antigen (HBsAg) and the hepatitis B "e" antigen (HBeAg). More than 90% of these women are chronic HBV carriers, although women acutely infected with the virus during pregnancy may also transmit it to their children. Infected newborns rarely develop acute hepatitis, although several reports of fatal fulminant hepatitis have been reported. These carriers are at high risk of death from cirrhosis or primary hepatocellular carcinoma (PHC) and they form a pool of infectious individuals who will infect others in the community, and eventually their own offspring (Integration of hepatitis B vaccine in the EPI, 1990).

Three possibilities for transmission of HBV from carrier mothers to infants are suggested: transplacental transmission of HBV in utero (prenatal transmission); transmission during delivery; postnatal transmission from mothers to infants during child care or through breast milk.

Although most specialists think that in general perinatal HBV infection occurs during delivery as the infants pass through the birth canal, intrauterine infection of HBV may be recognized in some cases. It was estimated that intrauterine transmission of HBV from HBeAg-positive mothers to the fetus occurred in 5–15% (Wong et al., 1980; Beasley et al., 1983).

The exact mechanism of infection of newborns during labor and delivery is uncertain. It was supposed that transmission of HBV could take place through microhematologic leaks across the placenta, precipitated by trauma associated with the birth process, and/or exposure of the infant to maternal secretions in the birth canal. In carrier mothers HBsAg can be found in different fluids. HBsAg was detectable in 33% of amniotic fluid samples, 50% of cord blood samples, 98% of vaginal fluid samples, 71% of breast milk samples, and 95.3% of samples of gastric contents from newborns (Lee et al., 1978).

The HBsAg-positive mothers continue to be infectious after delivery but most specialists believe that postnatal infection from mother to infant is not common because most high-risk infants have already been infected. The breast milk of HBsAg-positive mothers is often found to be positive for HBsAg, but it does not seem to play an important role in the disease transmission. There are apparently no differences in infection rates between breast-fed and bottle-fed infants of infected mothers (Lee et al., 1978).

As noted above, the transmission of HBV from mothers to babies takes place also in the case of acute HB infection of mothers. Acute HB is an unusual complication of pregnancy and often results in premature labor. If the acute disease occurs in the third trimester of pregnancy, there is a 50–70% chance that the infant will become HBsAg-positive (Tong et al., 1981). HB acquired in pregnancy was not found capable of causing congenital defects or malformations of the fetus (Hansher et al., 1985).

As mentioned above, the factors determining transmission from mother to infant are only partially understood, but the maternal factor that appears to be important in determining whether infection will occur or not is the presence of HBe antigen in mothers' blood (Stevens et al., 1975; Hwang et al., 1985). Infants born to HBsAg carrier mothers are at high risk for becoming chronic HBsAg carriers: about 40% of newborns become chronic carriers (Stevens et al., 1975). When the carrier mothers also are HBeAg-positive, 70–90% of infants become chronic carriers of HBV within

3 months of birth (Okada et al., 1975; Stevens et al., 1979; Tong et al., 1981; Lo et al., 1985).

Various data show that genetic factors can be involved in perinatal transmission of HBV (see Ghendon, 1987).

Transmission from child to child, so called horizontal transmission, is responsible for the majority of HBV infections and carriers. Although the relative importance of the various modes of transmission from child to child has not been established, many hepatitis researchers believe that skin lesions such as impetigo, scabies, abrasions, and infected insect bites play an important role. These lesions provide a route for the virus to leave the body of infectious children, and a route into the body of susceptible children with whom they have skin to skin contact such as wrestling or sharing the same bed. Other modes of transmission include reuse of unsterile needles and other medical and dental equipment, tattooing and other scarification procedures, sharing of household items such as toothbrushes, and sexual activity. Premastication of food and insect transmission have been postulated as modes of transmission but remain unproven (Integration of hepatitis B vaccine into the EPI, 1990).

HBV transmission to adults is the primary type of transmission in regions of lower endemicity where large populations of susceptible adults are found. About one-third of infected adults develop clinical hepatitis B with jaundice, and 6–10% become chronic HBV carriers with a subsequent risk of chronic active hepatitis, cirrhosis, and PHC. Sexual transmission, both heterosexual and homosexual, accounts for the majority of adult transmission (Piot et al., 1990). In some western countries, needle sharing by drug abusers is also important. Hepatitis B is the major infectious occupational hazard to health care workers in areas of low and intermediate endemicity (Hadler, 1990). Transmission to patients by contaminated blood product and unsterilized reused medical and dental instruments also occurs. In addition, any of the modes of transmission discussed for child to child transmission may also occur.

IV. VACCINES

As noted above, HB is now preventable with safe and effective vaccines. As stressed at the WHO meeting of the Technical Advisory Group on Viral Hepatitis, the most important means of controlling HB on a global scale and of reducing mortality from its sequelae is mass immunization of infants with HB vaccines (Progress in control of viral hepatitis, 1988).

HB vaccines are alum-adjuvanted, highly purified preparations of hepatitis B surface antigen (HBsAg), the glycoprotein that forms the outer coat of the hepatitis B virus. HBsAg can either be purified from the plasma of HBV carriers (plasma derived vaccines) or produced in yeast by recombinant technology (recombinant vaccines).

The first hepatitis B vaccines were licensed in 1981 in France and the United States. These vaccines were the first such products to be manufactured from human plasma and possessed the additional attribute of being the first anticancer vaccines to become available for human use.

Plasma-derived HB vaccine is prepared by purifying HBsAg particles from the plasma of HBsAg-positive donors. In natural HBV infections, liver cells produce much more HBsAg than is needed to coat viral particles, and the excess HBsAg forms 22 nm spherical and tubular particles. Plasma-derived vaccine is inactivated to ensure that no infectious viral or other micro-organisms are present and then is alum adjuvanted.

Although vaccine supplies were initially limited, and available primarily in private sector markets, by the beginning of 1990 there were several manufacturers of plasma-derived HB vaccines and more than 50 million doses of product had been distributed globally.

Many studies found that the vaccine can induce protective anti-HB antibodies in 90–95% of healthy individuals, depending primarily on the age of the recipient. Efficacy in the range of 90–95% is regularly obtained for pre-exposure prophylaxis. For postexposure prophylaxis of infants born to HBsAg-positive mothers, efficacies of 75–85% are achieved (Progress in control of viral hepatitis, 1988; Integration of hepatitis B vaccine into EPI, 1990).

Hepatitis B also has the distinction of being the first disease for which vaccines have been produced by recombinant DNA (rDNA) technologies. The first such vaccines produced in yeast were licensed in 1986, and such products are now being manufactured in Europe, Japan, and the United States.

Recombinant HB vaccine is produced from HBsAg derived from yeast that have had a part of the viral genome coding HBsAg inserted into yeast genomes.

A synthesized HBV-specific protein is associated with a yeast cell and is extracted by homogenization, after which it undergoes several complex stages of purification. Purified particles of the surface antigen are chemically treated to transfer them into a complete form possessing disulfide linkages similar to that found in human blood plasma HBsAg. The final product is sterilized by filtration, treated with formalin and absorbed on aluminium hydroxide. Several research projects have shown that the resulting virus-specific product consists of particles morphologically identical to analogous particles from human blood plasma of HBsAg-positive carriers, although the average size of particles produced from yeast is somewhat smaller. Sodium dodecyl sulfate–polyacrylamide gel electrophoresis (SDS-PAGE) analysis has revealed HBV non-glycosylated p 24 protein that produced particles bound by disulfide linkages (see Ghendon, 1990b).

Examination of yeast-derived HBV protein for other physical, chemical, and antigen properties, including analysis involving monoclonal antibodies, has demonstrated its total identity to plasma-derived HBsAg. The final product is over 99% purified and clinical tests have not revealed any yeast protein antibodies in the serum of individuals vaccinated with recombinant yeast-derived HB vaccine (Emini et al., 1986; Jilg et al., 1984a).

The important epitopes on HBsAg designated as "a" and that induce broadly protective antibodies against HBV are three-dimensional conformation-dependent epitopes typical of those displayed on other globular proteins. These are best identified by monoclonal antibodies induced to intact HBsAg. The gene product of the HBsAg gene is a 226 amino acid peptide with a molecular weight of 24,000 daltons that lacks these important discontinuous "neutralizing" epitopes. A sophisticated mimicking of conformational epitopes is necessary to ensure the efficacy of recombinant HBsAg vaccine, since vaccine antigen molecules are composed of 100 or more copies of the gene product when assembled. Ensurance of correct assembly can be demonstrated by using monoclonal antibodies and by demonstration of clinical efficacy (Gerety, 1988).

Studies of recombinant yeast-derived HBsAg particles using a set of monoclonal antibodies and by immunization of chimpanzees and volunteers have shown that immune response to the recombinant HBsAg was identical to the response seen in subjects vaccinated with natural antigen or exposed to HBV (Hanser et al., 1988).

In wider studies of recombinant yeast-derived HB vaccine, it was found that the recombinant vaccine does not cause any significant adverse reactions (Andre and Safary, 1988; Andre, 1990). Many studies showed that the efficacy of recombinant HB vaccine is very high and is at least equivalent to plasma-derived HB vaccine (see Ghendon, 1990b; Andre, 1990).

In 1985 WHO held a meeting to discuss the requirements for production and control of yeast-derived recombinant HB vaccines. A regulation has been drafted on the production of yeast-derived recombinant HB vaccines (Hepatitis B vaccines, 1985). In 1986 the WHO Expert Committee on Biological Standardization adopted this document as a Requirement (Requirement for hepatitis B vaccines, 1987).

Recombinant HBsAg for HB vaccines may be produced in almost unlimited amounts in brewery-like fermentation vats, so there need to be no concern that availability of antigen will compromise future vaccine supply. Manufacturers could produce tens of millions of doses over the next few years, but will require firm commitments from vaccine purchasers before they make the investment to produce vaccine at the 100 million dose level necessary to provide vaccine for many of the world's children.

At the meeting of the WHO Technical Advisor Group on Viral Hepatitis, it was concluded that recombinant HB vaccines are equivalent to plasma-derived vaccines with respect of safety, immunogenicity, and efficacy, and neither vaccine currently offers any advantage over the other in these respects. It also noted that plasma-derived vaccines will continue to play an essential role in control programs worldwide for the foreseeable future (Progress in control of viral hepatitis, 1988).

V. WHO STRATEGY FOR CONTROL OF HB

The WHO has been actively involved in the field of viral hepatitis for almost 30 years and in 1984 a WHO Viral Hepatitis Control Programme was adopted. This Programme is implemented with the help of a Technical Advisory Group on Viral Hepatitis, 10 WHO Collaborating Centres for Reference and Research on Viral Hepatitis, and 54 National Institutions for Viral Hepatitis in 44 countries.

The recommendations of the WHO meetings on strategies for control and prevention of hepatitis B may be summarized as follows:

1. Elimination of HB as a cause of posttransfusion hepatitis
2. Reduction of infections through environmental control
3. Control of HB by active immunization
4. Elimination of the HBV persistent carrier state (see Ghendon, 1990c).

The screening of blood and blood products for HBsAg and the use of only products free from this marker should be a very important component of any strategy for control of HB.

The discovery of HBsAg and its specificity in identifying infections with HBV have made possible the testing of donors and screening of blood and certain blood products. Such screening has been routine in most developed countries since the early 1970s, with a dramatic reduction (up to 85–90%) in posttransfusion HB. Highly sensitive and specific tests for HBsAg are available and are widely used (radioimmunoassay [RIA], enzyme-linked immunosorbent assay [ELISA], and rapid phase hemagglutination assay [RPHA]).

Both the HBsAg carrier rate and the susceptibility of the population to infection with HBV vary in different countries and regions. In most of the countries of central Europe and North America, the HBsAg carrier rate is low (0.1–0.5%) but susceptibility of the population is high (about 95%). On the other hand, in many countries of southern Asia and tropical Africa, the HBsAg carrier rate ranges from 8 to 20% but only 5–30% of adults are susceptible to HBV infection. Because most of the population in these highly endemic areas is already infected with HBV, some specialists suggest that blood screening in such areas is not very important. However, an analysis with a special formula shows that such an opinion is incorrect (Ghendon and Kane, 1991). It was established that for areas of low endemicity (HBsAg carrier rate about 0.3%) with high susceptibility (about 95% of population susceptible to HBV infection), the probability that a blood transfusion of a single unit of unscreened blood will cause posttransfusion HBV infection (p) is 0.26%. For areas of high endemicity (HBsAg carrier rate about 14%) but low susceptibility to infection among adults (about 17%), $p = 2.14\%$. It should be noted that transfusing blood to children in such hyperendemic areas carries a much higher risk since many more children are susceptible to HB infection (about 40%). For children in this area $p = 4.9\%$.

This analysis clearly shows the need to screen donors and samples of blood for HBsAg in countries and regions with a high prevalence of HBsAg carriers.

The WHO requirements for the collection, processing, and quality control of blood, blood components, and plasma derivatives (1989) state that "each unit of blood or plasma collected shall be tested for HBsAg by an approved method and only those giving a negative result shall be used." Unfortunately, the blood used for transfusions in many developing countries does not meet such requirements. Of 108 developing countries from which data about blood screening for HBsAg are available, only one-half screened all blood samples for HBsAg. In 37% of countries only some of the blood samples were screened for HBsAg, and in 14% no samples of blood were tested for HBV markers (Ghendon and Kane, 1991).

The prevention of transmission of infectious agents through blood transfusion can be controlled at three levels: at the source, involving donor requirements and selection; after collection, involving testing of blood for transmissible agents; after transfusion, involving patient review. The first two levels are the most important for preventing transmission of HBV through blood transfusion.

The WHO Requirements for the collection, processing, and quality control of blood, blood components, and plasma derivatives (1989) stated:

"Donors shall not have a history of positive laboratory test results for viral hepatitis or corresponding symptoms and signs, of close contact with an individual with hepatitis within the past 6 months, or receipt within the previous 2 years of human blood or any blood component or fraction that might be a source of transmission of infectious agents." In most developed countries donors with a history of viral hepatitis or of a positive test for HBsAg are permanently excluded. But these procedures are not carried out as yet in many developing countries. Costs are often the main reason for inadequate screening of donors, additional factors being inadequate laboratory facilities and difficulties in procuring imported reagents.

There is no doubt that the most important way to prevent the transmission of HBV through blood transfusion is, as recommended by WHO, to screen all blood samples and use for transfusion only samples giving negative results for HBsAg. At the moment, the situation in regard to the screening of blood for HBsAg in many developing countries is unsatisfactory. It is now time to increase efforts to help developing countries avoid infection with HBV by blood transfusion.

At the moment in the WHO Programme on Control of HB, attention is mainly focused on active immunization as the most effective method for preventing acute HB infection and the development of its chronic sequelae (see Ghendon, 1990a,c).

The first stage of the implementation of the WHO programme was the organization of several collaborative studies to investigate the safety, immunogenicity, and efficacy of HB vaccines on volunteers and in field trials. WHO has also held several meetings to discuss the efficacy of HB vaccines and the optimal strategy for vaccination to control the disease. WHO headquarters coordinates activity with its Regional Offices in the implementation of the of the programme (see Ghendon, 1990c; Kane et al., 1991).

The last meeting of the WHO Technical Advisory Group on Viral Hepatitis, which took place in Geneva in November 1987 (Progress in control of viral hepatitis, 1988), reiterated that the most important means to control HB on a global scale and to reduce mortality due to its sequelae is mass immunization of infants and young children. The strategy for the control of HB in countries with different prevalences of HB infection and carrier rates that was recommended in 1987 is as follows: in hyperendemic regions where most infections are acquired early in life, the vaccine should be administered shortly after birth. Vaccination of all infants should be considered for all population groups with chronic carrier rates of HBV over 2% and vaccination of all infants should be a major public health priority for populations with carrier rates above 10%. In countries with a low carrier rate, vaccination should be directed to high-risk groups and to newborns of HBsAg-positive mothers.

To high-risk groups belong health-care workers who are exposed to blood; staff and residents of institutions for the developmentally disables; staff and patients in hemodialysis units; male homosexuals; parenteral drug abuse; and members of families with an HB carrier.

As to high-risk groups, it should be stressed that because HBV infection is the major infectious occupational hazard for health care workers, immunization of this group should receive high priority. All health care workers with exposure to blood should be informed of the risk of HBV infection, the availability of a safe and effective vaccine, and be actively offered HB vaccine free of charge by their employers.

Universal infant immunization with HB vaccine is the basic strategy for long-term control of HB in areas of high and intermediate endemicity. Infection during infancy and early childhood plays a disproportionate role in generating the HBV carrier pool, and in much of the world the infant immunization programs are the only functioning vaccine delivery systems. Countries with additional resources may wish to add additional programs once infant immunization is established. These programs may include "catch up" immunization of older children, maternal screening and treatment of infants of carrier mothers with HBIG and HB vaccine, and immunization of health care workers and other high-risk groups.

As to the control of HB in areas of low endemicity, it should be noted that in these areas perinatal and child-to-child transmission is relatively uncommon. Most infections occur in adults through sexual activity, needle sharing during drug abuse, or during occupational exposure to blood. As noted above, strategies for HBV control in these areas have stressed the immunization of high-risk groups, the screening of pregnant women, and treatment of the infants of HBV carrier mothers. There is now serious doubt that this strategy will lead to the control of HB.

Analysis done in the United States (Kane et al., 1989) has shown that there are about 300,000 annual infections of HB, up from 200,000 in the early 1980s. This increase has occurred despite the availability of a safe and effective HB vaccine since 1982. HB occurs primarily in young adults because of their lifestyle or occupationally related exposure. Cases due to heterosexual transmission and intravenous drug use are increasing. The proportion of cases in health-care workers has decreased, possibly because 30–40% of high-risk health workers have been vaccinated. But it should be noted that cases of HB in health-care workers represent less than 5% of reported cases of HB in the United States (Changing patterns of groups at high risk for Hepatitis B in the United States, 1988). Because of the increase in HB infection, the strategy of controlling this disease by vaccinating only high-risk groups, including infants of HBV carrier mothers, must be reconsidered. Immunization of all infants, and possibly adolescent immunization for an interim period before they begin life styles and behaviors that put them at risk for HBV infection, is being proposed by a number of experts as the only strategy that will provide long-term control of HBV infection even in areas of low prevalence.

It is likely that universal infant immunization is the proper strategy for long-range control of HBV infection everywhere and should receive highest priority, because these strategies will lead to the long-term control of HB in the population.

Recommended HB immunization strategies can be different in various regions of the world because of the different epidemiologic patterns of HBV infection.

In the hyperendemic areas of Asia, 7–10% of pregnant women are HBsAg-positive chronic carriers, and about 40% of these women are also HBeAg positive. Since 2.5–4% (40% of 7–10%) of Asians have an HBeAg-positive carrier mother, and since 10–15% of the population are carriers, it follows that 25–40% of carriers may have been infected by perinatal transmission. The majority of infection in the community, and the majority of the carriers, come from childhood infection.

The need to treat infants of HBV carrier mothers soon after birth poses a problem in areas where there is no contact with immunization services until several weeks or months after birth. In such areas born to HBeAg-positive carrier mothers may not receive protection from the vaccine. Immunization programs in Asia will need to provide HB vaccine near birth to maximize the prevention of HBV carrier children.

The problem is much less important in other areas of the world where perinatal transmission is less common. Two potential solutions to this problem include "stimulated" birth registration with a home visit by a vaccinator soon after birth, and the provision of vaccine (with appropriate training) to traditional birth attendants.

In sub-Saharan Africa, 10–15% of the population are HBV carriers, and 70–95% of the population show serologic evidence of period HBV infection. These prevalence figures are consistent in this region, and most experts do not believe that serologic studies need to be done in each country before HB vaccine programs are begun. It may be necessary, however, to do such studies to convince health authorities that their country has an HB problem of this magnitude.

The risk of newborn infants acquiring HB infection perinatally in Africa is much reduced compared with their Asian counterparts.

Although about 10% of women of childbearing age in Africa are HBsAg positive, only 10–15% of them are also HBeAg positive, so only 1–1.5% of African children are born to HBeAg-positive mothers. For this reason perinatal transmission is uncommon. In contrast, 70–90% of children become infected before the age of 17. In many sub-Saharan African countries PHC is the number one cause of cancer-related death in males.

Because perinatal transmission is uncommon, and because most African children are passively protected by maternal antibodies for about 6 months, the timing of the first HB vaccine injection is not critical. About 95–98% of fully immunized children would be protected whether the first dose is given at birth or at 3 months of age. There is some evidence that higher geometric mean titers of antibody may be achieved when the first dose is given at 3 months rather than at birth, and several studies in progress in Africa are designed to examine this question.

Less attention has been paid to HB control in areas of intermediate and low endemicity than in areas of higher or lower prevalence. Public health officials in these areas often believe that immunization of health care workers and maternal screening with treatment of newborns of carrier mothers is the proper strategy for control of hepatitis B. However, for reasons that have been discussed above, immunization of all newborns with HB vaccine is the only strategy that will provide long-term control. In areas of intermediate and low endemicity, if no maternal HBsAg screening is done, the first dose of HB vaccine should be given at birth.

Vaccination of all newborns will lead to a dramatic decrease in the number of new cases of acute and chronic HB. Nevertheless, particular attention should be paid to the protection of young children against HB. In fact, by 1991 there will be about 500 million infected children in various parts of the world where the disease is most endemic. Of these, up to 25%, or 7–15 million, will die in adulthood of liver cancer and cirrhosis.

Adolescent immunization should be added to the infant immunization program where economically feasible and where an appropriate infrastructure for delivery exists. A combined program of infant and adolescent immunization will provide optimal and timely long-term control of HBV infection.

There are numerous publications on the cost-effectiveness of HB immunization (Arevalo and Washington, 1988; Lahayne et al., 1987; Margolis et al., 1990; Mulley et al., 1982). Lahayne et al. (1987) concluded that immunization of all high-risk health care workers was cost beneficial when only the cost of work-loss was examined. Mulley et al. (1982) concluded that immunization of populations with an attack rate of 1–2% was cost-effective when direct and indirect costs were included. In both analyses the cost of hepatitis B vaccine was estimated at $100 for the three-dose series. In studies by Margolis et al. (1990), the cost of HB was analyzed in 16,000 persons who were hospitalized in the United States in 1986 with a primary or secondary diagnosis of acute HB. This analysis showed an expenditure of at least $197 million for direct medical costs and $126 million for the associated cost of work-loss.

Several studies predict a cost per HBV carrier prevented ranging from $100, and a cost per death prevented ranging from $260 to $400 at a vaccine cost of $1.00–$1.40 per dose; the cost per death prevented drops to $75.00 if vaccine costs drop to $0.50 per dose (see Integration of hepatitis B vaccine into EPI, 1990). However, all authors concluded that vaccination against HB should be cost-beneficial.

A. Integration of Hepatitis B Vaccine into EPI

At the meeting of the WHO Technical Advisory Group on Viral Hepatitis in 1987, it was recommended that HB vaccine be integrated into the WHO Expanded Programme of Immunization (EPI) (Progress in the control of viral hepatitis, 1988). This recommendation was strongly reiterated in 1989 at the Global Advisory Group of EPI.

Recently, within the framework of EPI, children are vaccinated with 6 vaccines: bacille Calmette-Guérin (BCG); oral polio vaccine (OPV), measles, and diphtheria/pertussis/tetanus (DPT).

The schedule for vaccination with the six WHO/EPI vaccines recommended for national consideration is the following: BCG, one dose at birth; OPV, four doses, at birth and with each DPT; DPT, three doses, at 6, 10, and 14 weeks; measles, one dose at 9 or 12 months.

This is not an absolute scheme, and the EPI recommends that each country determine its own schedule to fit best its own needs.

The meeting of the WHO Technical Advisory Group on Viral Hepatitis recommends that if the HB vaccine is integrated into the EPI, vaccination with the first dose of HB vaccine at birth or during the first month of life with BCG and OPV, and the second dose of HB vaccine after 4–12 weeks with the first vaccination of DPT could be acceptable. The third dose of HB vaccine is currently recommended to achieve high levels of antibody and prolonged protection. There is considerable latitude regarding the timing of this dose, which can be administered 2–12 months after the second dose, at a time most convenient to the EPI schedule in the country.

At the moment there are several publications on the simultaneous administration of HB vaccine with other EPI vaccines. It was found in experiments on laboratory animals that HB vaccine does not interfere with BCG, DPT, or measles vaccines (Mazert et al., 1983). In studies on children, it was found (Chiron et al., 1984; Coursaget et al., 1986, 1990) that immune responses to the combination of HB vaccine and DPT+ inactivated poliomyelitis vaccines were similar to the immune responses observed after administration of each vaccine alone.

Data indicating that EPI antigens do not interfere with the immune response to HB vaccine and, conversely, that HB vaccine does not interfere with the response to BCG, DTP, polio, and measles antigens is available from laboratory animal studies as well as from human trials in Senegal, Burma, and China. Additional studies designed to confirm these findings are in progress (Integration of hepatitis B vaccine into the EPI, 1990).

The use of high-titer Edmonston-Zagreb measles vaccine at 6 months is now recommended in some areas, and there is no documentation of the effect of administering this vaccine with HB vaccine. While there is no reason to expect Edmonston-Zagreb vaccine to behave differently, research needs to be undertaken to clarify the issue.

Several authors consider that HB immunization should be a part of routine childhood immunization (Hoofnagle, 1989; Maynard, 1990). Such integration of HB vaccine with the existing childhood immunization programs has been made in several countries.

In the Gambia, HB vaccine has been integrated into the national EPI without major changes to the schedule of immunization or to the mechanisms of delivery (The Gambia Hepatitis Study Group, 1989). The HB vaccine project was part of the Gambia Hepatitis Intervention Study, a collaborative project of the Gambia Government, the International Agency for Research on Cancer (WHO), and the Medical Research Council of the United Kingdom. The study has three phases: first integration of HB immunization in the EPI; second, evaluation of the immunogenicity of the vaccine and the duration of protection, which requires the long-term follow-up of a cohort of 1000 immunized children; and third, determination of the incidence of chronic liver disease in vaccinated and unvaccinated subjects. The schedule for vaccination in Gambia is the following: at birth, BCG, HB/1; at 2 months, DPT/1, OPV/1, HB/2; at 3 months, DPT/2, OPV/2; at 4 months, DPT/3, OPV/3, HB/3; at 9 months, measles, OPV/4, HB/4, yellow fever.

Serologic results on a sample of more than 700 children at 1 year of age show that the strategy has been effective in providing a significant titer of anti-HBs antibody. The antibody concentrations attained in responding children should give adequate protection when they are at high risk of persistent hepatitis B infection.

In Singapore the program of HB immunization within the framework of EPI started in mid-1973 with the immunization of health care workers on a volunteer basis (Goh et al., 1989). Immunization of babies born to carrier mothers was not started until October 1, 1985, when laboratory facilities for the routine screening of pregnant women for HBsAg and HBeAg became available. On September 1, 1987 the program was extended to include all newborns and has been fully integrated into the existing national childhood immunization programmes. The schedule for vaccination in Singapore is the following: at birth, BCG, HB/1; at 2 months, HB/2; at 3 months, DPT/1, OPV/1; at 4 months, DPT/2, OPV/2; at 5 months, DPT/3, OPV/3, HB/3; at 12 months, measles; at 18 months, DPT/4, OPV/4.

Several factors could contribute to a wider use of HB vaccines within the framework of EPI. First is the price of HB vaccines. Countries outside of Europe, North America, and Australia are able to obtain HB vaccine for public sector programs for $0.90–$2.00 per pediatric dose. Although this represents a dramatic improvement over the $30 per pediatric dose price of a few years ago, $3 per child is more than UNICEF pays for BCG, OPV, DPT, and measles vaccine combined. Introduction of HB vaccine at current prices would more than double the cost of infant vaccines in many parts of the world, money that many governments, UNICEF, and other international agencies do not have, and money that most donors have not yet been willing to give.

WHO and UNICEF have held discussions about the possibility of UNICEF procuring HB vaccine in an attempt to develop a global revolving fund for hepatitis B vaccine. UNICEF has agreed to do this if donors can be found to purchase the vaccine, or if countries who wish to purchase vaccine ask UNICEF to do the procurement. Pooling of orders from a number of countries and competitive bidding with large orders should lead to significantly lower prices, which in turn would allow more countries to afford HB immunization. One can assume that a mass vaccination campaign against HB coordinated by WHO and UNICEF would be able to use a much cheaper vaccine, as was the case with other components of the EPI (e.g., measles). The price of measles vaccine for the private sector is $4–6, but the EPI is charged only $0.13.

Because HB vaccine administration presently requires at least three doses, the implication is that the child must be seen the same number of times. It is known that drop-out rates from second and third doses of DPT are significant, and a similar drop-out rate must be expected with HB vaccine. Any device that would reduce this drop-out rate would be an advantage.

One approach utilizes combined DPT-HB vaccines. Such a combined vaccine, which is presently under development, would reduce additional storage and delivery costs, and would spare the recipient several additional injections. In Asia, an additional univalent HB vaccine could be delivered at birth to prevent perinatal infection, or an additional "booster" dose could be given with measles vaccine if extremely high titers of antibody are deemed important.

A second approach to reducing drop-out is the development of a slow-release product that can provide solid long-lasting immunity only with one injection. Various controlled-release systems include biodegradable synthetic polymers, liposomes, microsponges, and biodegradable glasses. A WHO project is developing a slow-release tetanus toxoid incorporated into injectable and biodegradable polymers. These microspheres will release the antigen in predetermined intervals over a long period of time, thus mimicking repeated injections (Programme for Vaccine Development and Transdisease Vaccinology, 1989). The concept of a slow-release product may apply, in general, to any vaccine that requires more than one injection, including HB vaccine.

B. Elimination of New Cases of Hepatitis B

Despite the relatively high prices of HB vaccines, more and more countries are starting an HB control program. At the beginning of 1990, 22 countries, primarily in the western Pacific and eastern Mediterranean have a policy of vaccinating all newborns with HB vaccine or plan to do so in the near future. Twenty-three additional countries have pilot infant immunization projects underway in selected regions of the country or plan to begin such projects in 1990 or 1991. Several such projects are supported and conducted by WHO. Twenty-seven other countries have selective immunization programs in place or planned. Selective programs may include screening of pregnant women and vaccination of newborns of carrier mothers, immunization of health-care personnel, and/or immunization of other high-risk groups (Integration of hepatitis B vaccine into the EPI, 1990).

It is possible to predict that in 5–7 years most of the countries in the world, especially in the areas of high and intermediate endemicity of HB, will use HB vaccines for mass vaccination of infants.

If we take into account that HB virus infects humans and has no known animal vectors for human HBV, that there are effective vaccines against this disease and sensitive tests for screening blood and blood products for HBsAg, and that these vaccines can be used within the framework of the EPI, it is probably timely to consider the initiation of a global program to eliminate new cases of HBV infection and its sequelae (e.g., chronic hepatitis and HBV-induced cirrhosis), and reduce primary hepatocellular carcinoma. If it became possible to immunize all babies and children in all countries and also those individuals belonging to high-risk groups, it is possible to assume that all new cases of acute and chronic HB could be eliminated in the next 20–30 years.

However, for successful implementation of the program of elimination of new cases of HB, several problems must be solved. As it was noted above, the chief obstacle to realizing the program of mass vaccination of infants and children is the price of HB vaccine. We must also determine the best strategy to use this vaccine within the framework of EPI. It is likely that these problems will be solved in the next 3–5 years.

Another very important problem in the control, and especially the elimination, of HB is the duration of immunity and the need for booster immunization. The duration of protection from HB vaccine is a crucial issue that will only be understood by carefully evaluating long-term HB vaccine trials.

It is generally assumed that immunity to HB persists for as long as at least 10 IU/L of anti-HBs can be detected in serum. A recent evaluation of the long-term protection (>5 years) afforded by vaccination indicates that vaccine-induced antibody levels decline significantly (Coursaget et al., 1986; Hadler et al., 1986). Antibody may decrease to low levels in 30–40% of vaccinated adults who initially develop adequate antibody levels during the first 5 years after vaccination, and may become undetectable in 10–15% of these persons. The duration of antibody persistence is directly related to the peak level achieved after the third dose of vaccine (Jilg et al., 1984b).

Studies of the plasma-derived HB vaccine in American adults have demonstrated that despite declining levels of antibody, protection against clinical HBV infection persists for >5 years (Hadler et al., 1986). It was suggested that among adults who have responded to the vaccine, protection against clinically significant HBV infection appears to outlast detectable anti-HBs, and booster doses following immunization may not be necessary for many years, if at all (Hadler et al., 1986).

For infants born to mothers who are HBV carriers, a 7 year study in Senegal has demonstrated that protection against viremic HBV infection can decline within 6 years in infants vaccinated between 6 months and 2 years of age. It was therefore concluded that children in endemic areas should be given a booster dose 5 years after the initial vaccination (Coursaget et al., 1986).

It is unclear how long clinical protection will persist against disease and the development of the carrier state. Some experts believe that long-term, even lifelong, protection against significant infection will occur following the immunologic "prime" provided by the initial vaccine series.

Others disagree, and consider that loss of protection against significant disease will occur at some point and booster doses may be necessary. Further research in this area is indicated.

Several studies found that in those regions and countries where perinatal transmission of HBV is the main mode of infection, immunization with HB vaccine alone will prevent development of infection in 75–80% of infants born to highly infectious HBeAg-positive mothers. Concurrent use of HB immunoglobulin (HBIg) and HB vaccine in such infants appears to increase the rate of protection to as high as 95% (see Ghendon, 1987). Unfortunately, HBIg is too expensive for most developing countries. Protection of 75–80% of newborn babies of HBsAg-positive mothers would represent a significant milestone in the control of hepatitis B, but fall short of eliminating HB.

One article recently reported achieving approximately 90% efficacy in preventing the carrier state in infants of HBeAg-positive mothers by use of recombinant HB vaccines without HBIg (Poovorawan et al., 1989). Further studies are necessary to confirm this finding.

It was also found recently that experimental HB vaccines containing S and pre-S1 proteins after one injection induced antibodies in 100% of adults who were previous nonresponders to standard plasma-derived or recombinant HB vaccines (Thoma, 1990). It is unclear if this vaccine could improve on the postexposure efficacy of current vaccines in vaccinating infants born to HBeAg-positive mothers.

Much more attention should be paid to devising the best strategy for protecting nonresponding newborns and adults and to investigate the reasons why these cannot be protected with HB vaccine alone.

The next and extremely important problem of elimination and even eradication of HB is that of HBV carriers. As noted above, it is estimated that there are nearly 300 million HBV carriers worldwide. These carriers are permanent source of infection. For example, it was found recently in Cyprus that the carrier rate reached 18.3% among family contacts of carriers (Papaevangelou et al., 1988). To eliminate new cases of HB, all members of families in which one of the members is an HB carrier should be vaccinated. It is also clear that eradication of hepatitis B can only be achieved if a cure can be found for the 300 million HBV carriers of the disease in the world today.

VI. CONCLUSION

Hepatitis B is one of the major disease of humans. More than 2 billion individuals have been infected with the hepatitis B virus globally, of whom some 300 million are chronically infected carriers at high risk of serious illness and death from cirrhosis of the liver and primary liver cancer. HB is now preventable with an extremely safe and effective vaccine: the first vaccine against cancer. A total of 22 countries have a policy of vaccinating all newborns with HB vaccines or plan to do so in the near future.

Epidemiologic data from a number of developed countries indicate that even in areas of low endemicity, strategies targeting HB vaccine to high-risk groups will not effectively control HBV infection in the population, and that universal immunization of infants with HB vaccine is the proper strategy for long-term control in all areas of the world.

The most important step in the global control of HB will be the integration of this vaccine into the EPI.

HB vaccines have proven themselves to be stable, safe, immunogenic, and effective. There are no technical or scientific impediments to their immediate use. Indeed, the dimensions of the global problem of HBV infection make it clear that their use is a matter of urgency. As with all vaccines, research and development efforts must continue to improve the vaccine and its preparations, determine the most cost-effective strategies for delivering it, and lower the costs of production. The paramount task is to develop national programs and obtain financial resources to provide this important antigen to the world's children.

Global control of hepatitis B is within reach. WHO will be working toward the following goals:

Universal infant immunization with HB vaccine through complete integration into the EPI.

Immunization for persons subject to occupational exposure and those with high-risk lifestyles.

Reduction in price of HB vaccine to the same order of magnitude as other EPI antigens.

Appropriate local production of HB vaccine through transfer of technology.

Development of HB vaccines that are effective with a single injection and stable in a warm climate.

Universal HBsAg screening of blood and blood products.

Development of "secondary prevention" strategies for HBV carriers. This would include effective antiviral chemotherapy and determination of the efficacy of alpha-fetoprotein screening for early detection of liver cancer.

As noted above, human HBV has no known animal reservoir or vectors. Therefore, a systematic vaccination program could theoretically eliminate and even eradicate HBV infection and its sequelae. The problem of control and especially eradication of hepatitis B may be more complicated than predicted and many important and difficult obstacles need to be overcome before the eradication of hepatitis B can be realized.

REFERENCES

Advances in viral hepatitis. (1977). WHO Tech. Rep. Ser. 602.

Andre, F. (1990). *Vaccine 8*(Suppl):S74–S78.

Andre, F., and Safary, A. (1988). In *Viral Hepatitis and Liver Disease,* A. Zuckerman (Ed.). Alan R. Liss, New York, pp. 1025–1030.

Arevalo, J., and Washington, A. (1988). *JAMA 259*:365–369.

Beasley, R., Hwang, L., Stevens, C., Lin, C., Hsich, F., Wang, K., Sun, T., and Szmuness, W. (1983). *Hepatology 3*:135–141.

Beasley, R., and Hwang, L. (1984). In *Viral Hepatitis and Liver Diseases.* G. Vias, G. Dienstag, and J. Hoofnagle (Eds.). Grune and Stratton, New York, pp. 209–224.

Chiron, J., Coursaget, P., and Yvonet, B. (1984). *Lancet 1*:623–624.

Coursaget, P., Chotard, J., Vincelot, P., Dior-Mar, J., Yvonet, B., Sarr, M., N'doye, R., and Chiron, J. (1986). *Lancet 2*:1143–1144.

Coursaget, P., Yvonet, B., Relyveld, E., Brizard, A., Bourdil, C., Bringer, L., Jeannee, E., Guindo, S., Dior-Mar, I., and Chiron, J. (1990). *Coll. INSERM 194*:319–324.

Deinhardt, F., and Gust, I. (1982). *Bull. WHO 60*:661–691.

Deinhardt, F., Able, I., and Assaad, F. (1983). *WHO Chron. 37*:203–207.

Emini, E., Ellis, R., Miller, W., McAleer, W., Scolnic, E., and Gerety, P. (1986). *J. Infect. 13*(Suppl.):3–9.

Fay, O. (1990). *Vaccine 8*(Suppl.):S100–S106.

Gerety, R. (1988). In *Viral Hepatitis and Liver Disease.* A. Zuckerman (Ed.). Alan R. Liss, New York, pp. 1017–1024.

Ghendon, Y. (1987). *J. Virol. Methods 17*:69–79.

Ghendon, Y. (1990a). *Vaccine 8*(Suppl.):S129–S133.

Ghendon, Y. (1990b). *Progr. Clin. Med. 5*:247–259.

Ghendon, Y. (1990c). *Progr. Clin. Med. 5*:99–107.

Ghendon, Y., and Kane, M. (1991). In *Viral Hepatitis and Liver Disease.* F. Hollinger, S. Lemon, and H. Margolis (Eds.). Williams and Wilkins, Baltimore, pp. 722–724.

Goh, K., Doraisingham, S., Tan, K., Oon, C., Ho, M., Chen, A., and Chan, S. (1989). *Bull. WHO 67*:65–70.

Goudeau, A. (1990). *Vaccine 8*(Suppl.):S113–S116.

Hadler, S. (1990). *Vaccine 8*(Suppl.):S24–S28.

Hadler, S., Francis, D., Maynard, J., Thompson, S., Judson, F., Echenberg, D., Ostrow, D., O'Malley, P., Penley, K., Altman, M., Braft, E., Shipman, G., Coleman, P., and Maudd, E. (1986). *N. Engl. J. Med. 315*:209–214.

Hanser, P., Walters, T., Simoen, E., Voet, P., and DeWilde, M. (1988). In *Viral Hepatitis and Liver Disease*. A. Zuckerman (Ed.). Alan R. Liss, New York, pp. 1031–1037.

Hepatitis B vaccines prepared from yeast by recombinant DNA technique. (1985). *Bull. WHO 63*:57–61.

Hollinger, F. (1990). *Vaccine 8*(Suppl.):S122–S128.

Hoofnagle, J. (1989). *N. Engl. J. Med. 321*:1333–1334.

Hwang, L., Roggendorf, M., Beasley, R., and Deinhardt, F. (1985). *J. Med. Virol. 15*:265–269.

Integration of hepatitis B vaccine into the EPI. (1990). WHO Document EIP/GAG/90/WP.14.

Jilg, W., Schmidt, G., Lorbeer, B., Wilske, B., and Deinhardt, F. (1984a). *Lancet* 2:1174–1175.

Jilg, W., Schmidt, M., Deinhardt, F., and Zachoval, R. (1984b). *Lancet* 2:458.

Kane, M., Alter, M., Hadler, S., and Margolis, H. (1989). *Am. J. Med. 87*(Suppl. 3A):S11–S13.

Kane, M., Ghendon, Y., and Lambert, P.-A. (1991). In *Viral Hepatitis and Liver Disease*. B. Hollinger, S. Lemon, and H. Margolis (Eds.). Williams and Wilkins, Baltimore, pp. 706–708.

Kiire, C. (1990). *Vaccine 8*(Suppl.):S107–S112.

Lahayne, D., Strauss, P., Baleux, C., and van Ganse, W. (1987). *Lanceat* 2:441–443.

Lee, A., Ip, H., and Wong, V. (1978). *J. Infect. Dis. 136*:668–671.

Lo, K., Tsai, Y., Lee, S., Wu, T., Wang, I., Chen, G., Yeh, C., Chiang, B., Yeh, S., Goudeau, A., Coursaget, P., and Tong, M. (1985). *J. Infect. Dis. 152*:817–822.

Margolis, H., Schatz, G., and Kane, M. (1990). *Vaccine 8*(Suppl.):S81–S85.

Maynard, J. (1990). *Vaccine 8*(Suppl.):S18–S20.

Maynard, Y., Kane, M., Alter, M., and Adler, S. (1988). In *Viral Hepatitis and Liver Disease*. A. Zuckerman (Ed.). Alan R. Liss, New York, pp. 967–969.

Maynard, J., Kane, M., and Hadler, S. (1989). *Rev. Infect. Dis.* 2(Suppl. 3):S574–S575.

Mazert, M., Chabanier, G., Adamovicz, P., and Gerfaux, G. (1983). *Dev. Biol. Stand. 54*:53–62.

Mulley, A., Silverstein, M., and Dienstag, J. (1982). *N. Engl. J. Med. 307*:644–652.

Obayashi, A., Okochi, K., and Mayumi, M. (1972). *Gastroenterology 62*:618–625.

Okada, K., Yamada, T., Miyakama, Y., and Mayumi, M. (1975). *J. Pediatr. 87*:360–367.

Papaevangelou, G., Roumeliotou, A., Chartziminas, M., Kotsianopoulou, M., Ioannou, P., Tricopoulou, E., and Nestoridou, A. (1988). *Eur. J. Epidemiol.* 4:150–153.

Piot, P., Goliav, C., and Kegels, E. (1990). *Vaccine 8*(Suppl.):S37–S40.

Poovorawan, Y., Sanpavat, S., Pongpunlet, W., Chumdermpadetsuk, S., Sentrakul, O., and Safary, A. (1989). *JAMA 261*:3278–3280.

Progress in control of viral hepatitis: Memorandum from a WHO meeting. (1988). *Bull. WHO 66*:443–455.

Programme for Vaccine Development and Transdisease Vaccinology. (1989). WHO, MIM/EXBUD/89.1.

Requirements for hepatitis B vaccine made by recombinant DNA techniques in yeast. (1987). *WHO Tech. Rep. Ser. 760*:106–138.

Requirements for the collection, processing and quality control of blood, blood components and plasma derivatives. (1989). *WHO Tech. Rep. Ser. 786*:94–175.
Stevens, C., Beasley, R., Tsui, J., and Lee, W. (1975). *N. Engl. J. Med. 229*:771–774.
Stevens, C., Neurath, R., Beasley, R., and Szmuness, w. (1979). *J. Med. Virol. 3*:237–241.
Sung, J. (1990). *Vaccine 8*(Suppl.):S95–S99.
The Gambia Hepatitis Study Group: Hepatitis B Vaccine in the Expanded Programme of Immunization. (1989). *Lancet 1*:1057–1060.
Thoma, H. (1990). International Symposium on Viral Hepatitis and Liver Disease, Houston, p. 118.
Tong, M., Thursby, M., and Lin, J. (1981). *Progr. Med. Virol. 27*:137–147.
Toukan, A. (1990). *Vaccine 8*(Suppl.):S117–S121.
Wong, V., Lee, A., and Ip, H. (1980). *Br. J. Obstet. Gynaecol. 87*:958–965.

Part III

Measles and Global Control

7

MEASLES VIRUS AND DISEASE
Old and New Problems

Raymond G. Marusyk *University of Alberta, Edmonton, Alberta, Canada*

I. INTRODUCTION

Measles was first clinically described in the Middle Ages, and early writings indicate the disease seen in those times was not unlike that seen by physicians today (Greenhill, 1848; cf. Norrby and Oxman, 1990).

Measles is ubiquitous. No sector of our world has not experienced childhood measles. Although largely eradicated in developed countries with good immunization programs, the children of developing countries are still very much the target of this virus disease. Approximately 2 million children die each year as a direct result of measles infection (Cutts et al., 1991). Unfortunately, measles is a tenacious and highly infectious disease. The high transmission rate of measles makes herd immunity difficult to achieve. Measles is also associated with such serious complications as otitis media, pneumonia, encephalitis, prolonged diarrhea, and, rarely, subacute sclerosing panencephalitis (Norrby and Oxman, 1990).

In countries where a vaccine program has been developed and implemented, there has been a striking change in the incidence and average age of incidence of measles infection. Where the latter has occurred, it is often thought to be a result of failure of the vaccine delivery programs (not all the target population was immunized), vaccine failure, or the loss of natural circulating measles virus as a booster agent in the population. However, it is well established that a major short-term reduction in measles incidence following the introduction of a mass immunization program can be followed by new measles epidemics at increasing intervals (Cutts et al., 1991).

II. THE DISEASE

Measles is defined clinically as a generalized maculopapular rash persisting for 3 or more days, with an accompanying temperature of 38.3°C or higher and a cough and/or coryza and/or conjunctivitis. Such clinical diagnoses do not have to be confirmed virologically or serologically if good clinical or epidemiologic data are available.

Some authorities have suggested that measles cases should be classified as suspect cases, probable cases, or confirmed cases dependent upon the availability of clinical or epidemiologic data.

Measles is usually associated with a typical skin rash, other body tissues may be involved in virus multiplication (cf. Norrby and Oxman, 1990). A 10–12 day incubation period usually follows infection with measles virus but may, in some cases, be as short as 2–3 days. Virus can be isolated from the throat, tears, nasal secretions, and urine during the prodromal period and has been isolated from the blood. As the prodromal period ends, typical Koplik spots may be seen within the oral cavity. The Koplik spots reportedly contain viral structural components (Surinaga et al., 1970). When the typical measles rash becomes evident, IgM and IgG titers rise, the levels peaking at 10 days and 30 days, respectively. The immunity developed against natural measles infection is believed to be lifelong (Black, 1989).

Occasionally, measles virus infection can lead to clinically unusual forms of disease. Atypical measles was described in partially immunized individuals by Rauk and Schmidt (1965). This manifestation is seen in patients who have received killed vaccine and then been exposed to live virus. The disease is associated with a variable skin rash: macropapular becoming petechial or hemorrhagic. The rash usually begins on the limbs (unlike typical measles) and spreads to the body trunk. Individuals diagnosed as having atypical measles are often more seriously ill than if they had typical measles infection. Atypical measles infection is not often seen because of the direct association with the use of killed vaccine preparations, but more than 2000 cases were reported during a measles epidemic in Canada in 1979 (cf. Marusyk, 1984). This consequence of the use of killed vaccine in many countries is still very much a problem. The administration of the killed virus product has now been shown to have interfered with the subsequent live vaccine programs, even as long as 20 years after the initial immunization program (Mäkelä et al., 1989). Of particular interest, is the difficulty in obtaining measles virus isolates in these new outbreaks of measles virus infection (Marusyk and Tyrrell, 1984).

Other unusual host responses such as measles encephalitis and subacute sclerosing panencephalitis are seen relatively infrequently in immunized populations, and a description of these manifestations is not within the scope of this review.

III. THE VIRUS

Measles is the prototype virus of the genus morbillivirus, family paramyxoviridae. The genus also includes the canine distemper, rinderpest, and peste des petits ruminants viruses (Fenner, 1976). Although members of this genus reportedly do not possess detectable neuraminidase activity (Choppin and Compans, 1974), newly developed highly sensitive assays can detect viral-specific neuraminidase activity at a level of 10^{-18} M (R. Marusyk and G. Armstrong, unpublished observations).

The measles virion is composed of an outer lipoprotein envelope that contains two glycoprotein peplomers, the hemagglutinin (designated H) and the hemolysin or fusion factor (HL or F; Tyrrell and Norrby, 1978). The internal nucleocapsid contains a single-stranded RNA genome of unit length. The size of the RNA genome has been variously reported to be between 4.6 and 6.2 million daltons, but is now generally accepted to be 5.2 million daltons (45–48 S; Hall and Martin, 1973; Lund et al., 1986).

Analytic electrophoresis techniques have shown that there are seven constituent polypeptides within the virion. These polypeptides range in size from 36,000 to more than 200,000 daltons (Tyrrell and Norrby, 1978). Several of the components have associated biological activities: H (hemagglutinin), F (cell membrane fusion), and P (RNA polymerase).

The replication process of measles virus has not been well studied. All events take place intracytoplasmically, however (Portner and Bussell, 1973). Of interest is the observation that production of measles virus defective-interfering particle is temperature-dependent and that the presence of such particles enhances the development of persistent infections at 37°C (Tsang et al., 1981). Since current measles vaccine strains are attenuated, temperature-sensitive mutants and the presence of defective-interfering particles in such preparations should be closely monitored.

IV. ANTIGENIC COMPOSITION AND DETERMINANTS

Although data are available concerning the possible antigenic variation of measles virus through the use of monoclonal antibody (cf. Norrby and Oxman, 1990), there is, as yet, no strong evidence to indicate that such changes occur in antigenic sites responsible for the induction of neutralizing antibody. However, in light of the recent observation that consistent genome variation does exist among measles virus isolates (Rota and Bellini, 1990), earlier observations relative to inconsistencies in observed virus-associated biological activity (high infectious titer vs. no hemagglutinating titer) may, in fact, be correct observations related to genomic differences between virus isolates (Marusyk and Tyrrell, 1984).

The two surface glycoproteins of measles virus, the H and F peplomers, are relatively stable antigenically. Minor antigenic differences have been observed in neutralization tests with laboratory strains and fresh isolates from natural infections (Albrecht et al., 1981). Monoclonal antibodies directed against specific epitopes on a number of different strains have shown minor antigenic variation on the H peplomer (Birrer et al., 1981; Carter et al., 1982; Sheshberadaran et al., 1984; ter Meulen et al., 1981). No strong evidence exists for the presence of epitopic variations on the F peplomer (Sheshberadaran et al., 1984), although the work of Rota and Bellini (1990) would indicate that these do exist and could play a major role in the disease process.

Of the four internal components of measles virus, three have been well characterized antigenically. The NP and P components are relatively stable, although variation in the NP protein has been detected (Giraudon and Wild, 1988; Sato et al., 1985). The M protein shows considerable variation (cf. Norrby and Oxman, 1990).

There appears to be a strong antigenic relationship between the NP and F proteins within the members of the genus *Morbillivirus*, family Paramyxoviridae. The remaining major structural components, M, P, and H, show a lesser relationship. Norrby et al. (1985) have speculated on the evolutionary relationship between the morbilliviruses and postulated that rinderpest is the progenitor of the *Morbillivirus* genus.

V. THE IMMUNE RESPONSE

The immune response to measles virus can be measured easily. However, evidence indicates that this immune reaction is likely very complicated. Activated T cells and stimulated B cells produce antibody of several classes and subclasses, with each type of T or B cell responding to one or more epitopes on the virions internal and external structural components. Most infections produce a number of specific immune responses, each of which may be modulated by the previous antigenic experience of the infected individual. The significance of these immunologic events in measles virus infection is not clearly understood.

Measles has long been considered to be a stable, monotypic virus, that is, antibody developed against a specific strain will neutralize the infectivity of another strain. It is now accepted that there are likely to be several "strains" or multiple lineages of measles virus coexisting (Rota and Bellini, 1990; Taylor et al., 1991). The evidence points to differences at the genome level that are apparently reflected in noticeable (detectable) differences in antigenic composition of the virus. Measles virus strains differ in their reactivity with component specific monoclonal antibodies, but do not differ in reactivity with human immune serum.

The extensive antigenic stimulation caused by the disseminated measles virus infection that occurs before the onset of rash activates a variety of host immune responses (Black and Rosen, 1962; Krugman, 1977; Panum, 1939; Preblud and Katz, 1988).

Most of the major measles virus components elicit an immune response from T and B cells (Ilonen et al., 1988). The T-cell response usually declines below the detectable level within a few months of infection and tests give results indicative of an immune status. The B cell response includes IgM and IgA class antibodies as well as IgG, but the IgM response is transient. The IgA is not essential to protection and wanes in a few years. Immunity to measles in humans can be assessed by examination of the specific IgG and IgM response alone (Black, 1989).

Since cell-mediated immunity cannot be readily measured and interpreted, the response to measles infection or immunization is generally determined by assessing the humoral immune response. The antibody response to vaccination is similar to that caused by natural infection: an initial short-lived rise in serum IgM followed by a later rising IgG level (Markowitz et al., 1990). As with natural infection, IgG antibody induced by vaccination decreases over time. Individuals who have experienced primary antigenic stimulation from either natural measles or vaccine generally exhibit an anamnestic or secondary response after either revaccination or exposure to natural measles. This secondary response is characterized by a rapid and often transient increase in IgG antibody but little or no detectable IgM production.

Several different assays are available for measuring measles antibody. The most commonly used tests are the hemagglutination inhibition (HI) and virus neutralization (NT) tests, with the latter providing a good evaluation of immunity (Neumann et al., 1985; Chui et al., 1991). The plaque-reduction assay is even more sensitive than the virus neutralization test and many times more sensitive than the HI test, and is, therefore, considered the optimal measles antibody test. Enzyme immunoassays (EIA) are widely available and also are much more sensitive than the HI test.

There is reportedly a close correlation between the HI and NT tests, and some authors have claimed that the HI test results are indicative of NT titers, and by inference, protection (Black, 1989). Others, however, have shown that such relationships are not consistent (Mäkelä et al., 1989; Chui et al., 1991; R. Marusyk, A. Salmi, and D. Tyrrell, submitted for publication).

The minimum antibody titer necessary for protection against measles virus infection is not known, nor is it known which particular component-specific antibodies are crucial to mounting an adequate protective response. The detection of any amount of HI antibody after live measles vaccination has been accepted as evidence of immunity to measles (Black, 1989). However, recent evidence suggests that some persons with small concentrations of antibody detected by the plaque reduction assay may not be protected (Mäkelä et al., 1989).

Maternal antibodies are believed to provide protection during the first 6 months of life and often longer. Interference with the replication of vaccine virus is frequently still seen at the age of 12 months (Albrecht et al., 1977; Archibald et al., 1971; Nader et al., 1968). The entire question of the longevity of maternal antibodies is being investigated, since evidence suggests that the implementation of successful vaccine programs has resulted in much lower levels of antibody being transferred transplacentally, and with many infants having no protective virus-specific antibodies until they are themselves vaccinated (Chui et al., 1991). This observation indicates that, in some populations at least, infants at an early age have very low or no immunity of maternal origin to measles.

Cell-mediated immunity is required to clear measles virus infection. However, both humoral and cell-mediated immunity appear to be capable of preventing infection in normal individuals exposed to the virus. In situations in which long-term immunity appears to be based upon antibody production, there is a need for antibodies against the fusion factor (F or HL) as well as against the hemagglutinin. This is evidenced by experience with atypical measles in recipients of inactivated measles vaccine (Frey and Krugman, 1981; Fulginiti et al., 1967; Norrby, 1975; Norrby et al., 1975). The frequent failure of postexposure prophylaxis with immune serum globulin to prevent severe measles infection in patients with deficient cell-mediated immunity suggests that the participation of some cell type is required for antibody to be protective.

Cell-mediated immunity to measles virus is measured with antigen-specific T-cell proliferation or cytotoxic T-lymphocyte assays. Cytotoxic T cells can be identified both in peripheral blood (Kreth et al., 1979; Ruckdeschel et al., 1975) and after in vitro culture of peripheral blood lymphocytes (Gordon and Knighton, 1941; Wright and Levy, 1979). However, reactivity is generally weak and short-lasting. The nature of the histocompatibility restriction of measles virus-specific cytotoxic T cells is a matter of controversy (Ilonen et al., 1977). In early studies it was concluded that the restriction was class I antigen-specific (Kreth et al., 1979; Lucas et al., 1982) but in more extended studies it was found to be class II antigen-restricted (Jacobson et al., 1984, 1987; Richert et al., 1985, 1986). This has been demonstrated both with separated peripheral blood lymphocytes and with T cell clones. The cytotoxic T cells show specificity not only for measles virus surface antigens but also for internal antigens, especially the NP component.

VI. CONTROL OF MEASLES

Measles virus infections can be controlled through the use of vaccines. Killed vaccines were found to confer temporary immunity to measles, but unknown to the distributors of the vaccine was the fact that the inactivation procedure used had destroyed the antigenicity of the hemolysin (F) component of the virus (Norrby and Golmar, 1975). Upon exposure to wild-type measles virus, individuals who have received the killed virus vaccine may develop atypical measles (described above), with an associated anamnestic response to the hemagglutinin (as measured by hemagglutinin-inhibition antibody titers) and nucleocapsid. It is apparent that an immunologic response to the hemolysis component is necessary for the development of long-term immunity (Norrby and Golmar, 1975).

Currently available attenuated measles vaccines have none of the problems associated with the first such available products (Katz et al., 1960). Little if any virus is spread via excretion from vaccine recipients. Black (1989) has suggested that there is no need for revaccination programs other than in individuals who earlier received only the killed virus vaccine or in very young children who may have been selected for immunization. However, in North America where numerous measles virus outbreaks have occurred in well-immunized populations, evidence shows that vaccine-induced immunity to measles has, in fact, waned to very low levels over 20 years (Mäkelä et al., 1989).

Consequently, recent outbreaks of measles virus in the United States among college students have led authorities in a number of jurisdictions to begin area-wide immunization programs to increase the level of measles immunity among the very large population of college and university students. The high susceptibility of certain segments of this particular age group may be related to several factors, including that many children may not have been immunized with measles vaccine during the period immediately following its approval; many children/students may have entered schools without the legislated immunization now in effect; similarly, many advanced education institutes lacked immunization requirements for new registrants; many children/students may have escaped natural measles infection because of decreasing transmission; vaccine-induced immunity is not as long-lived as that induced by natural infection.

In other areas, measles has been reported in older age groups, confirming the observation that the average age at infection has moved upward. In recent cases reported in a number of North American centers, the mean age of measles infection is now approaching 20 years (Mäkelä et al., 1989). This observation is in strong contrast to the mean age of less than 2 years in areas where vaccine programs have not been introduced (Black, 1989).

Regulations concerning the administration of virus vaccines vary greatly between countries. There is agreement, however, that measles vaccine should be given, it at all possible, to young children between the ages of 9 and 15 months (even as young a 6 months), the exact age to be determined by particular circumstances.

In those areas where measles vaccine is used, there has been a dramatic effect on the incidence of measles and its associated complications (Black, 1989). A measles elimination program must be based on three major premises: achievement and maintenance of high immunization levels; development of strong and effective surveillance systems; and aggressive response to the occurrence of the disease. Such goals are not difficult to set and attain in a country with a highly efficient health delivery and protection system.

Similarities have been made between the programs to eradicate smallpox and measles: both viruses produce rashes, confer life-long immunity, have no known animal reservoir (other than humans), and do not induce a chronic carrier state. There are, however, sufficient points of difference that must be considered before drawing parallels between the eradication of these two viruses: the highly infectious nature of measles virus and the average age of infection with the two viruses (4–5 years for smallpox and less than 2 years for measles).

What are the prospects for the eradication of measles? An early constraint on the success of such a program previously was the lack of a heat-stable vaccine and the inherent cost of cold-handling and delivery of the available vaccines. The development of relatively heat-stable, lyophilized vaccines and relatively inexpensive low-temperature storage containers has addressed these problems. Properly administered measles vaccine is capable of inducing immunity in more than 90% of the recipients.

Thus far, no serious side effects or contraindications have been associated within the currently available vaccines.

VII. CONCLUSION

There is no question that in those areas of the world where well-developed and implemented measles virus immunization programs have succeeded, there has been a substantial drop in the number of measles cases. Debate still continues, however, over the choice of a single- or multiple-dose immunization schedule and whether the initial vaccine dose should be given to infants at less 9 months of age.

The situation in less fortunate areas of the world is more basic. How can the measles virus immunization program be implemented in a manner to ensure complete (adequate?) coverage? Is a better vaccine indicated? Can combined virus vaccine programs be introduced? The World Health Organization has recently stated (Cutts et al., 1991) that the success of any measles immunization program will require the introduction of high-dose measles vaccines that can be given at 6 months of age, and recognition of predictable changes in measles epidemiology following the introduction of a new immunization program.

REFERENCES

Albrecht, P., Ennis, F., Salzman, F., and Krugman, S. (1977). *J. Pediatr. 91*:915–918.
Albrecht, P., Hermann, K., and Burns, R. (1981). *J. Virol. Methods 3*:251–260.
Archibald, R., Weller, R., and Meadow, S. (1971). *J. Pathol. 103*:27–34.
Birrer, M., Bloom, B., and Udem, S. (1981). *Virology 198*:381–390.
Black, F., and Rosen, L. (1962). *J. Immunol. 88*:725–731.
Black, F. (1989). *Prog. Med. Virol. 36*:1–33.
Carter, M., Willcocks, M., Loffler, S., and ter Meulen, V. (1982). *J. Gen. Virol. 63*:113–120.
Choppin, P., and Compans, R. (1974). In *Comprehensive Virology*, volume 4. F. Fraenkel-Conrat and R. Wagner (Eds.). Plenum Press, New York, pp. 95–178.
Chui, L., Marusyk, R., and Pabst, H. (1991). *J. Med. Virol. 33*:199–204.
Cutts, F., Henderson, R., Clements, C., Chen, R., and Patriarca, P. (1991). *Bull. WHO 69*:1–7.
Fenner, F. (1976). *Intervirology 7*:1–116.
Frey, H., and Krugman, S. (1981). *Am. J. Med. Sci. 281*:51–55.
Fulginiti, V., Eller, J., Downie, A., and Kempe, C. (1967). *JAMA 202*:1075–1080.
Giraudon, P., and Wild, T. (1985). *Virology 144*:46–58.
Gordon, H., and Knighton, H. (1941). *Am. J. Pathol. 17*:165–176.

Greenhill, W. (1848). *A Treatise on the Smallpox and Measles.* A translation of the original Arabic text of Abu Becr Mohammed Ibn Zacairiya (Rhazes). Sydenham Society, London.
Hall, W., and Martin, S. (1973). *J. Gen. Virol. 19*:175–182.
Hinman, R., Brandling-Bennett, A., and Nieburg, P. (1979). *JAMA 242*:1157–1162.
Ilonen, J., Herva, E., Reunanen, M., Panelious, M., Meurman, O., Arstila, P., and Tiilikainen, A. (1977). *Acta Neurol. Scand. 55*:299–309.
Ilonen, J., Salonen, R., Marusyk, R., and Salmi, A. (1988). In *Virus Diseases in Asia.* P. Thongcharoen and E. Kurstak (Eds.). Mahidol University Press, Bangkok, pp. 301–304.
Jacobson, S., Richert, J., Biddison, W., Satinsky, A., Harzman, R., and McFarland, H. (1984). *J. Immunol. 133*:754–757.
Jacobson, S., Rose, J., Flerlage, M., McFarlin, D., and McFarland, H. (1987). *Viral Immunol. 1*:153–162.
Katz, S., Kempe, C., and Black, F. (1960). *N. Engl. J. Med. 263*:180–184.
Kreth, H., ter Meulen, V., and Eckert, G. (1979). *Med. Microbiol. Immunol. 165*: 203–214.
Krugman, S. (1977). *J. Pediatr. 90*:1–13.
Lucas, C., Biddison, W., Nelson, I., and Shaw, S. (1982). *Infect. Immun. 38*:226–232.
Lund, G., Tyrrell, D., Bradley, R., and Scraba, D. (1984). *J. Gen. Virol. 65*:1535–1542.
Mäkelä, M., Marusyk, R., Norrby, E., Tyrrell, D., and Salmi, A. (1989). *Vaccine 7*:541–545.
Markowitz, L., Preblud, S., Fine, P., and Orenstein, W. (1990). *Pediatr. Infect. D is. 9*:101–110.
Marusyk, R., and Tyrrell, D. (1984). In *Control of Virus Diseases.* E. Kurstak and R. Marusyk (Eds.). Marcel Dekker, New York, pp. 67–78.
Marusyk, R. (1984). In *Applied Virology.* E. Kurstak (Ed.). Academic Press, New York, pp. 211–219.
McFarland, H., Pedone, C., Mingioli, E., and McFarlin, D. (1980). *J. Immunol. 125*:221–225.
Nader, P., Horwitz, M., and Rousseau, J. (1968). *J. Pediatr. 72*:22.
Neumann, P., Weber, J., Jessamine, A., and O'Shaughnessy, M. (1985). *J. Clin. Microbiol. 22*:296–298.
Norrby, E. (1975). *J. Biol. Stand. 3*:375–380.
Norrby, E., and Golmar, Y. (1975). *Infect. Immun. 11*:231–239.
Norrby, E., and Oxman, M. (1990). In *Fields Virology.* B. Fields and D. Knipe (Eds.). Raven Press, New York, pp. 1013–1044.
Norrby, E., Enders-Ruckle, G., and ter Meulen, V. (1975). *J. Infect. Dis. 132*:262–269.
Norrby, E., Sheshberadaran, H., McCullough, K., Carpenter, W., and Orvell, C. (1985). *Intervirology 23*:228–232.
Panum, P. (1939). *Med. Classics 3*:839–886.
Portner, A., and Bussell, R. (1973). *J. Virol. 11*:46–53.
Preblud, S., and Katz, S. (1988). In *Vaccines.* S. Plotkin and E. Mortimer (Eds.). W. Saunders, Philadelphia.
Rauk, L., and Schmidt, R. (1965). *Am. J. Dis. Child. 109*:232.

Richert, J., McFarland, H., McFarlin, D., Johnson, A., Woody, J., and Hartzman, R. (1985). *J. Immunol. 134*:1561–1566.
Richert, J., Rose, J., and Reuben-Burnside, C. (1986). *J. Immunol. 137*:2190–2194.
Rose, J., Bellini, W., McFarlin, D., and McFarland, H. (1984). *J. Virol. 49*:988–991.
Rota, P., and Bellini, W. (1990). In Proceedings and Abstracts of the VIIIth International Congress of Virology, Berlin.
Ruckdeschel, J., Graziano, K., and Mardiney, M. (1975). *Cell. Immunol. 17*:11–18.
Sato, T., Fududa, A., and Sugiura, A. (1985). *J. Gen. Virol. 66*:1397–1409.
Sheshberadaran, H., Chen, S.-H., and Norrby, E. (1984). *Virology 128*:341–353.
Surinaga, D., Bank, L., and Ackerman, A. (1970). *N. Engl. J. Med. 238*:1139–1142.
Taylor, M., Godfrey, E., Baczko, K., ter Meulen, V., and Rima, B. (1991). *J. Gen. Virol. 72*:83–88.
ter Meulen, V., Loffer, S., Carter, M., and Stephenson, J. (1981). *J. Gen. Virol. 57*:357–364.
Tsang, L., Chang, N., and Marusyk, R. (1981). *J. Gen. Virol. 56*:195–198.
Tyrrell, D., and Norrby, E. (1978). *J. Gen. Virol. 39*:219–229.
Wright, L., and Levy, N. (1979). *J. Immunol. 122*:2379–2387.

8

GLOBAL CONTROL OF MEASLES

New Strategies for the 1990s

Christopher John Clements *World Health Organization, Geneva, Switzerland*

M. Strassburg *Los Angeles County Department of Health Services, Los Angeles, California*

Felicity T. Cutts *London School of Hygiene and Tropical Medicine, London, England*

Julie B. Milstien and Carole Torel *World Health Organization, Geneva, Switzerland*

I. INTRODUCTION

The eradication of smallpox from the world in 1977 proved the feasibility of eradicating infectious diseases. Since that time, public health officials, researchers, politicians, and others have been systematically evaluating other candidates for potential eradication. In May, 1998, the World Health Assembly (WHA) selected poliomyelitis as the next disease to be targeted for eradication. Many agree that measles, with its far greater impact on child mortality throughout the world, should also be considered, if not for eradication, at the very least for a well-coordinated global control program.

To date, measles has not been successfully controlled globally. The disease has already proved to be a formidable adversary. Twice in the last 20 years, a program has been put forward to eliminate measles from the United States and twice it has failed (Sencer et al., 1976; Hinman et al., 1979). This chapter surveys key issues in the global control of measles and identifies reasons why increased attention to the subject is needed. It is to be hoped that when such control programs are in place, there will be a great reduction in disease incidence during the 1990s, paving the way for eventual eradication of this disease.

II. GLOBAL SITUATION

A. Expanded Programme on Immunization

With global measles immunization coverage now at 80% for 1990, the next stage of the attack on this virus is clear: to find and immunize those children who are continually missed by immunization services. Simply maintaining the same levels of services will not succeed in reaching those who have been missed. The focus of the Expanded Programme on Immunization (EPI) is now firmly on closing this coverage gap during the next 5 years.

Before the EPI, virtually all children contracted measles: an estimated 130 million cases with about 16 million deaths each year. The activities of the EPI have resulted in a dramatic reduction in both measles morbidity and mortality. In 1990, it is estimated that approximately 80% of the world's children under 1 year of age received measles vaccine, and more than 1,952,000 deaths were prevented.

The estimated total number of measles cases occurring in the developing world for 1990 was 45 million cases and a staggering 842,000 deaths. Thus measles is still responsible for more deaths than all of the other EPI target diseases combined. Complications from measles include diarrhea, pneumonia, otitis media, blindness, and encephalitis, which leave many thousands of children disabled. Actual numbers dying as a result of measles may be twice the estimated 842,000 if the delayed effect of the disease is taken into account. Measles ranks as one of the leading causes of childhood mortality in the world. In one study in Kenya (Spencer et al., 1987), measles accounted for 35% of reported deaths in infants 1–12 months of age and for 40% of deaths in children 1–4 years old. The impact of measles on the lives of millions of young children every year, particularly in developing countries, indicates the urgent need for further reduction in measles incidence.

B. WHA Global Measles Goal

The EPI has its basis in resolution WHA 27.57, adopted by the WHA in May, 1974. General program policies include the EPI goal of providing immunization services for all children of the world (resolution WHO 30.53, 1977) with a target of at least 90% coverage by the year 2000 with all antigens. In 1989, the WHA defined a specific goal for measles control: "A reduction in measles incidence of 90% from preimmunization levels by 1995."

In order to achieve the WHA goal, EPI has set specific measles control objectives:

By 1995 measles incidence will be reduced by 90% from preimmunization levels.

By 1995 measles coverage of at least 90% will be achieved at the national regional, and district levels, and

By 1995 all countries will have a disease surveillance system in place capable of the timely reporting of measles from all districts.

Although some countries have already achieved these objectives, and others are well on the way to achieving them, there are many countries where these objectives are still out of reach. Unfortunately, often the same countries that have problems achieving high coverage levels also have other major health problems and have difficulties in obtaining necessary resources.

The EPI goals were endorsed by heads of states and other world leaders who attended the World Summit for Children in New York in September, 1990. The meeting resulted in the "World Declaration on the Survival, Protection and Development of Children and Plan of Action for Implementing the World Declaration." Here a new dimension was added to the above goals with the following resolution:

> Reduction by 95% in measles deaths and reduction by 90% of measles cases compared to preimmunization levels by 1995, *as a major step to the global eradication of measles in the long run.*

The goals announced by the World Health Assembly and other international organizations set the tone for global efforts to control measles over the next decade. However, intermediate objectives will need to be worked out on the way to achieving these measles control goals.

Procedures for measuring the attainment of the disease reduction goal remain to be identified. At present, a combination of improved accuracy in coverage and more sensitive surveillance data may be the best option.

Improved vaccine coverage has had a clear impact on disease incidence. This impact can be seen in Figure 1, which shows the global trend of decreasing numbers of reported cases between 1974 and 1990. However, problems in sensitivity of surveillance systems between countries and between years make it difficult to quantify the precise relationship between coverage and disease reduction.

The European Region of WHO has adopted the target of no indigenous measles by the year 2000. In April, 1990, the English Speaking Caribbean countries, supported by PAHO/WHO, adopted a Plan of Action for the elimination of indigenous transmission of measles virus in their subregion by 1995. There are good grounds for optimism: measles transmission has already been greatly reduced with only reasonably high immunization coverage, with many countries achieving only 60–70%. Western Pacific island communities have experienced little or no poliomyelitis for a

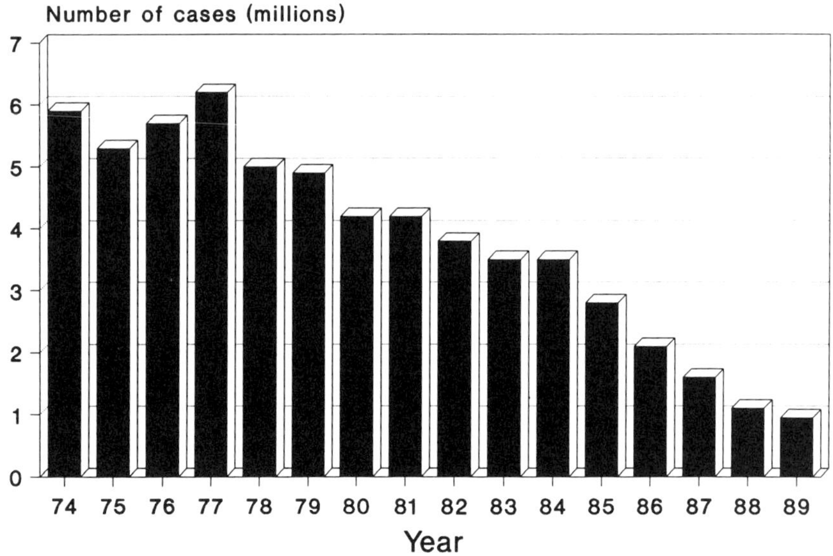

FIGURE 1 Number of cases of measles reported globally, 1974–1989. (Source: World Health Organization.)

decade. By analogy, it would appear that such an epidemiologic situation would be ideal to stop the transmission of measles as well. Lessons learned in the Caribbean should be of value to the rest of the world as other nations take up the challenge of measles elimination.

It must be stressed that for the present, the global target is disease reduction and not eradication. There is still much to be learned about the natural history of measles, especially with regard to elimination.

III. THE DISEASE

A. A Highly Successful Virus

Measles infection is caused by a virus that is extraordinarily uniform, wherever it occurs around the globe (Black, 1989). No major strain variations appear to occur, and the genotype is stable with little evidence of geographical variation in antigens. Virus strains can be made to vary only in the laboratory, where such strains react to specific monoclonal antibodies but do not differ appreciably in their reaction with whole serum (Sheshberadoran et al., 1983). Thus, a single vaccine is effective against all strains. The virus has been highly successful and continues to cause unparalleled morbidity and mortality in many parts of the world, despite the availability of a vaccine for over 20 years (Assad, 1983; Foster, 1984; Black, 1989).

B. Basic Virology

The measles virus is classified as a member of the genus *Morbillivirus* in the family Paramyxoviridae. The virion consists of about 2000 units of nucleocapsid wound into a single helix. The virus enters the body through the respiratory tract mucous membrane. The conjunctiva may also act as a portal of entry. Primary multiplication occurs in the epithelial cells, with spread to regional lymph nodes and reticuloendothelial cells throughout the body (Kingsbury et al., 1988).

C. Synergistic Impact of Measles and Diarrhea

In a study in Bangladesh, measles and diarrhea acted to increase mortality and the irreversible effects of nutritional deprivation. The effect seemed to be greater than either would have exerted in isolation (Koster et al., 1981). This study underlines the complex interaction between measles infection and diarrhea, but may be equally applicable to the virus's interaction with vitamin A deficiency and other serious childhood diseases.

D. Nutrition and Crowding

The relationship between measles and malnutrition is not entirely clear. It has been reported that measles is more severe and produces higher mortality rates in undernourished populations (Morley, 1983). However, in studies in Bangladesh and Guinea-Bissau, the pre-existing nutritional status of children who died from measles was not significantly different from those who survived (Aaby et al., 1985). Aaby and colleagues (1984) suggested that overcrowding rather than undernutrition may be more strongly associated with both increased risk of measles infection at an early age and greater severity of the disease (Sinha, 1977).

E. Vitamin A

In addition to protein energy undernutrition, measles rapidly depletes stores of vitamin A in young children, leading to complications such as xerophthalmia and blindness from corneal damage (Barclay et al., 1987). WHO has recommended incorporating vitamin A supplementation along with vaccine delivery (WHO/UNICEF, 1987). Treatment with vitamin A reduces both morbidity and mortality in children with severe measles. Children with measles in high-risk areas should be given large doses of vitamin A supplementation following WHO/UNICEF guidelines.

F. A Pattern of Outbreaks

Despite improved immunization levels, measles remains endemic in most countries. In addition to continuous background cases, typically measles erupts into outbreaks. These outbreaks still occur in both developing and developed countries, and are generally due to the accumulation of susceptible cases, consisting largely of unimmunized children. However, these may include immunized children in whom the immunization has failed to protect for some reason (see below).

IV. CHANGING EPIDEMIOLOGY

The epidemiology of measles changes rapidly in the face of increasing coverage. Despite additional efforts being placed behind measles control, outbreaks of measles are expected to continue to occur and do not necessarily indicate program failure. After high coverage levels are reached, a period of low measles incidence should follow for a number of seasons. This low incidence, or "honeymoon" period, may be followed by a resurgence of cases or even epidemics of considerable size. Interepidemic periods are likely to become increasingly long. Due to the highly infectious nature of measles virus, even small pockets of susceptibles are capable of sustaining outbreaks. Nevertheless, with control programs in place, these expected outbreaks can be minimized and the average number of cases over a given period greatly reduced from that of the preimmunization era.

Reported measles cases have declined since the introduction of the first measles vaccines in the 1960s (Fig. 1). Some countries (developed and developing) experienced more than 99% reduction in incidence of reported disease. However, in recent years, the number of cases in some of those countries has increased, although the levels are still far below those of prevaccine eras. Outbreaks have occurred among school-aged children, due to a number of causes. In developing countries, measles remain endemic in most areas, with the largest proportion of cases reported to occur in children under 5 years, and up to 27% in those less than 9 months of age (Taylor et al., 1988). Transmission continues in some urban settings due to a combination of factors including crowded conditions. Transmission also occurs in younger children before they reach the recommended age for immunization. It was previously thought that the coverage in older children would automatically protect younger ones, but this has not been observed due to the highly infectious nature of measles virus.

Measles vaccine has been one of the last EPI antigens to be introduced on a wide scale. Live attenuated measles vaccine was introduced during the late 1960s, and by 1982 virtually all countries had incorporated measles vaccine into their EPI activities. Since 1983, coverage with measles vaccine has increased annually, so that by 1990 the overall estimated coverage with measles vaccine was 70% (Fig. 2).

As coverage rates increase, the proportion of measles cases occurring among children who have been immunized previously is expected to increase. This by itself does not necessarily imply that vaccine efficacy is low; the evaluation of such cases requires careful methods that take into account individuals in the same community who received the vaccine and did not develop the disease (Orenstein et al., 1985).

A. Pockets of Low Coverage

In areas of high coverage, small pockets of susceptibles may persist. Immunization programs will increasingly be faced with potentially embarrassing situations: outbreaks continuing to occur despite high coverage. While the explanation may be clear in epidemiologic terms, it is likely to pose considerable difficulties for public relations and establishing program credibility.

If, for example, 90% of children are immunized every year, 10% will remain unimmunized and an additional 5–10% will fail to seroconvert, either due to administration of impotent vaccine or vaccine failure. Thus,

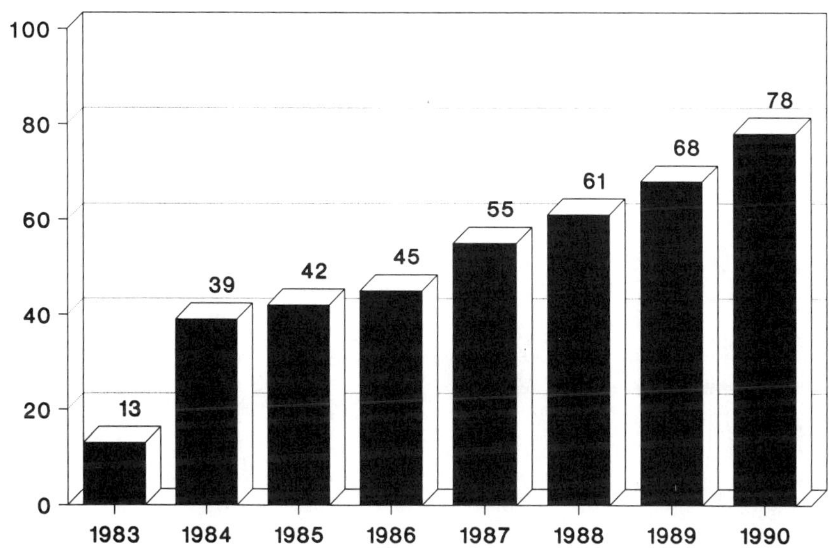

FIGURE 2 Global coverage with measles vaccine, 1983–1990. (Source: World Health Organization.)

the highest level of protection that can be expected in such a population is 85%. Therefore, a proportion of each year's birth cohort will accumulate until there is a sufficient number of susceptibles of various ages who can sustain an outbreak. Such an outbreak ended the "honeymoon period" of low incidence in Hong Kong in 1988 (Fig. 3; measles outbreak in Hong Kong, 1990).

Densely populated urban areas are particularly at risk, where the virus may be kept circulating by pockets of low coverage even when surrounded by communities with excellent coverage (Coetzee et al., 1990). Such pockets may be made up of largely urban poor who have less access to immunization services than other groups. There may be ethnic or other cultural barriers to children being immunized. There is a tendency to label pockets of the population as socially hard to reach, even before efforts have been made to find approaches to providing services in a way that is acceptable to such groups.

B. Age Distribution of Cases

Maternal antibodies protect an infant to varying degrees in the first few months of life. Thereafter, the attack rates for measles increase to a

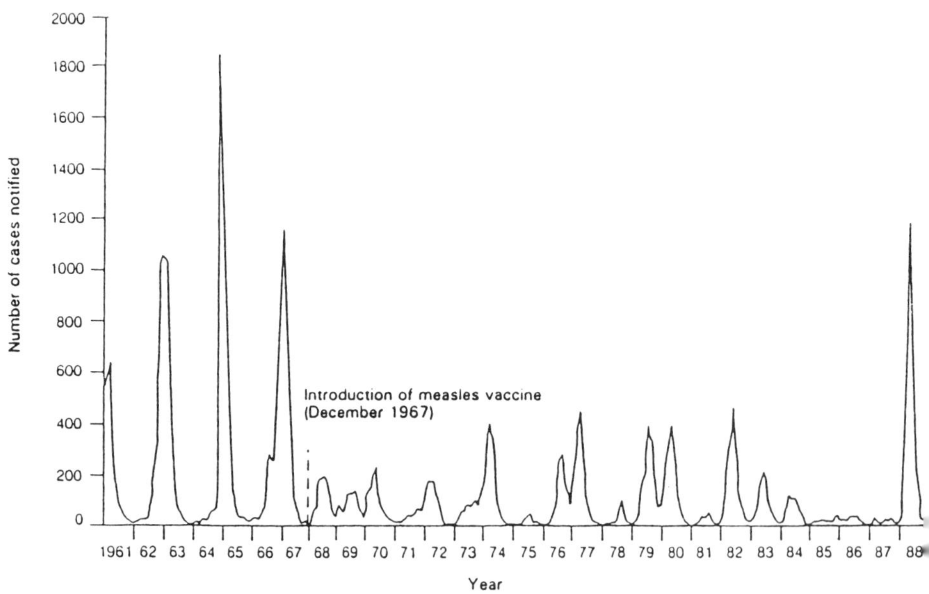

FIGURE 3 Monthly measles notifications, Hong Kong, 1961–1988. (From [*Wkly. Epidemiol. Rec. 101.* (1990). *49*:379–381].)

maximum between 1 and 2 years of age in developing countries. In Afghanistan, one study reported a typical picture of age distribution of cases, with 74% of cases occurring in children between 4 months and 3 years (Arya et al., 1987).

Up to a quarter of all cases are now occurring before 9 months of age in some developing countries. While this may not represent an absolute increase, the proportion of cases in the younger age group has increased over preimmunization days and is due to a higher proportion of children over 9 months of age being protected by immunization (Spencer et al., 1987; Taylor et al., 1988). This observation has served as a critical impetus for researchers to find a measles vaccine that could successfully immunize infants earlier in life.

Many countries with good immunization programs are now experiencing a shift in age distribution, with a second peak occurring in later childhood or even in college-age students (MMWR, 1990).

V. MEASLES IN UNIMMUNIZED POPULATIONS

A. Unimmunized Areas and Populations

The highly infectious nature of measles and the explosive nature of outbreaks have been well documented. One study among an unimmunized population in India (Nairu et al., 1989) reported that measles affected 80% of children under 10 years of age. The present strategy of improving coverage not only at the country level but also at the local level should ensure that outbreaks among older age groups are unlikely to happen again.

Crowded conditions have been found to be associated with higher case fatality rates (Aaby, 1988). Large urban agglomerates present ideal conditions for measles transmission, especially among dense populations of poor who are not only underimmunized but also experience high rates of other infectious conditions and reduced access to medical care. Up to 80% of those exposed in households who are nonimmune are likely to contract measles. In contrast to densely populated areas, nomads and other groups in sparsely populated areas experience very little disease transmission (Louton and Paillard, 1991). However, when such peoples come together for festivals or markets, explosive outbreaks may occur.

There appears to be an interrelationship between continuous urban transmission and rural outbreaks. Bartlet (1957) and Black (1966) suggest that a minimum population of 400,000–500,000 susceptible individuals is required to sustain measles endemicity. If this is correct, rural transmission may need to be maintained by repeated seeding from nearby cities.

Special consideration needs to be given to improving coverage in highly urbanized areas where large segments of the population do not routinely receive immunization. If measles is to be prevented from infecting and reinfecting such populations, problems of access to care will require creative approaches. One approach is to divide urban areas into zones of responsibility and to focus activities on the population in these problem areas. Involvement of representatives from the urban poor is essential in planning and implementing urban programs.

B. Explosive Outbreaks

Among highly susceptible populations in crowded settings, the opportunity of explosive point source outbreak is great. In one study in the United States, one infected person was believed to have transmitted measles to many others at a sports meeting (Chen et al., 1989), again emphasizing the highly infectious nature of measles.

C. Secondary Cases

Whether measles is more severe in secondary cases or in so-called "intense exposure" situations remains to be determined. A number of confounding variables makes interpretation and comparison between studies difficult.

For example, if secondary cases are younger than primary cases, this might explain the higher observed case fatality rates. In addition, large households may have other contributing factors such as lower nutritional status of children, or the presence of other bacterial or viral infections that might complicate the course of measles.

From a study in Machakos District, Kenya, Aaby and colleagues (1991) showed that in families with several cases of measles, children infected in the home (secondary cases) had a higher risk of dying than those who were infected from outside. Older children whose mobility increased the opportunity for infection outside the home tended to have lower case fatality rates.

Another study from The Gambia showed that measles mortality was strongly associated with more than five measles cases in a household (Hull, 1981). Intense exposure to measles virus may be a secondary risk factor for death following measles. In contrast, in a developed country, no difference in severity between primary and secondary cases was found (Sutter et al., 1991).

D. Herd Immunity

The required level of immunization needed to achieve herd immunity for measles is not clearly defined. It has traditionally been assumed that once a population reaches a certain level of immunity, the remaining unimmunized individuals will be protected by the immunity of the surrounding "herd." However, due to the highly infectious nature of the measles virus, the level is thought to be high, probably in excess of 90% in cities. Other unanswered questions, such as the effect on herd immunity of birth rate, mass immunization programs, and other demographic factors, need to be studied to help assist health planners in developing appropriate strategies for their given areas (Anderson and May, 1990).

Even in highly immunized communities, outbreaks can occur. In 1988, Harare, Zimbabwe, experienced an outbreak when coverage was known to be 83% (Kambarami et al., 1991). Another study from Texas reported an outbreak that occurred with 99% coverage, and the same population had a 95% level of demonstrable antibodies to measles (Gustafson et al., 1987). There are other examples of outbreaks occurring in populations with reported high coverage, such as the outbreak in Hungary in 1988, at a time when coverage was 98% (Measles outbreak, 1988). It is difficult to ascertain the herd immunity with a high degree of certainty based on such reports, since a large number of factors may have contributed to these outbreaks. Reported coverage may not have reflected the true levels of immunity in the community.

It appears that the level of herd immunity needed to interrupt transmission will vary with the epidemiologic situation. A rural or island population may need much lower herd immunity, whereas 83% coverage was not sufficient for a city like Harare. In crowded conditions, even 95% vaccine coverage may not be sufficient to interrupt transmission completely.

E. Spread in Health Care Settings

Health care settings have been the foci of a number of measles outbreaks. It is paradoxical that the immunization clinic, where parents bring their children to be protected against disease, becomes the place where the child acquires a life-threatening illness.

A study in the United States confirmed that in 1984 nearly 3% of measles cases were acquired in a health care setting (Davis et al., 1987). A study in Côte d'Ivoire revealed that two-thirds of measles cases treated in a health center were nosocomial in origin (Klein-Zabban et al., 1987). Prevention of measles must include routine immunization of children brought to clinics and improvements in waiting areas so that patients with measles can be isolated easily. In some settings, medical personnel have been the source of measles spread. Policies requiring immunization or proof of immunization among health workers may need to be implemented in such settings.

VI. MEASLES VACCINE PROTECTS

Before the administration of measles vaccine, measles was a major cause of death in young children in certain populations. Today, measles remains an important cause of death in young children in areas where vaccine coverage is less than optimal. It is surprising that relatively few studies have demonstrated the effectiveness of intervention with measles vaccine. Several studies, including those from Senegal (Aaby et al., 1981) and Bangladesh (Koenig et al., 1990), have shown convincingly that measles vaccine has produced a major impact on childhood mortality when used in programs of mass immunization. In the Bangladesh study, there was a pronounced impact on both short and long-term survival. The mortality rates for immunized children were as much as 46% lower than those for unimmunized children.

In a study from Haiti (Holt et al., 1999), children were more likely to survive if they had received measles vaccine, regardless of other factors such as socioeconomic status, maternal level of knowledge, or maternal literacy. These studies confirmed measles immunization as one of the most important components of any child survival program.

VII. MEASLES IS A SERIOUS DISEASE

A. Complications

Contrary to popular belief, measles carries with it the risk of complications of varying degrees of seriousness. Complications from measles can affect virtually any organ. Even in countries with good health care and healthy child populations, around 10% of cases can be expected to develop some form of complication (MMWR, 1990). The most common complications in industrialized countries are otitis media (around 5%), pneumonia (around 2.5%), diarrhea (around 2.5%), and encephalitis (around 0.1%).

The picture is significantly different in developing countries, where many children are already experiencing a background of viral, bacterial, and parasitic infections and may additionally be malnourished. One study from India showed that 76% of children with measles had complications (Nairn et al., 1989). These were pneumonia 39%, diarrhea 32%, and dysentery 20%. Measles was more severe in young children. In a study from Mexico, half the cases with complications were less than 1 year of age, and 70% of these were malnourished (Avila-Figuera et al., 1990).

Due to complications of measles, a large number of children become handicapped with deafness, impaired vision, or blindness. A less common but devastating complication is subacute sclerosing panencephalitis (SSPE), which develops in 1–5:100,000 cases several years after the initial measles infection.

B. Case Fatality Rates

There is a wide range in the reported measles case fatality rates (CFRs). There are intercountry, interregional, and even interepidemic variations in CFRs. The CFRs in industrialized countries are estimated to be less than 0.01%. This is partly due to the difference in age-specific attack rates, underlying good nutrition, supportive treatment, and other environmental and sociologic factors. In particular, supportive treatment for bacterial chest infections and diarrhea appears to be the most important contributor to this difference between CFRs in developed and developing countries.

Quantifying CFRs is difficult since most information is obtained from potentially biased sources. Hospitals tend to admit and report the more serious cases who are at an increased risk of dying. Recognizing such difficulties, WHO/EPI has until now estimated the CFRs for acute measles infection among persons of all ages in the developing world as 2–4%. Such point estimates must be viewed with caution: more recent community-based studies suggest that this may be a significant underestimate (Aaby et al., 1991), and there may be a need to redefine how CFRs are calculated. For instance, an outbreak in Afghanistan resulted in an overall CFR of 28% and of 42% in the children 0–4 years. This underlines the added danger of acquiring measles at a younger age (Wakeham, 1978).

C. Delayed Impact on Mortality

In addition to well-documented complications and mortality associated with the acute illness, the long-term impact of the infection is now being reported (Hull et al., 1983; Aaby and Clements, 1989). Several African studies have now been documented that for many months after the acute attack, there is a reduced survival rate in affected infants. Thus, it appears that those infected with measles virus who survive the acute disease have a greatly increased chance of dying after the acute illness compared with those not infected with measles. Death may result from a variety of apparently unrelated conditions in the months following measles infection. This may be accounted for by a reduced cell-mediated immune response as a result of measles infection.

The younger the age of infection, the more dramatic the effect of this delayed mortality phenomenon, and the more urgent the need to protect children at the youngest possible age. Therefore, based on such studies, it is now thought that the true impact of measles virus infection is much greater than is actually recorded in the number of deaths generally attributed to measles, making the control of this disease an even greater priority. Studies describing delayed mortality have all been African. It would be important to confirm these observations in Asia and the Americas.

D. Treatment

At present there is only symptomatic treatment available for infection with measles virus. However, there may be a variety of complications for which appropriate treatment should be provided, such as antibiotics to combat bacterial infection and oral rehydration salts for dehydration following diarrhea. Case fatality rates can be lowered if patients reach health care facilities where appropriate care is offered. For uncomplicated cases, supportive fluids, antipyretics, and nutritional therapy may be required. Many children need 4–8 weeks to recover their premeasles nutritional status.

VIII. VACCINES

The major strains of live attenuated measles vaccines presently in use throughout the world include Schwarz, Moraten, Connaught, (standard titer) Edmonston Zagreb, Leningrad-16, CAM-70, AIK-C, and Shanghai strains. These vaccines are recommended for use at or later than 9 months of age. They are inexpensive, have an excellent record of seroconversion, safety, and lasting immunity, as well as demonstrating high levels of protection against clinical illness. Such vaccine strains should not be discarded lightly. Newer, more antigenic, candidate vaccines need to be evaluated carefully over long periods of time before their widespread use is begun.

All measles vaccines should meet WHO requirements regardless of strain, potency, or recommended age of recipients. Experience from administration of millions of doses of measles vaccine proves this to be a very safe vaccine.

A. Meeting WHO Requirements

WHO publishes production requirements for a number of vaccines including measles vaccine (WHO, 1988). To meet WHO requirements, a measles vaccine must be produced in accordance with good manufacturing practices, using certified virus seeds and cell substrates. Moreover, all vaccines manufactured must be continually subjected to control testing, and certified by a competent national control authority that confirms that it has been produced according to established requirements. All vaccines supplied to countries by UNICEF have been subject to this certification, and are, in addition, continually checked for compliance with WHO potency and stability requirements.

To meet WHO potency and stability requirements, measles vaccine must show a potency of more than 1000 infectious units after being exposed continuously for 7 days at 37°C. In addition, when compared to vaccine that has been maintained frozen, the loss of potency when incubated at this high-temperature storage must not be more than 1 order of magnitude ($\log_{10}$). Both requirements for potency and stability must be met.

B. Meeting WHO and UNICEF Potency Requirements

Although the WHO Requirements specify a minimum potency of 1000 infectious units, the current UNICEF tender (through which UNICEF makes massive bulk purchasing of vaccines) requires a higher potency for measles vaccines. That is, the vaccines must have a minimum potency of 10,000 infectious units when titered relative to the International Reference Reagent for Measles Vaccine. In addition, the stability requirement described above must be met. The rationale for this specification is that maternal antibody may be present at 9 months, interfering with a good immune response by the infant. Higher doses of measles vaccine are better able to overcome the interfering effect of maternal antibody. This potency requirement applies to all strains of measles vaccine virus supplied to UNICEF, including Schwarz, CAM-70, and Edmonston Zagreb.

C. Special Cases: High-Potency Vaccines

Data are now available using the Edmonston Zagreb (EZ) strain. This strain appears to be more immunogenic and therefore better able to overcome interference from maternal antibody. Thus EZ vaccine can be given to infants younger than nine months of age. The lower age limit has yet to be established; however, it now appears that infants as young as 6 months of age exhibit good antibody response. The current specification in the UNICEF tender in effect during 1991 for the titer of the measles vaccine for use at 6 months is that the vaccine must have a potency of 50,000 infectious units when determined relative to the International Reference Reagent for Measles Vaccine (EPI, 1991). Vaccines for use before nine months of age continue to be evaluated.

D. Storage

Freeze-dried measles vaccine should be kept below +8°C and, if possible, below –20°C in central and regional stores. It should be protected from light. Due to marked improvements in stabilizer technology, the vaccine will not degrade between deep storage and reconstitution. In addition, the vaccine can remain potent for 36 hr at ambient temperatures up to 40°C. A color marker is now being introduced on the vaccine vial that will indicate by a change in color if the vaccine is no longer sufficiently potent for use.

E. Vaccine Efficacy

Since the introduction of the Schwarz vaccine in the 1960s, there have been a number of opportunities to study the field efficacy of this measles vaccine strain (Kenya, 1982; Tanzania, 1981). Vaccine efficacy rates (VE) are typically determined by comparing the rate of measles in immunized children with that of measles in unimmunized children (Orenstein et al., 1985). The results of these studies are in general agreement, although a wide variety of values have been reported in the literature. For instance, it was found to be 84–90% in a field study in Haiti (Holt et al., 1990). Under most field conditions, the VE is thought to be about 85% for children receiving the vaccine at 9 months of age or older. At present it is not clear what the VE will be for the newer measles vaccines now being used for infants at 6 months of age.

In addition to testing the clinical and field effectiveness of new vaccines, VE studies may be useful for identifying problems with the cold chain or with the vaccine's ability to produce protection.

F. Duration of Immunity and Waning

It is generally assumed that an infection with wild measles confers lifelong protection in virtually every individual. A carefully studied measles outbreak in the Faroe Islands in 1846 revealed that those who had been infected 65 years earlier were still immune (Panum, 1940). Given that the measles vaccine virus is an attenuated strain of the live virus, there is the possibility that the antigenic capabilities of the vaccine strain are not equal to that of the wild virus. The development and persistence of serum antibodies following administration of measles vaccine have been lower but parallel to the response following natural measles. Peak antibody responses occur 6–8 weeks after infection or immunization (Lian, 1979). Since the vaccine is a relatively recent development, the precise duration of protection remains uncertain. However, studies from Iceland (Black and Gudnadottir, 1966) and the Amazon (van Mazjik et al., 1982) confirmed that immunity from the vaccine lasted at least 15 years. More recent studies now show that protection lasts at least 21 years (Miller, 1987).

When an immune individual is exposed to the wild virus, an amnestic response occurs, usually with a resulting boost to antibody levels. As outbreaks of measles become rarer, exposure to wild virus diminishes, and therefore the boosting effect by the wild virus will diminish also. The net result will be that an individual's protection against measles will be solely dependent on the long-lasting antigenicity of the vaccine.

If measles could be controlled effectively in a country in a relatively short period of time, the issue of duration of immunity would not play a critical role. It was previously thought that if children were protected during the first few years of life (the usual time of peak transmission), the likelihood of future exposure would be low. However, in some countries a second peak of transmission is now occurring in older children and young adults (Measles, US, 1989). Young people exposed to this peak in their second decade of life will need protection using a vaccine with the ability to confer immunity lasting at least 20 years.

Duration of immunity is considered a critical factor in the new generation of measles vaccines for use at 6 months of age. Using the more immunogenic EZ vaccine, Whittle et al. (1990) have so far shown persistence of antibody for up to 36 months.

The effect is not fully known on subsequent immunization and duration of antibody to infants of immunized mothers compared with infants born to mothers naturally infected. However, several studies reported that antibody titers are lower in infants born to immunized women (Lennon and Black, 1986). It is therefore assumed that infants born to immunized mothers are more likely to be susceptible to measles earlier in life. However, it may also mean that early immunization could be more successful in such children as the maternally derived antibodies may disappear in such children sooner than in children born to mothers with natural immunity.

G. Route of Administration

Because measles virus enters the body through the respiratory mucosa of the nose, oropharynx, and conjunctiva, there has been interest for a number of years in administration of the vaccine by routes other than parenteral injection. A number of successes have been noted by Sabin et al. (1983), Ekunwe (1990), and others. At least one public health program is using an inhaled vaccine preparation on a regular basis. As demonstrated by the oral polio vaccine, an easily administered vaccine that does not need a syringe is attractive for mass administration. Further research is needed on the subject. Meanwhile EPI/WHO remains interested in this approach.

H. Impact of Human Immunovirus

In response to a rising prevalence of human immunovirus (HIV) infection in infants in many parts of the world, guidelines have been developed by WHO/EPI for immunizing affected children (WHO/UNICEF, 1989; Consultation, 1987). Such infants are at increased risk of contracting measles and dying from complications. Measles vaccine appears safe and at least partially effective in protecting these infants.

I. Contraindications

In a public health setting there are virtually no contraindications to providing measles vaccine (Galazka, 1984). Sensitivity to some ingredients of the vaccine, such as the antibiotic used for maintaining sterility of the vaccine, is often quoted by manufacturers. In reality, vaccinators almost never know in advance of the existence of such a sensitivity in infants of immunizable ages. While HIV infection is not a contraindication, severe immune deficiency of other types may be.

J. Adverse Reactions

Severe adverse reactions following administration of measles vaccine have been reported at the rate of less than 1:3 million doses administered. Such reactions are usually in the form of encephalitis. Approximately 5–15% of infants immunized with standard vaccine develop fever, while approximately 5% develop a generalized rash lasting 1–3 days beginning 5–7 days after immunization. These reactions are generally mild and well tolerated (Halsey and Stetler, 1983).

In any discussion of adverse reaction rates, it is important to stress that the benefits of administering the vaccine far outweigh the disadvantages associated with contracting the disease, in terms of both human suffering and cost.

K. Primary Vaccine Failure

Children who do not successfully seroconvert after immunization are considered to have experienced primary vaccine failure. This occurs in an estimated 3–5% of immunized children in developed countries. Age of immunization was found to be critical in one study in Haiti, where seroconversion rates increased from 45% when children were immunized at 6 months of age to 100% at 12 months (Halsey et al., 1985). The use of impotent vaccine, due either to problems with vaccine production, or the cold chain, raises the number of vaccine failures.

In industrialized countries, outbreaks in older children are now occurring principally among those who have been immunized and who have not been exposed to measles due to the reduction of circulating wild measles virus in their community. The role of vaccine failures in developing countries is difficult to assess since documentation of immunization may be difficult, especially among older children. Breaks in the cold chain may add to the problems of protecting children with measles vaccine, thus further complicating the evaluation of vaccines.

L. Secondary Vaccine Failure

Children who received measles vaccine, seroconverted, and subsequently either lost their detectable antibodies or contracted measles disease are considered to have experienced secondary vaccine failure. It is not fully understood to what degree loss of detectable antibody correlates with loss of protection (Mathias et al., 1989).

M. Administration with Other Antigens

Measles vaccine may be given simultaneously with bacille Calmette-Gúerin (BCG), oral poliovirus (OPV), injectable poliovirus (IPV), and diphtheria/pertussis/tetanus (DPT) vaccines (Galazka, 1991). As other vaccines are added to the schedule, such as hepatitis B and yellow fever, simultaneous antibody response to all vaccines will have to be reassessed. However, there is no theoretical reason to expect a problem, nor has field experience to date given any cause for concern.

N. Killed Vaccine

Formalin-inactivated vaccine was one of the first measles vaccines. Its use was discontinued when it was realized that immunity was not long-lasting and that many recipients were likely to develop atypical measles when exposed to the live virus (Krugman and Ward, 1973).

IX. AGE AT ADMINISTRATION OF MEASLES VACCINE

A. Standard Measles Vaccines

One key factor in determining the appropriate age for immunization is the epidemiology of measles in a given country. Standard vaccines should be administered at or as soon as possible after 9 months of age in any developing country where measles is a public health problem. Industrialized countries (where cases do not usually occur before 12 months, and where the CFR is almost zero) are recommended to delay immunization until 12–15 months to obtain the best possible seroconversion rates. If measles before 9 months of age is not a problem in a country using standard measles vaccines, there would seem little indication to change to another strain or schedule at present.

B. Immunization at Younger Ages

The high-titer Edmonston Zagreb measles vaccine for use at 6 months of age has been described elsewhere (WHO, 1990). After careful review of the relevant literature, the Global Advisory Group, meeting in Tokyo in 1989, recommended:

> High titer, Edmonston Zagreb measles vaccine be administered at 6 months of age or as soon thereafter as possible in countries in which measles before 9 months is a significant cause of death.

Several other vaccines have also been evaluated for use at early ages. Two Japanese vaccines, CAM-70 and AIK-C vaccine strains, the Connaught strain and the Leningrad-16 strain are presently undergoing comparison trials. Developments in measles vaccines over the coming decade, however, could result in different recommendations regarding use of these vaccines early in the first year of life.

X. STRATEGIES FOR CONTROL

A. Schedule

The adverse effects of measles on the mortality and morbidity of young children are well documented, particularly when measles is contracted in the first year of life. Therefore, where measles is endemic, the vaccine should be administered as early in life as recommended with a vaccine of appropriate potency. The exact age of immunization will be determined by the available vaccines and epidemiologic situation in a country. The Global Advisory Group of the EPI periodically advises on the availability of vaccines and recommended schedules.

B. Primary Target

Within the context of existing strategies for vaccine delivery, improvement in coverage in the defined primary target age group, usually children 9 to 12 months of age, is needed. In particular, we must address the major problems of "missed opportunities" (including excessive use of vaccine contraindications), reduce drop-out rates, and solve problems associated with minority groups, such as nomads, who are not usually reached by fixed health care services.

The use of national or regional immunization days can be a useful adjunct to routine services. These usually result in a rapid rise in coverage. The use of all the EPI antigens is essential on such occasions, allowing a broader benefit to be gained from these activities. Special "mop-up" operations, or house-to-house immunization, have been shown to be effective in raising polio vaccine coverage when programs are close to interrupting transmission.

Regardless of the stage of a country's measles control program, the first essential requirement of the strategy will be to achieve and maintain immunization coverage with a potent measles vaccine in the target group of at least 90%. The primary target age group will be infants in the first year of life, the upper age limit being determined by the local epidemiology of measles (see above).

C. Secondary Target Groups and the Concept of "High Risk"

When epidemiologic information indicates that children outside the primary target group are a major source of circulating measles virus, or a significant proportion of older children are found to be susceptible, targeting such groups is indicated. Efforts to immunize such secondary groups play a role mainly in intermediate or late stages of control. Such efforts should not, however, jeopardize reaching high coverage or maintaining coverage in the primary target group.

Secondary targets are essentially the same as high-risk populations, and their identification is vital in the control of measles. A number of approaches can be used to determine where high-risk populations are located. These populations might be identified through noting low reported coverage, high incidence of reported cases, or the presence of known high-risk population groups such as the urban poor. Identification of high-risk groups by geographical and demographic characteristics is important to the control of measles, and will help set priorities for each stage of a measles control program. The ability to concentrate control efforts on such groups will substantially reduce the foci of transmission of measles.

The following high-risk groups are reviewed in greater detail.

Preschool Children

In countries where measles coverage has been low, a large proportion of preschool-aged children have not received measles vaccine, and may not have had measles disease.

School Children

Because in some countries measles coverage has been low and these countries may have experienced a long period of temporary low incidence, considerable numbers of school-aged children may be unimmunized and not yet have been infected with measles virus. In areas where school immunization records are maintained, periodic audits can be conducted, with the subsequent provision of missing immunizations.

Ethnic Minorities

These groups are sometimes underserved, or have cultural beliefs that restrict their access to health services or inhibit their acceptance of immunization services. Such groups may form large pockets of susceptibles, and require special attention.

Hospitals

When children with measles are admitted to hospital, there is the danger of nosocomial outbreaks. To avoid such outbreaks and the potential spread to the community, children admitted to hospitals where there are patients with measles should be immunized beginning at 6 months of age. Infants receiving the Schwarz vaccine before 9 months of age should be given a second dose of measles vaccine at the nationally recommended age.

Refugee Camps

Due to crowded conditions in refugee camps, there is a high likelihood of transmission if measles is introduced. When one or more cases occur in such special settings, it is advisable to broaden the target age group for immunization. In such instances, all children aged 6 months to 5 years should be immunized with measles vaccine as soon as they enter an organized camp or settlement. Depending on the availability of vaccine and the epidemiologic indications, older children may need to be included (Toole et al., 1989). Infants receiving the Schwarz vaccine before 9 months of age should be given a second dose of measles vaccine at the nationally recommended age.

D. Two-Dose/Reimmunization Strategy

The question of whether a two-dose regimen is needed has often been posed. Such a strategy should not be confused with the need for a catch-up round of immunization in a subgroup of the population found to be at particular risk. Whether the two-dose schedule should be adopted as a routine in all epidemiologic situations is less clear.

Initial attempts to use a two-dose schedule were motivated by the need to protect children before 9 months of age, the recommended age of measles immunization. Some programs tried giving a first dose at 6 months with a second at 9 or 12 months (Wood et al., 1980). This practice was not encouraged after studies revealed that few children who had received a first dose before 9 months actually returned for a second dose.

There have been suggestions that an early dose of measles vaccine might blunt the immune response to subsequent doses (Black et al., 1984; Wilkins and Wehrle, 1989). The issue seems to have been resolved by Krugman et al. (1965), Bass et al. (1976), and Shasby et al. (1977), who uniformly found that additional doses resulted in a booster or amnestic effect. The body of literature seems to support these findings (Stetler et al., 1986).

Whether it is necessary to provide a second dose of Schwarz or Moraten vaccine when the first dose has been administered before 9 months of age has been somewhat resolved by the availability of strains that can be administered at 6 months of age. Nevertheless, some still argue in favor of a two-dose schedule. The justification given includes boosting the level of antibody in order to prolong the duration of immunity, increasing coverage by catching children previously missed by the first round, and the production of seroconversion in vaccine failures.

An outbreak of measles was shown to be due to primary vaccine failure when it was demonstrated that 98% of a group of U.S. college students had evidence of measles immunization before contracting measles (Hersh et al., 1991). In 1989, in response to a large number of measles outbreaks, the United States recommended that a two-dose schedule be adopted in problem measles areas, with the first dose at 9 months and the second at 15 months as triple vaccine (Measles Prevention, 1989).

Tulchinksy et al. (1990) examined an outbreak in Israel in which outbreaks in older children continued despite high coverage. They concluded that a two-dose schedule would be needed if the country was to achieve eradication by the target date of 1992. Such a policy would cost an additional $1 million and save around $4.5 million (Ginsberg and Tulchinsky, 1990).

Much interesting work has been done by mathematical modeling of different possibilities regarding the number of doses administered and the timing of the doses (Anderson and May, 1985). The use of such models assist for projected levels of vaccine coverage. This method of forecasting has been of limited use to date, but as interest increases in two or more doses of vaccine, much more attention is likely to be paid to modeling.

EPI/WHO gives priority to achieving the highest possible coverage with a single dose of potent vaccine as near to the target age as possible. In terms of reducing the impact of measles globally, this policy claims precedent over a two-dose regimen. However, in countries with high coverage already achieved, there may be justification for using a two-dose regimen. At a time when eradication is targeted, even *multiple* doses of a *multiple antigen* vaccine may become the strategy of choice. Such a strategy would increase seroconversion rates to the maximum possible.

E. Strategies for Delivery

Experience in many countries indicates that the control of measles will require the use of flexible strategies along with a combination of several tactics. Control activities will need to be aimed at all sectors of the target population, including those that do not have easy access to health services. The ultimate goal is to eliminate transmission by relying on the routine delivery of immunization services within the context of primary health care and, when necessary, the use of special immunization delivery strategies. There are undoubted advantages in developing an infrastructure in which vaccine is offered from fixed clinics on a regular basis, but this is not ideal in every instance.

Fixed Services

Clinic-based services should offer immunization at times and frequencies appropriate for and convenient to the target population. Other antigens such as tetanus toxoid for the mother and other services such as prenatal care can be offered simultaneously.

Outreach Services

These services may need to be offered at fixed locations for populations at less than a day's travel from the base clinic.

Mobile Teams

Mobile teams may need to operate in areas too remote to be served easily by fixed or outreach services.

Special Activities

The campaign approach should be considered if the health infrastructure has not been successful in dramatically raising the level of coverage. Such activities may take a variety of forms; they may consist of publicity campaigns alone or be coupled with the provision of immunization and other services. When possible, measles campaigns should be linked with polio campaigns, and all antigens should be offered. Such campaigns have been nationwide or targeted. Approaches to delivery include use of existing clinics, adding special community-based clinics, and even door to door visits by teams. One such program in São Paulo, Brazil, carried out over 10 days, reached over 4 million children aged 9 months to 14 years: 86% of the target population. As a result, 98% of participating children subsequently tested had antibodies to measles (Pannuiti et al., 1991). Campaigns by themselves will not sustain high coverage and will either need to be repeated regularly or be supported by the development of routine programs.

Rural and Urban

In large urban areas, special consideration needs to be given to ways to improve coverage. Problems of access to care will require creative solutions (e.g., providing outreach activities in villages). In contrast, dispersed rural populations and nomads will require equally imaginative but different approaches. Services at watering holes and markets are possible solutions.

F. Legislation

Reports from countries with high measles coverage show that many measles cases are now occurring in school- and college-aged young people (Hersh et al., 1991). In response to this, some countries are passing legislation that requires proof of completed immunization with DPT, polio, and measles vaccines for school entry. This provides a checkpoint at which to catch and immunize those children who have not yet been reached. It is recognized, however, that such action may not be applicable in some countries.

XI. SURVEILLANCE

Improving the surveillance system is a basic requirement in any measles control program and must be a prominent feature of immunization programs in the 1990s. It is, however, not an activity that can be separated from improving surveillance for the other EPI target diseases. Steps taken to improve measles surveillance can only complement the improvement of the surveillance system in other areas.

In the early stages of measles control, improving coverage in infants under 1 year and improving routine surveillance are the cornerstones of the program. As coverage rises, increasing the sensitivity of surveillance systems becomes even more critical in the control and evaluation of antimeasles activities.

A. Revitalizing Routine Surveillance

The central framework for measles surveillance is the existing routine reporting system. In some instances this system is already well defined and in place. However, in many countries this system is not operational; therefore, together with the efforts being made for polio eradication, it will be necessary to revitalize or re-energize this routine reporting system.

Routine reporting forms the basis of surveillance for measles control as well as all other infectious and notifiable diseases. Because of the difficulties inherent in reporting measles cases, most countries will need to improve existing routine surveillance systems. Improvements may need to be made in the areas of training health personnel and revising existing reporting systems, including the development of appropriate forms. In addition to the routine system, new methods of surveillance, such as sentinel site reporting, may need to be introduced.

B. Case Definition

Whatever the source of reporting, it is important that the definition of a case be consistent within a country and between countries. All staff concerned with reporting measles cases should be aware of the case definition. Private doctors and health workers also need to be aware of the program goals and case definitions being used. The following definitions are proposed:

At least one of the following: cough, coryza, or conjunctivitis
History of fever 38°C (101°F) or more (if not measured, HOT to touch)
Generalized maculopapular rash of 3 or more days' duration.

C. Sites for Routine Reporting

Health Clinics and Hospitals

These sites should form the basis of the routine surveillance system. Most immunizations are given at special immunization clinics, designated parts of hospital outpatient facilities, or by special teams of vaccinators who offer outreach services. The personnel running these services should be the ones providing the basic information on the number of immunization doses given. To some extent they will also know about cases of measles occurring in the population they serve, and should be encouraged to report this information routinely.

Sentinel Reporting

Sentinel sites may be selected based upon a review of the most common source for reporting measles cases. The most likely sources of notification of suspected cases of measles in an area should be incorporated into the surveillance activities and contacted on a regular basis. Facilities might include all acute care hospitals (public and private, general and specialized), as well as outpatient units at the same facilities.

Sentinel sites can provide accurate and timely information to health officials regarding measles. Such information will allow officials to respond in a timely manner with action that can help control outbreaks. Figure 4 shows how a children's hospital in Istanbul reported measles

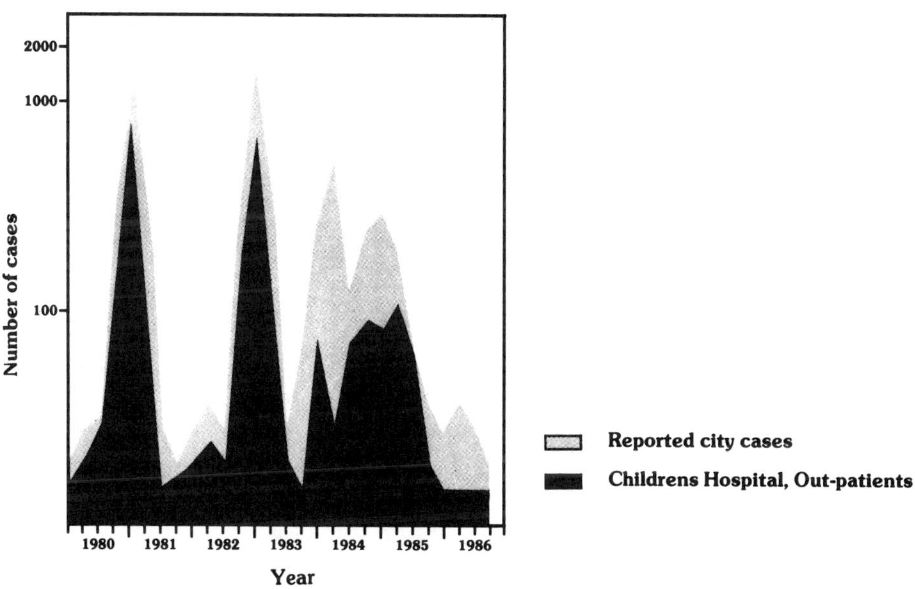

FIGURE 4 Sentinel reporting: cases of measles per quarter, Istanbul 1976–1987. (From *Wkly. Epidemiol. Rec.* (1987). *62*:325–327.)

cases admitted to the infectious diseases or pediatric wards. The trends in the inpatient cases matched well the trends in the reported cases in the community. Frequent reporting from such sites can provide a valuable addition to routine reporting as well as an early warning system.

Private Practitioners

In many cities, private practitioners see a majority of cases of measles (and indeed may immunize more children than government clinics). They should be considered an important source of surveillance information.

Reporting from the Community

In many countries, measles is still considered to be a normal childhood occurrence. When parents suspect measles, the child is often kept at home without seeking medical assistance. To stimulate reporting of the disease. It will be necessary to educate the population about the importance of informing health care providers as soon as possible when a case of measles occurs. The mass media should be used for this purpose. Families, neighbors, nursery schools, kindergartens, and school teachers will need to be encouraged to report suspected cases to a health worker as early as possible.

D. Information to Collect

Number of Cases

At a minimum, the number of cases for each district should be reported and presented monthly. This information should be reviewed and organized geographically. Simple rates can be calculated by using population data.

Additional Information

As routine reporting improves and coverage increases, countries will want to start collecting additional information on each case, including patients' name, address, age, date at onset of disease, immunization status, and age at immunization.

E. Use of Surveillance Data

The principal uses of surveillance data are to document program progress, identify potential problems, and direct program activities to the areas of greatest need. As coverage and surveillance improve, additional information obtained about cases may be used to evaluate the age distribution of cases and to assess whether vaccine policies are targeting the appropriate age groups. Such data may also help in evaluating the adequacy of the cold chain.

F. Measuring Coverage

Coverage data need to be collected on a regular basis and organized and presented at the district level. When analyzed appropriately, such coverage data can be used to assign priorities to program activities. Recent developments in specially designed computer programs can assist countries in analyzing their data.

Because of the difficulties inherent in routine information systems, special coverage surveys, such as cluster sample surveys, may need to be performed. Such special surveys should be directed particularly at high-risk populations, such as the urban poor, who are likely to be underserved by existing health services. Methods need to be developed to measure small changes in coverage or small areas.

XII. OUTBREAK RESPONSE

While surveillance is an unquestioned program priority, outbreak response may not be. Although outbreaks should be analyzed in situations of medium or high coverage, programs should not react to all outbreaks with extensive control methods. Outbreaks are to be expected in unimmunized populations. The effectiveness of control measures, particularly if applied late in an epidemic may be negligible. There is the risk of diverting resources needed to maintain or extend routine immunization services into a continual chase after epidemics that occur because of the lack of routine immunization.

A. Developing a Plan

Nevertheless, in many countries, immunization programs have reduced measles incidence, so that health workers and the public expect measles outbreaks not to occur. When outbreaks do occur in such countries, they generate strong political and social pressure for a response. Therefore, such countries will need to develop plans for the investigation of outbreaks.

Precise criteria remains to be developed for determining exactly when and how to respond to an outbreak. There may be special circumstances, such as in refugee camps, where even a few cases constitute an emergency that must be responded to at once with vigor.

It may be appropriate to respond to reports of one or two outbreaks early in the measles season, and not only to attempt to control them but also to inform the public about measles disease and immunization as well as to gain valuable information for future prevention. For instance, it is relatively simple and inexpensive to undertake a vaccine efficacy study in an outbreak to establish whether potent vaccine has been administered. Knowing that the cold chain is successfully delivering vaccine with an efficacy of 80% or greater gives managers confidence in responding appropriately to other outbreaks.

B. Data Analysis of Outbreaks

All surveillance information must be reviewed and analyzed at a local level so that action can be taken as soon as possible. Although it is important that information about outbreaks be transmitted to higher levels of the system, this must not delay an appropriate response at a local level. Reports on all outbreaks and case importations should subsequently be published and disseminated.

Analysis of data generated by an outbreak may identify a particular age group, social or ethnic subgroup as being at special risk of acquiring measles. Success of an immunization program requires knowledge of this age and subgroup distribution of susceptibles in order to focus control efforts on these groups.

Estimates from studies on the percentage of immunization coverage required to achieve herd immunity indicate that no single level of coverage will eliminate measles in all situations. The coverage required to interrupt transmission varies with the epidemiologic situation in a given country.

A reduction in the incidence of measles cases may be accompanied by a shift to higher attack rates in older children. This change in age distribution of cases is a strong indicator that an effective program of measles control is in place.

ACKNOWLEDGEMENTS

Material for this chapter was drawn from document EPI/GAG/90/WP.10, "Acceleration of the EPI towards 1995 to reach the measles control goal." The article is published with the permission of the Director-General of the World Health Organization.

REFERENCES

Aaby, P. (1988). *Rev. Infect. Dis. 10*:451.

Aaby, P., and Clements, C. J. (1989). *Bull. WHO 67*:443–448.

Aaby, P., Bukh, J., Smits, I. M., and Smedman, A. J. (1984a). *Lancet* 2:93.
Aaby, P., et al. (1981). *Am. J. Epidemiol. 120*:49–63.
Aaby, P., Coovadia, I., Bukh, J., et al. (1985). *Med. Hypotheses 18*:93–112.
Aaby, P., Clements, C. J., and Orinda, V. (1991). In press.
Anderson, R. M., and May, R. M. (1985). *J. Hyg. 94*:365–436.
Anderson, R. M., and May, R. M. (1990). *Lancet 335*:641–645.
Arya, L. S., et al. (1987). *J. Trop. Med. Hyg. 90*:117–122.
Assad, F. (1983). *Rev. Infect. Dis. 5*:452–459.
Avila-Figuera, C., Navarette-Mavarro, S., Martinez-Aguilar, M., Ruiz-Gutierrez, E., and Santos, J. I. (1990). *Bull. Med. Hosp. Inf. Mexico 47*:520–524.
Barclay, A. J. G., et al. (1987). *British Med. J. 294*:294–296.
Bartlet, M. S. (1957). *J. R. Stat. Soc. A 120*:48–70.
Bass, J. W., Halstead, S. B., Fisher, G. W., Podgore, J. K., et al. (1976). *JAMA 253*:31.
Black, F. L. (1966). *J. Theor. Biol. 11*:207–211.
Black, F. L. (1989). *Prog. Med. Virol.* Basel, *36*:1–33.
Black, F. L., and Gudnadottir, M. (1966). *Bull. WHO 35*:955–957.
Black, F. L, Berman, L. L., Libel, M., et al. (1984). *Bull. WHO 62*:315.
Chen, R. T., Goldbaum, G. M., Wassiklak, S. G. F., Markowitz, L. E., and Orenstein, W. A. (1989). *Am. J. Epidemiol. 129*:173–182.
Coetzee, N., Yach, D., Blignaut, R., and Fisher, S. A. (1990). *S. Afr. Med. J. 78*:733–737.
Consultation on Human Immunodeficiency virus (HIV) and routine childhood immunization. (1987). *Wkly. Epidemiol. Rec. 62*:297–299.
Davis, R. M., Whitman, E. D., Orenstein, W. A., et al. (1987). *Am. J. Epidemiol. 126*:438–449.
Ekunwe, E. O. (1990). *Ann. Trop. Pediatr. 10*:145–149.
Expanded Programme on Immunization. Global Advisory Group. (1990). *Wkly. Epidemiol. Rec. 65*:5–11.
Expanded Programme on Immunization. Global Advisory Group. (1991). *Wkly. Epidemiol. Rec. 66*:9–12.
Foster, S. O. (1984). *Pop. Dev. Rev. 10*:119–140.
Galazka, A. (1984). *Bull. WHO 62*:357–366.
Galazka, A. (1991). WHO/EPI Research and Development Group Meeting, Geneva.
Ginsburg, G. M., and Tulchinsky, T. H. (1990). *J. Epidemiol. Commun. Health 44*:274–280.
Gustafson, T. L., Lievens, A. W., and Bourell, P. A. (1987). *N. Engl. J. Med. 316*:717–774.
Halsey, N. A., and Stetler, H. C. (1983). In *Recent Advances in Immunization*, N. A. Halsey and C. A. de Quadros (Eds.). Pan American Health Organisation, Washington, D.C., Scientific Publication No. 451, 90–102.
Halsey, N. A., et al. (1985). *N. Engl. J. Med. 313*:544–549.
Hersh, B. S., Markowitz, L. E., Hoffman, R. E., Hoff, D., Doran, M., Fleishman, J. C., Preblud, S. R., and Orenstein, W. A. (1991). *Am. J. Public Health 81*:361–364.
Hinman, A. R., Brandlin-Bennett, A. D., and Nieburg, P. I. (1979). *JAMA 242*:1157–1161.

Holt, E. A., Boulos, R., Halsey, N. A., Boulos, L. M., and Boulos, C. (1990). *Pediatrics* *85*:188–194.

Hull, H. (1981). *Rev. Infect. Dis. 10*:463–467.

Hull, H. F., Williams, P. J., and Oldfield, F. (1983). *Lancet 1*:972–975.

Kambarami, R. A., Nathoo, K. J., Nkruma, F. F., and Pirie, D. J. (1991). *Bull. WHO* *69*:213–219.

Kenya. The optimal age for measles immunization. (1982). *Wkly. Epidemiol. Rec.* *57*:89–92.

Kingsbury, D. Q., Bratt, M. A., Choppin, P. E., et al. (1988). *Intervirology 10*:137–152.

Klein-Zabban, M. L., et al. (1987). *Bull. WHO 65*:197–201.

Koenig, M. A., Khan, M. A., Wojtyniak, B., Clemens, J. D., Chakraborty, J., Fauveau, V., Phillips, J. F., Akbar, J., and Barua, U. S. (1990). *Bull. WHO 68*:441–447.

Koster, F. T., et al. (1981). *Bull. WHO 59*:901–908.

Krugman, S., and Ward, R. (1973). *Infectious Diseases of Children and Adults.* C. V. Mosby, St. Louis.

Lennon, J. L., and Black, F. L. (1986). *J. Pediatr. 108*:;671–676.

Lian, J. F. (1979). Dissertation, Yale University, New Haven, CT.

Loutan, L., and Paillard, S. (1991). In press.

Mathias, R. G., et al. (1989). *Am. J. Public Health 79*:475–478.

Measles outbreak. (1988). *Wkly. Epidemiol. Rec. 18*:137–138.

Measles, United States. (1989). *MMWR 38*:601–605.

Measles outbreak in Hong Kong. (1990). *Wkly. Epidemiol. Rec. 49*:379–381.

Measles prevention: Recommendations of the Immunization Practices Advisory Committee. *MMWR* (1989) *1*:11–14.

Miller, C. (1987). *Br. Med. J. 295*:22–24.

MMWR (1990). *38*:863–871.

Morley, D. (1983). *Rev. Infect. Dis. 5*:460–462.

Nairn, J. P., Khare, S., Rana, S. R. S., and Banegee, K. B. (1989). *Int. J. Epidemiol.* *18*:952–957.

Orenstein, W. A., et al. (1985). *Bull. WHO 63*:1055–1067.

Pannuiti, C. S., Moraes, J. C., Souza, V. A. U. F., et al. (1991). *Bull. WHO 69*:557–560.

Panum, P. I. (1940). Observations made during the measles epidemic in the Faroe Islands in the year 1846. American Publishing Association, New York.

Sabin, A. B., Arechiga, A. F., de Castro, F., et al. (1983). *JAMA 249*:2651–2662.

Sencer, D., Dull, H. B., and Langmuir, A. D. (1976). *Public Health Rep. 1967*: 253–256.

Shasby, D. M., Shope, T. C., Down, H., et al. (1977). *N. Engl. J. Med. 296*:585.

Sheshberadaran, H., Chen, S. N., and Norrby, E. (1983). *Virology 128*:341–353.

Singapore measles control. (1986). *Wkly. Epidemiol. Rec. 61*:165–168.

Sinha, D. P. (1977). *Trop. Georg. Med. 29*:125–134.

Spencer, H. C., et al. (1987). *Ann. Trop. Parasitol. 81*(1):36–45.

Stetler, H. C., Orenstein, W. A., Bernier, R. H., Herrmann, K. I., Sirotkin, B., Hopfenspeger, D., Schuh, R., et al. (1986). *Pediatrics 77*:471–476.

Sutter, R. W., Markowitz, L. E., Bennetch, J. M., Morris, W., et al. (1991). *J. Infect. Dis.* *163*:12–16.

Tanzania. (1981). Seroconversion after measles immunization. *Wkly. Epidemiol. Rec.* *56*:234–237.

Taylor, W. R., Kalis, R., ma-Disu, M., and Weinman, J. M. (1988). *Am. J. Epidemiol.* *127*:788–794.

Toole, M. J., Stecketee, R. W., Waldman, R. J., and Nieburg, P. (1989). *Bull. WHO* *67*:381–388.

Tulchinsky, T. H., Abed, Y., Ginsburg, G., Shaheen, S., Friedman, J. B., Schoenbaum, M. L., and Slater, P. E. (1990). *Rev. Infect. Dis. 12*:951–958.

van Mazjik, J., Pinheiro, F. P., Black, F. L. (1982). *Trop. Geog. Med. 34*:3–6.

Wakeham, P. F. (1978). *J. Trop. Pediatr. 24*:87–88.

Whittle, H. C., Campbell, H., Rahman, S., and Armstrong, J. R. M. (1990). *Lancet* *336*:1048–1050.

WHO. (1988). *Tech. Rep. Ser.* 771.

WHO. (1990). Measles control in the 1990s: immunization before 9 months of age. Geneva, WHO/EPI/GEN/90.3.

WHO/UNICEF. (1987). Joint statement on vitamin A for measles. *Wkly. Epidemiol. Rec. 19*:133–134.

WHO/UNICEF. (1989). Joint statement on early immunization for HIV-infected children. *Wkly. Epidemiol. Rec. 64*:48–49.

Wilkins, J., and Wehrle, P. F. (1979). *J. Pediatr. 94*:865.

Wood, P. B., Sohendra, K. S., Branken, P. M., and Houser, N. E. (1980). *Trans. R. Soc. Hyg. 74*:381–383.

Part IV

Poliomyelitis and Rabies

9

THE ROLE OF VIROLOGIC SURVEILLANCE IN THE GLOBAL INITIATIVE TO ERADICATE POLIOMYELITIS

Olen Kew, Lina De, Chen-Fu Yang, Baldev Nottay, and Mark Pallansch *Centers for Disease Control, Atlanta, Georgia*

Edson da Silva *Fundação Oswaldo Cruz, Rio de Janeiro, Brazil*

I. INTRODUCTION

For the second time in this century, a broad alliance has formed to achieve the eradication of a viral disease (Fenner et al., 1988; World Health Assembly, 1988; Reid, 1989; Lemon and Robertson, 1991; Task Force for Child Survival, 1991). Paralytic poliomyelitis, which has afflicted children of every generation since the dawn of civilization (Paul, 1971), is being driven into extinction. Following the introduction of effective vaccines, first the inactivated polio vaccine (IPV; Salk et al., 1954) and subsequently the live, attenuated oral polio vaccine (OPV; Sabin et al., 1960), poliomyelitis was quickly controlled in most developed countries (Kim-Farley et al., 1984; Varughese et al., 1989; Strebel et al., 1992). By 1974, the sharp contrast in the incidence of poliomyelitis and other infectious diseases between the developed and developing worlds called for the establishment of the Expanded Programme on Immunization (EPI) of the World Health Organization (Henderson et al., 1988). The major goal of the EPI is to provide protective immunization for every child on Earth. The centerpiece of the EPI is the Poliomyelitis Eradication Initiative, first launched by the Pan American Health Organization (PAHO) in 1985 (Pan American Health Organization, 1985). The dramatic success of the Initiative in the Americas (de Quadros et al., 1991; Pan American Health

Organization, 1991a,b) set the stage in 1988 for a commitment to global eradication by the year 2000 (World Health Assembly, 1988).

Since the preparation of our previous chapter in this series (Kew et al., 1990), important milestones along the way to eradication have been reached. The entire region of the Americas is now nearly polio-free (de Quadros et al., 1991; Pan American Health Organization, 1991a,b), and the few remaining pockets of endemicity are currently under intensive immunization and surveillance (Pan American Health Organization, 1992). Elsewhere, immunization coverage for poliomyelitis and other EPI-targeted diseases (measles, neonatal tetanus, diphtheria, pertussis) is steadily increasing (World Health Organization, 1991). Current estimates suggest that many more cases of poliomyelitis are being prevented (440,000/year) than are still occurring (130,000/year). Nonetheless, most of Asia and Africa, and parts of Europe, remain endemic for poliomyelitis (World Health Organization, 1991).

Eradication of endemic poliomyelitis requires the extinction of the causative agents, wild polioviruses (Evans, 1984). Consequently, virologic surveillance is a central activity within the Poliomyelitis Eradication Initiative. New surveillance methods, developed through the collaboration of epidemiologists and virologists, have been integrated into the Initiative. Improved technical and analytic approaches continue to be developed, in order to promote optimal utilization of the very limited world resources currently available for public health, infectious disease control, and poliomyelitis eradication.

In this chapter, we review recent developments in virologic surveillance as implemented in the Poliomyelitis Eradication Initiative. Emphasis will be placed on the lessons learned in the American region. New lessons await us as the coalition broadens to conquer poliomyelitis worldwide. It is hoped that the insights into viral disease control obtained through the eradication of poliomyelitis will endure long after the last case of endemic poliomyelitis has been recorded.

II. EPIDEMIOLOGIC AND VIROLOGIC BACKGROUND

A. Poliomyelitis and Acute Flaccid Paralysis

Poliomyelitis is a disease of acute flaccid paralysis following febrile illness (Paul, 1971; World Health Organization, 1989; Melnick, 1990). Surveillance for acute flaccid paralysis is the primary means for detecting poliovirus transmission. Unfortunately, this approach, by itself, is neither highly specific nor highly sensitive. Many other conditions, including Guillain-Barré syndrome and infections with non-polio enteroviruses (NPEV), may also be associated with acute paralytic disease (Figueroa et al., 1989; Hayward et al., 1989; Melnick, 1990; Morens et al., 1990). Paralyses associated with NPEV infections are generally transient, but the early clinical signs can be indistinguishable from poliomyelitis (Gear, 1984; Grist and Bell, 1984; World Health Organization, 1989). Thus, the underlying cause cannot be definitely identified without virologic analyses. Large outbreaks of paralytic illness are associated nearly exclusively with polioviruses. However, as immunization programs develop and cases become more sporadic, the role of virologic studies assumes increased importance.

The sensitivity of surveillance for acute flaccid paralysis for detecting polioviruses is limited by the fact that only about 1% of wild poliovirus infections in unimmunized children are clinically apparent (Melnick, 1990; Morens et al., 1990). In populations with intermediate levels of immunity, widespread circulation of polioviruses may occur with the appearance of few or no paralytic cases (Pöyry et al., 1988). Thus, modified field and virologic methods are required to detect silent poliovirus transmission.

B. Polioviruses Found in Nature

Polioviruses occur as three serotypes. Full protection against poliomyelitis requires immunity to all three serotypes. Both OPV and IPV are capable of inducing durable protective immunity (Salk and Salk, 1977; Sabin, 1985; Faden et al., 1990). Antigenic variability within poliovirus serotypes has long been recognized (Nakano et al., 1963, 1978), and the genetic and structural bases for this variability are well understood (Minor et al., 1986a,b; Page et al., 1988; Kinnunen et al., 1990; Reynolds et al., 1990; Rombaut et al., 1990). However, the range of antigenic variability is sufficiently restricted to have prevented the emergence of wild polioviruses resistant to neutralization by antibodies found in well-immunized populations.

Polioviruses obtained from clinical or environmental samples are classified into two broad categories: vaccine-related or wild. Vaccine-related polioviruses are derivatives of the Sabin OPV strains (Sabin type 1, LSc 2ab; Sabin type 2, P712 Ch 2ab; Sabin type 3, Leon 12 a_1b; Sabin and Boulger, 1973). Wild polioviruses are independent of the poliovaccine strains, and are spread by continuous fecal–oral or person-to-person transmission among humans. Although the Sabin strains are derived from historical wild polioviruses endemic to the United States in the 1930s to 1950s, the lineages from which they descend now appear to be extinct (Kew et al., 1990; Yang et al., 1992). Contemporary wild polioviruses descend from multiple separate lineages, and are clearly distinguishable from vaccine-related polioviruses by molecular methods.

C. Physical and Biological Properties of Polioviruses

Polioviruses, members of the *Enterovirus* genus of the Picornaviridae family, are among the smallest of human viruses (Melnick, 1990; Rueckert, 1990). Poliovirions (8.4 mDa; ≈30 nm in diameter) consist of a highly structured protein capsid enclosing a molecule of single-stranded RNA. The capsid contains 60 identical subunits arranged in icosahedral symmetry. Each subunit contains four polypeptide chains: VP1 (35.5 kDa), VP2 (30.0 kDa), VP3 (26.4 kDa), and VP4 (7.4 kDa). The detailed architecture of poliovirions has been revealed by x-ray crystallography (Hogle et al., 1985; Filman et al., 1989). Most of the amino acid residues on the external virion surface are contributed by VP1, small loops from VP2 and VP3 also form the outer surface, while VP4 is completely internal. These surface residues form three or four major neutralizing antigenic sites (Minor et al., 1986b; Page et al., 1988).

The poliovirus genomic RNA is about 7450 nucleotides in length (Kitamura et al., 1981; Racaniello and Baltimore, 1981; Stanway et al., 1984; Toyoda et al., 1984), and has a 3′-terminal polyadenylated tract. The genome is organized into three major intervals: the 5′-noncoding region (≈740 nucleotides), a single open reading frame (≈6635 nucleotides), and the 3′-noncoding region (≈75 nucleotides; Fig. 1). Virion RNA serves directly as a messenger for viral protein synthesis, which involves the formation of a large polyprotein that is processed by viral proteases to generate functional viral proteins (Pallansch et al., 1984; Toyoda et al., 1986; Rueckert, 1990). Capsid proteins are derived from the amino terminal 40% of the polyprotein. Noncapsid proteins include the viral RNA replicase (Ward et al., 1988), an intracellular membrane protein, and two distinct viral proteases (Toyoda et al., 1986).

D. Rapid Evolution of Poliovirus Genomes

Like that of other RNA viruses (Smith and Inglis, 1987; Steinhauer and Holland, 1987), the polioviral replication machinery has a very high inherent error rate (Ward et al., 1988; Holland et al., 1990). Poliovirus populations, even those derived from a single infected cell, are genetically heterogeneous. Biological systems having an extreme degree of genetic diversity within clonal populations are described as "quasispecies" (Eigen and Beibricher, 1988). Mutational variation is distributed around an "average" genomic sequence, which is sampled when uncloned virus populations are analyzed by oligonucleotide fingerprinting or direct

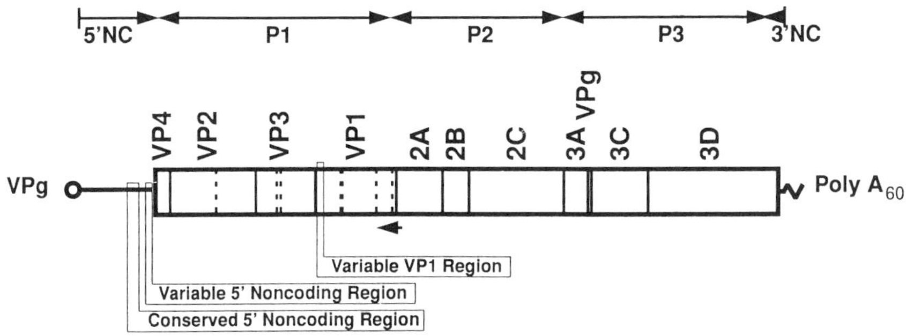

FIGURE 1 Schematic of organization of the poliovirus genome. Non-translated regions are shown as lines, the region of the translated polyprotein is represented by the rectangle. Nomenclature for viral proteins follows that of Rueckert and Wimmer (1984) except for the capsid proteins VP1, VP2, VP3, and VP4. Dashed vertical lines indicate location of sequences encoding virion surface residues. Arrow indicates the 150-nucleotide interval at the VP1/2A junction routinely analyzed by comparative sequencing. Variable and conserved sequences matching probes and PCR primer pairs are indicated.

sequencing of viral RNAs. Much of the population consists of variants that differ from the average genome at one or more nucleotide positions. Under equilibrium conditions (such as serial propagation of poliovirus in cell culture), the distribution of variants is usually quite stable, despite the high background of mutation (Nottay et al., 1981). Alteration of growth conditions may cause shifts in the genetic equilibrium, such that successive new distributions arise. Quite analogous evolutionary processes occur with foot-and-mouth disease viruses, as described in detail in the excellent review in this series by Domingo et al. (1990).

In contrast to their nearly static evolution in cell culture, polioviruses evolve rapidly during replication in humans (Nottay et al., 1981; Kew et al., 1981; Minor et al., 1982). The rates of evolution vary for different genomic regions. Much of the 5′-noncoding region is highly conserved (Toyoda et al., 1984), presumably because functional constraints limit variability. Within the coding region, variability occurs primarily by mutation to synonymous codons. This tendency towards amino acid conservation includes the residues forming the internal framework of the capsids. In contrast, the less structured (Hogle et al., 1985) surface residues forming neutralizing antigenic sites are quite variable (Minor et al., 1986a; Kinnunen et al., 1990), possibly in response to direct selection during replication in humans. Other highly variable intervals include the approximately 90 residues preceding the initiation codon and the first 30–32 codons of VP1 (Toyoda et al., 1984; da Silva et al., 1991; Yang et al., 1991, 1992).

When the oral polio vaccines replicate in humans, genomic evolution is initially quite rapid, occurring by both mutation and intertypic (and, presumably, intratypic) recombination (Kew et al., 1981; Kew and Nottay, 1984; Minor et al., 1982, 1986a). This initial burst of variability is thought to result from selection for reversion (by back mutation and suppression) of the attenuated phenotype (Minor et al., 1986a). The vaccine strains frequently undergo antigenic variation (Nakano et al., 1963, 1978; Crainic et al., 1983; Minor et al., 1986a), often involving mutations at more than one antigenic site.

Similar evolutionary processes occur when wild polioviruses replicate in humans, although the rates of change may in general be more uniform in the absence of strong functional selection (Rico-Hesse et al., 1987). For wild polioviruses, a typical rate for the fixation of mutations over the entire genome is one to two nucleotide substitutions per week (Nottay et al., 1981). Most of the mutations detected in the coding region generate synonymous codons, and probably confer little, if any, selective advantage. This suggests that the primary mechanism for the evolution of wild poliovirus genomes is by successive founder effects, occurring when virus populations decline to very small numbers (during cyclic replication in the human intestine or upon person-to-person transmission). Shifts in the genotypic distribution will occur whenever the surviving subpopulation of virus genomes differs from the "average" genome of the parental population. By this process, variability does not require functional selection, but only periodic random sampling of dilute populations. The rapid accumulation of mutations in poliovirus genomes permits chains of transmission to be inferred from the patterns of nucleotide variation among clinical isolates (Kew et al., 1990).

III. PRINCIPLES OF SURVEILLANCE FOR POLIOVIRUSES

A. Fundamental Epidemiologic Questions

From the perspective of poliomyelitis eradication, several central epidemiologic questions focus on identifying the sources of wild polioviruses and the conditions permitting their continued transmission. The key questions may be summarized as follows:

1. Which cases of paralytic illness are associated with wild polioviruses?
2. What is the relative proportion of cases associated with each serotype?

3. What are the epidemiologic relationships between cases and outbreaks in different regions and in different communities?
4. What are the pathways of transmission?
5. Where are the community reservoirs sustaining transmission of wild polioviruses?
6. Where and when are the chains of transmission sustaining endemicity most diminished?
7. Can wild polioviruses be isolated from the environment of communities that are free of clinical disease?
8. How do we know when transmission has been interrupted and the indigenous wild polioviruses eliminated?

Answers to these questions guide control activities towards the most effective strategies for breaking the chains of wild poliovirus transmission. In essence, poliomyelitis eradication is the permanent, worldwide interruption of all wild poliovirus transmission.

B. Methods for Characterizing Polioviruses

Poliovirus isolates are currently identified by either of two independent approaches (World Health Organization, 1990). The first differentiates vaccine-derived and wild polioviruses by their antigenic properties (Nakano et al., 1963, 1978). Serodifferentiation analyses have used both cross-absorbed antisera (van Wezel and Hazendonk, 1979) or panels of specific neutralizing monoclonal antibodies (Ferguson et al., 1982; Osterhaus et al., 1983; Crainic et al., 1983).

The second fundamental approach encompasses several different methods for comparing sequence relationships among poliovirus genomes. Molecular methods in current use include ribonuclease T_1 oligonucleotide fingerprinting (Nottay et al., 1981; Kew et al., 1984), partial genomic sequencing (Rico-Hesse et al., 1987; Kew et al., 1990; Pöyry et al., 1990), and hybridization with synthetic oligodeoxynucleotide probes (da Silva et al., 1991). These methods have been reviewed in the previous volume (Kew et al., 1990). More recently, the high sensitivity of in vitro amplification by the polymerase chain reaction (PCR; Saiki et al., 1985) has been used to identify polioviruses, either by amplification with genotype-specific primers (Yang et al., 1991, 1992) or by restriction fragment length polymorphism analysis of the products amplified with broadly reacting primers (Balanant et al., 1991).

The different methods have complementary applications. Antigenic analyses using cross-absorbed antisera are quite straightforward and rapid when adapted to enzyme-linked immunosorbent assay (ELISA) formats (Glikmann et al., 1987). This method is well-suited for laboratories that are more proficient in serologic, rather than molecular, procedures. The molecular methods, however, have greater accuracy, primarily because they are not confounded by the antigenic variation that frequently accompanies replication of the Sabin strains in humans. The most transferable of these methods is probe hybridization, which has been adapted to sensitive ELISA and histochemical assays widely used in diagnostic laboratories. The PCR method has excellent potential as a primary diagnostic procedure if the problem of template carryover can be overcome (Kwok and Sninsky, 1989). Genomic sequencing is most useful in molecular epidemiologic studies, while oligonucleotide fingerprinting is best applied in specialized surveys of total genomic variability.

C. Virus Identification and Programmatic Response

The identification of polioviruses by serotype and by whether they are vaccine-related or wild has important epidemiologic and programmatic implications. Vaccine-related isolates are commonly obtained from children who show signs of paralytic illness. The large majority of these isolates appear to be unrelated to the paralytic illness, which may be attributable to Guillain-Barré syndrome, co-infection with wild polioviruses, or underlying infections with the ubiquitous NPEVs (Parks et al., 1967). Identification of vaccine-related isolates associated with paralytic cases requires no programmatic response, since vaccine-derived polioviruses rarely spread beyond primary or secondary contacts (Benyesh-Melnick et al., 1967).

In contrast, detection of wild polioviruses clearly signals the need for programmatic action, because wild polioviruses are capable of explosive epidemic spread. Early detection of community transmission of wild polioviruses may permit the timely implementation of control measures. Identification of the serotypes of the wild polioviruses also provides important information on the status of control activities. Because seroconversion is most efficient for type 2 polioviruses and least efficient for type 3 viruses (Patriarca et al., 1988; Faden et al., 1990), detection of endemic type 2 polioviruses is evidence of serious deficiencies in vaccine coverages. Detection of type 3 polioviruses may indicate that population immunity has not yet attained sufficient levels to block endemic transmission.

While much can be learned from basic virologic characterization of clinical isolates, very detailed epidemiologic information is obtained from molecular epidemiologic studies.

D. Genomic Sequence Comparisons

The high rate of poliovirus genomic evolution makes it possible to monitor wild poliovirus transmission with precision. Sequence comparisons of comparatively small genomic intervals (e.g., 150 nucleotides, about 2% of the total genome) provide a reasonable initial survey of the natural distributions of different poliovirus lineages (Rico-Hesse et al., 1987). Further analyses, whether by oligonucleotide sequencing, probe hybridization, PCR, or additional sequencing, consistently support relationships detected by limited sequencing surveys (Rico-Hesse et al., 1987). The survey sequence comparisons are quite reliable because the number of combinations of synonymous codons that can occur within a 150-nucleotide coding interval is very large.

For our initial surveys, we selected an interval at the junction of the capsid and noncapsid domains (90 nucleotides encoding the carboxyl terminal residues of the largest virion protein, VP1, and 60 nucleotides encoding the amino terminal residues of the protease, 2A; Rico-Hesse et al., 1987). Since only a small fraction of the encoded residues reside on the virion surface (Minor et al., 1986b; Page et al., 1988), we reasoned that evolution of this domain probably occurs primarily by genetic drift rather than by antibody selection. We expected that the overall rates of evolution would be more uniform for selectively "neutral" mutations than for missense mutations whose rates of selection may vary in response to differing conditions (such as the immune status of human populations).

E. Dendrograms of Sequence Relatedness

Sequence comparisons among many independent genomes are conveniently summarized in dendrograms (Fitch and Margoliash, 1967; Figs. 2–5). The limit divergence (VP1/2A region) within each serotype (type 1, 23%; type 2, 23%; type 3, 26%) approaches the 29% divergence found for the three serotypes of Sabin poliovaccine strains (Toyoda et al., 1984). Viruses whose genomes share ≥85% nucleotide homology are defined as members of the same genotype, a grouping that is consistent with epidemiologic data (Rico-Hesse et al., 1987). The genetic relationships shown by the dendrograms provide an approximate measure of the epidemiologic relationships among cases and outbreaks. Because poliovirus genomes evolve rapidly, close genetic relationships among isolates is strong evidence for the existence of a recent common ancestral infection. The left sides of the dendrograms show the most direct and proportional relationships between genetic distance and epidemiologic linkage. At the right sides of the dendrograms, all independent genotypes appear to be equally divergent. The evolutionary relationships among different genotypes are difficult to discern because of the cumulative effects of additional mutations at the same site with continued genomic divergence. The algorithm used to construct the dendrograms is quite simple, scoring only whether nucleotides at equivalent positions in different genomes are identical. A more refined algorithm, evaluating the contributions of less frequent mutational events (such as transversion mutations or amino acid substitutions) and the cumulative

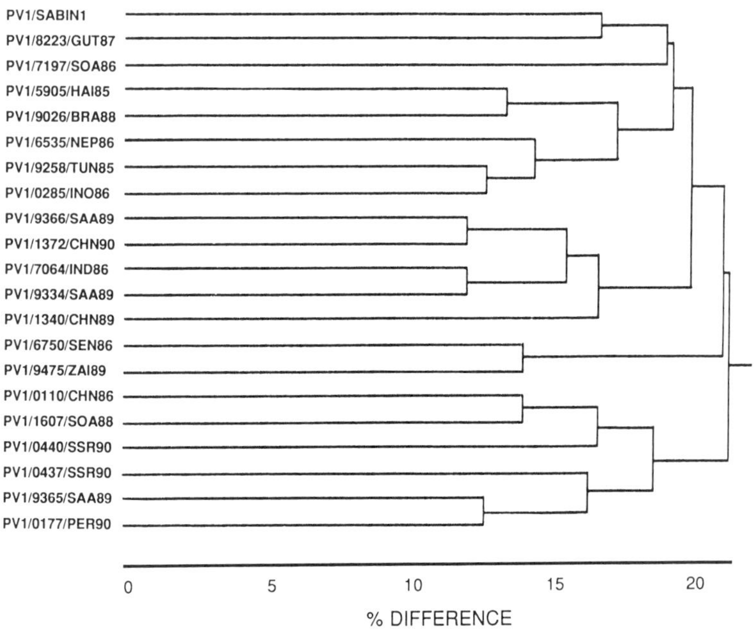

FIGURE 2 Dendrogram constructed according to sequence relatedness among 21 type 1 polioviruses across the interval of nucleotides 3296–3445 (VP1/2A region). All pairwise comparisons were performed using a computer program that assigned each nucleotide substitution an equivalent statistical weight. The percentage nucleotide sequence divergence between any two strains is the distance along the abscissa to the connecting node. Country abbreviations for Figs. 2–5 are: BRA = Brazil, CAM = Cameroon, CAN = Canada, CHN = China, COL = Colombia, DOR = Dominican Republic, EGY = Egypt, FIN = Finland, GUT = Guatemala, HAI = Haiti, IND = India, INO = Indonesia, ISR = Israel, JAM = Jamaica, JOR = Jordan, KEN = Kenya, MEX = Mexico, NEP = Nepal, NET = Netherlands, OMA = Oman, PER = Peru, ROM = Romania, SAA = Saudi Arabia, SEN = Senegal, SIN = Singapore, SOA = South Africa, SPA = Spain, SSR = USSR, SWE = Sweden, TUN = Tunisia, TUR = Turkey, USA = United States, VEN = Venezuela, YUG = Yugoslavia, ZAI = Zaire, ZIM = Zimbabwe.

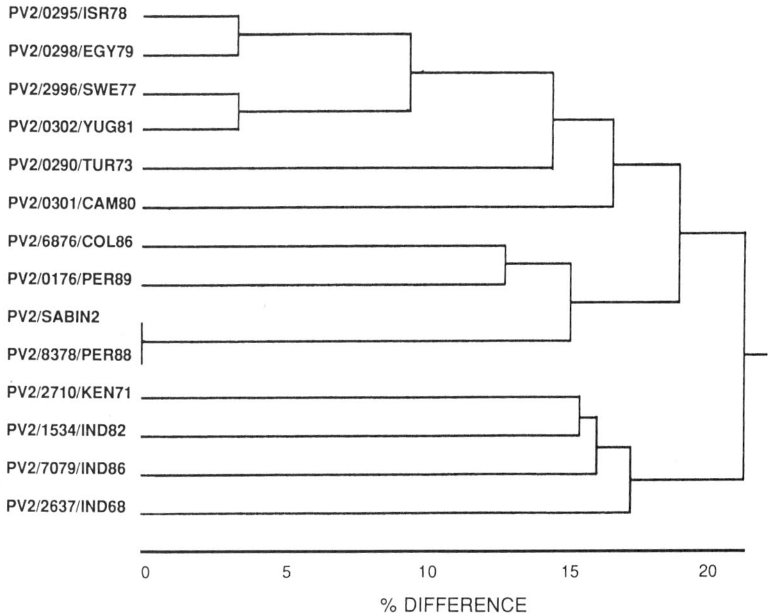

FIGURE 3 Dendrogram constructed according to sequence relatedness among 14 type 2 polioviruses across the interval of nucleotides 3295–3444 (VP1/2A region).

effects successive mutations at equivalent codon positions, must be used to obtain a broader evolutionary perspective. Inclusion of more sequence information per genome for the construction of the dendrograms rarely alters the structures of the major branches, but does increase resolution at the left sides of the patterns.

IV. MOLECULAR EPIDEMIOLOGIC VIEW OF POLIOVIRUS TRANSMISSION

Detailed virologic analyses provide insights into the patterns of poliovirus transmission that are unobtainable by any other means. We will review several molecular epidemiologic findings to illustrate application of this approach.

A. Geographic Distribution of Wild Poliovirus Genotypes

Many independent genotypes of wild polioviruses currently exist worldwide (Figs. 2–4). The number of surviving genotypes has been significantly reduced since the start of the Poliomyelitis Eradication Initiative. For

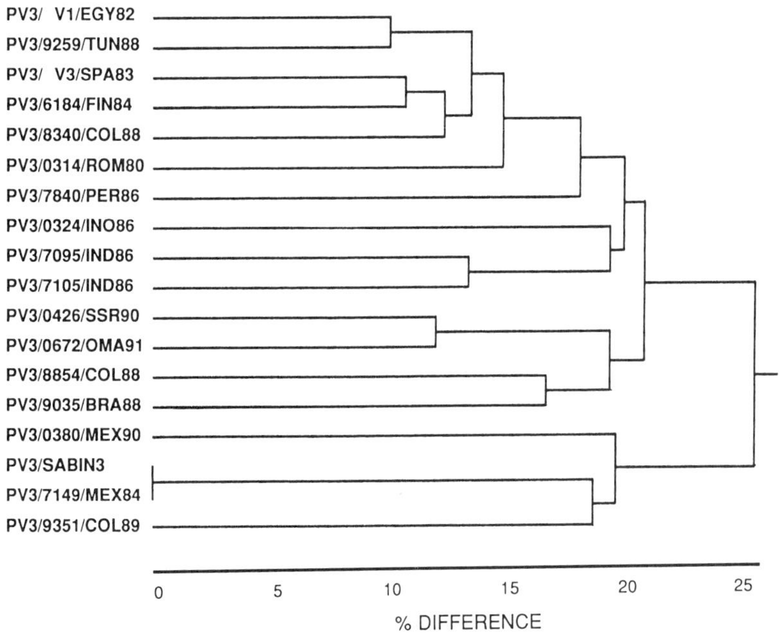

FIGURE 4 Dendrogram constructed according to sequence relatedness among 18 type 3 polioviruses across the interval of nucleotides 3287–3436 (VP1/2A region).

example, only one (type 1, Andean genotype) of the many genotypes (three type 1, two type 2, four type 3; Fig. 6) indigenous to the Americas in the 1980s could be found in 1991 (Fig. 7). In several other countries with high vaccine coverages (e.g., Oman, South Africa, Malaysia, and Thailand), the indigenous genotypes have all but disappeared in recent years. Unfortunately, in many other areas, poliovirus transmission continues largely unabated.

Type 1 polioviruses are most widely distributed, while type 2 polioviruses are most restricted in their range. When wild polioviruses are endemic to small, relatively isolated populations (such as island communities), they are usually type 1. Because humans seroconvert least efficiently to type 3 antigens (Salk and Salk, 1977; Sabin, 1985; Faden et al., 1990), the relative proportion of cases associated with type 3 polioviruses may increase at intermediate stages of control (Patriarca et al., 1988; Pan American Health Organization, 1991b).

Genetically related polioviruses cluster geographically (Fig. 6; Kew et al., 1990). This clustering has important implications for poliomyelitis

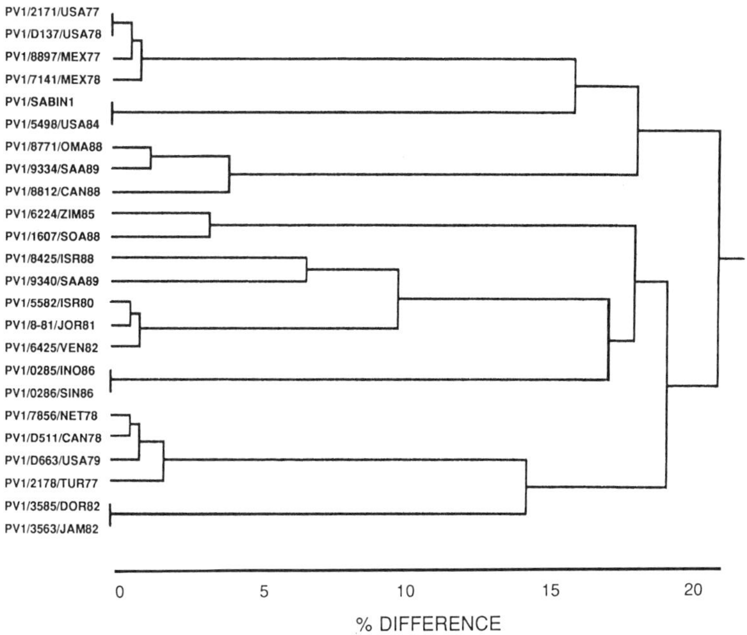

FIGURE 5 Dendrogram showing genetic relationships among 24 type 1 case isolates obtained from different regions of the world.

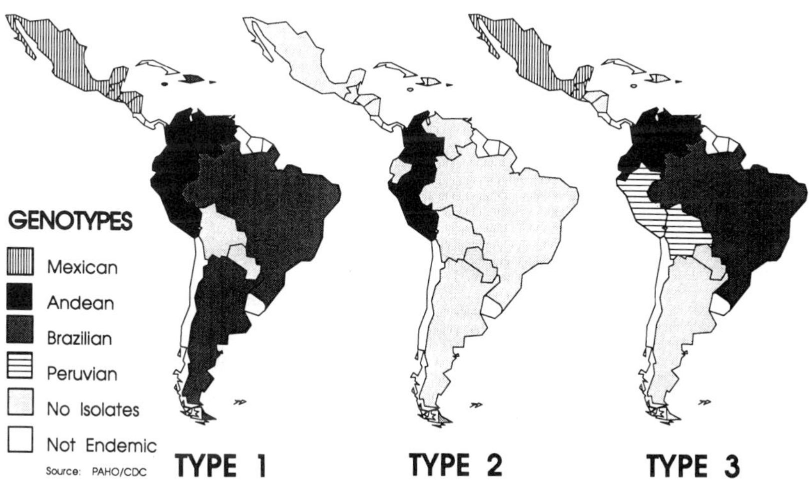

FIGURE 6 Geographic distribution by country of wild poliovirus genotypes obtained as clinical isolates in the American region since 1980. Each genotype is assigned a different pattern. Most assignments are based upon analyses of several independent case isolates from each country.

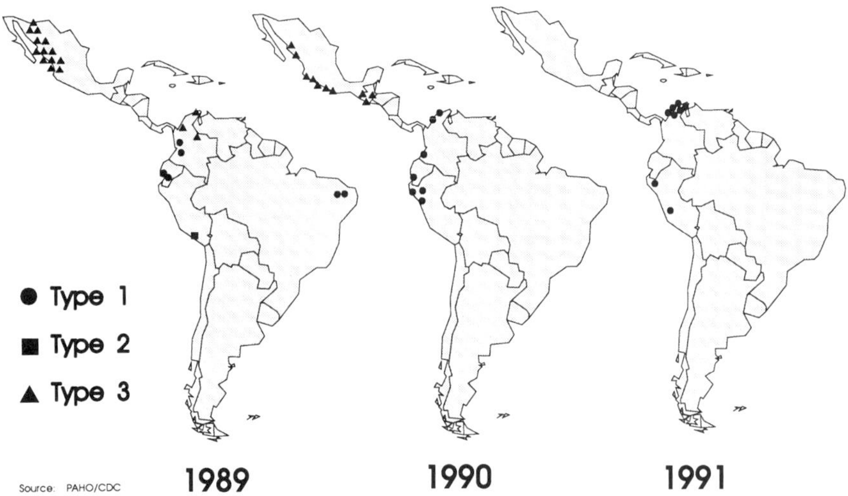

FIGURE 7 Locations of poliomyelitis cases from which wild polioviruses were obtained for the years 1989–1991. All isolates were shown to be representatives of the indigenous genotypes (Fig. 6) by sequence analysis. Dates of the most recent cases found to be associated with wild polioviruses were: Brazil, March 19, 1989 (type 1); Colombia, April 16, 1991 (type 1); Guatemala, September 23, 1990 (type 3); Mexico, October 18, 1990 (type 3); Peru, September 5, 1991 (type 1).

control, because it implies that local conditions (such as immunization coverages or patterns of human migration and interaction), rather than the specific properties of each virus (such as antigenicity), largely determine the extent of endemicity. Although some polioviruses have wider ranges than others, no pandemic genotypes have been recognized. When virus importations do occur, they usually originate from adjacent areas and do not establish endemicity in well-immunized populations.

Wild polioviruses are most prevalent in tropical latitudes, in areas with high population densities and poor sanitation (World Health Organization, 1991). Control of the disease has been most readily achieved in areas with temperate climates (which have the shortest seasons of peak poliovirus transmission), including tropical highlands (de Quadros et al., 1991; Pan American Health Organization, 1991b).

B. Poliovirus Genotypes in Highly Endemic Areas

Most countries have made good progress in immunizing against poliomyelitis, and the picture in many endemic areas is improving rapidly.

Even so, in some densely populated urban centers of Asia, for example, children have been co-infected with more than one serotype of wild poliovirus, and all three serotypes are present in the community (Enterovirus Research Centre, 1989). The isolation rates for different serotypes of wild polioviruses may vary by year, indicating separate cycles of epidemicity. Substantial genotypic heterogeneity may also be found in such regions (Kew et al., 1990), reflecting the presence of many independent community reservoirs that sustain continuous poliovirus transmission. Under such conditions, virologic surveillance is not a high priority, because the main task is implementation of good vaccine coverages.

C. Sources of Imported Genotypes

The sources of viruses imported into polio-free countries are often inferred from traditional case-contact investigations. However, the high proportion of silent poliovirus infections frequently conceals epidemiologic links. In the 1970s, Mexico was the primary source of case-associated viruses imported into the United States. During that same period, several distinct community reservoirs for type 1 polioviruses within Mexico could be identified from sequencing studies. Isolates from cases occurring in the United States frequently showed close sequence matches with viruses endemic to specific regions in Mexico (Fig. 5; Rico-Hesse et al., 1987). A similar situation may have occurred quite recently in the northern Andean region, where type 1 viruses closely matching those from endemic areas along the Caribbean coast of Colombia were associated with cases in Venezuela, which receives many migrants from those areas. Close sequence matches among type 3 viruses from Peru and Bolivia (1985-1986) were consistent with the view that southern Peru (with higher population densities and a tropical climate) was the endemic reservoir for the adjacent Bolivian highlands (isolated populations, cool climate).

The less frequent importations from very distant sources are often difficult, if not impossible, to detect by standard epidemiologic methods. Sequence analyses of case isolates from the Netherlands, Canada, and the United States provided independent evidence that Turkey was the endemic reservoir for the type 1 virus of 1978–1979 outbreaks in those countries (Fig. 5; Nottay et al., 1981; Rico-Hesse et al., 1987). Sequence matches among type 1 isolates from the 1988 epidemic in Oman (Sutter et al., 1991) and sporadic cases in Canada (1988; Varughese et al., 1989) and Saudi Arabia (1989; Sutter et al., in preparation) indicated the existence of a recent common progenitor infection (Fig. 5). The similarity of these viruses to earlier isolates from southern (but not western) India suggested that the large 1987 epidemic in the southern states of India was the source of the viruses found elsewhere. The type 3 virus of the 1984 epidemic in Finland appears to have originated from the eastern Mediterranean (Kew et al., 1990; Pöyry et al., 1990). The eastern Mediterranean also appears to have been the source of the type 1 polioviruses associated with 1982–1984 cases in Spain (Bernal et al., 1987; Kew et al., 1990). Interestingly, more recent type 1 isolates from Spain and Portugal (1987–1988) were most closely related to viruses endemic to northwest Africa (unpublished results).

D. Fine Structures of Epidemics

Local epidemics typically involve the clonal spread over short time periods of a specific genotypic variant (Kew et al., 1990). In endemic areas, substantial genotypic heterogeneity may exist prior to epidemics, with the epidemic genotype predominating afterwards. The net effect of each epidemic is the periodic reduction of genotypic diversity, which apparently accounts for why the catalog of wild poliovirus genotypes is not unmanageably large. Our experience in the Americas suggests that type 3 polioviruses tend to have greater genotypic diversity within a region than type 1 viruses, perhaps indicating that widespread outbreaks associated with type 3 are less frequent.

Epidemiologic links revealed by sequence analyses occasionally exclude hypotheses for transmission patterns suggested by epidemiologic data alone. Simple epidemic curves may mask complex transmission dynamics. Furthermore, epidemiologically unrelated cases may cluster temporally and geographically, while related cases may appear independent. For example, in the 1990 outbreak in Guatemala, the two type 3 viruses isolated in adjacent communities during September were not the most closely related pair, as one was more similar to a virus located in a more distant community in May. Type 1 isolates obtained in 1989 from adjacent communities in southern Saudi Arabia derived from two different endemic reservoirs [Fig. 2; southern India (probably via Oman) and the eastern Mediterranean; Sutter et al., 1991, in preparation]. A representative of a third type 1 genotype was associated with a 1988 case occurring in the northern part of the country (Fig. 2). Similarly, cases from the 1989–1990 epidemic in the Caucasus region were associated with two type 1 genotypes and a type 3 genotype (Figs. 2 and 4; G. Lipskaya, in preparation). When additional sequence information (such as complete VP1 sequences) is obtained for each isolate, it is sometimes possible to determine transmission patterns within communities (Slater et al., 1990; unpublished results).

E. Genotypic Indicators of Poliomyelitis Control

A landmark achievement of the Poliomyelitis Eradication Initiative in the Americas was the elimination of the indigenous genotypes of Brazil. The last case known to be associated with wild polioviruses occurred on March 19, 1989 (de Quadros et al., 1991). The success in tropical Brazil, the second most populous country in the Southern Hemisphere, clearly demonstrates the feasibility of global polio eradication. The immunization activities were accompanied by comprehensive case surveillance, supported by a strong network of laboratories within the country. Elimination of the poliovirus endemicity was associated with a progressive narrowing of the geographic range and genotypic diversity of the indigenous wild viruses (da Silva et al., 1991). Similar observations have been made throughout the American region (unpublished results; de Quadros et al., 1991).

F. Integration of Virologic Surveillance into Eradication Programs

PAHO and WHO have established networks of virology laboratories to support the Poliomyelitis Eradication Initiative. In addition to performing basic virologic investigations, the networks have also routinely applied molecular epidemiologic methods (da Silva et al., 1991; Pan American Health Organization, 1991b). Recognition that wild polioviruses are capable of spread from endemic areas to populations in distant continents has served to strengthen the commitment to global poliomyelitis eradication. Molecular epidmiologic findings have also helped focus efforts towards the high-risk areas that require intensified immunization action. For example, early detection of continued wild poliovirus circulation in Mexico and Guatemala confirmed the need for a final regional "mop-up" operation, which appears finally to have broken the last chains of wild poliovirus transmission. Similarly, identification of the surviving endemic reservoirs in Colombia and Peru, identified in part by virologic surveillance, was followed by very comprehensive mass immunization campaigns (Pan American Health Organization, 1991a).

While cases of acute paralytic illness still occur in the Americas, very few appear to be associated with wild polioviruses. By 1991, circulation of wild polioviruses appeared to be restricted to a few communities within the Andean region (Pan American Health Organization, 1991a). Virology laboratories in the American Regional Network are supporting increasingly intensive surveillance using very powerful molecular methods, yet only eight cases associated with wild polioviruses were detected in 1991 (Pan American Health Organization, 1992). A large mass campaign in western Peru in February 1992, may at last free the Americas of endemic poliomyelitis.

V. DEVELOPMENT OF NEW MOLECULAR REAGENTS

A. Nucleic Acid Probes

Among the molecular methods currently available, nucleic acid probe hybridization appears to have the widest diagnostic potential. Probe hybridization, especially when adapted to the dot-blot format, is technically straightforward, rapid, and readily adapted to routine diagnostic work. To apply these advantages to the identification of polioviruses, we developed sets of probes that specifically hybridize to poliovirus RNAs (Kew et al., 1990; da Silva et al., 1991). The first probes developed were synthetic oligodeoxynucleotides, 21–27 nucleotides in length. Because the oligodeoxynucleotide chains were short, hybridization reactions were rapid, effectively reaching completion in 2–4 hr. Two categories of probes were prepared: (1) a group probe that hybridized to RNAs of all polioviruses (and most NPEVs) and (2) poliovirus genotype-specific probes. The group probe complemented highly conserved sequences in the 5′-noncoding region (Fig. 1). The genotype-specific probes matched variable sequences encoding the amino terminal residues of VP1, or in the 5′-noncoding region interval immediately preceding the initiation codon for the polyprotein (Fig. 1). Because the group probe hybridizes with equal efficiency to all poliovirus templates, the intensity of the hybridization signal provides an approximate measure of the amounts of poliovirus (or NPEV) RNA applied to the filters.

Sabin-related isolates are directly identified using the Sabin strain-specific probes. Wild polioviruses are recognized by the inabilities of their genomes to form stable hybrids with the Sabin strain-specific probes. However, no information about the relationships among wild isolates could be obtained from such analyses. Consequently, we prepared several sets of probes specific for different genotypes of wild polioviruses, permitting important epidemiologic information to be obtained from rapid, reliable, routine tests (Fig. 8; da Silva et al., 1991). The synthetic oligodeoxynucleotide probes have been used extensively in the Americas to characterize case isolates (Pan American Health Organization, 1991b).

Despite the many advantages of synthetic oligodeoxynucleotide probes, several practical considerations limited their widespread applicability to a global program. Chief among the limitations were: (1) the continued requirement for organic synthesis for preparation, (2) the intermediate stabilities of the hybrids formed with short probes, (3) the

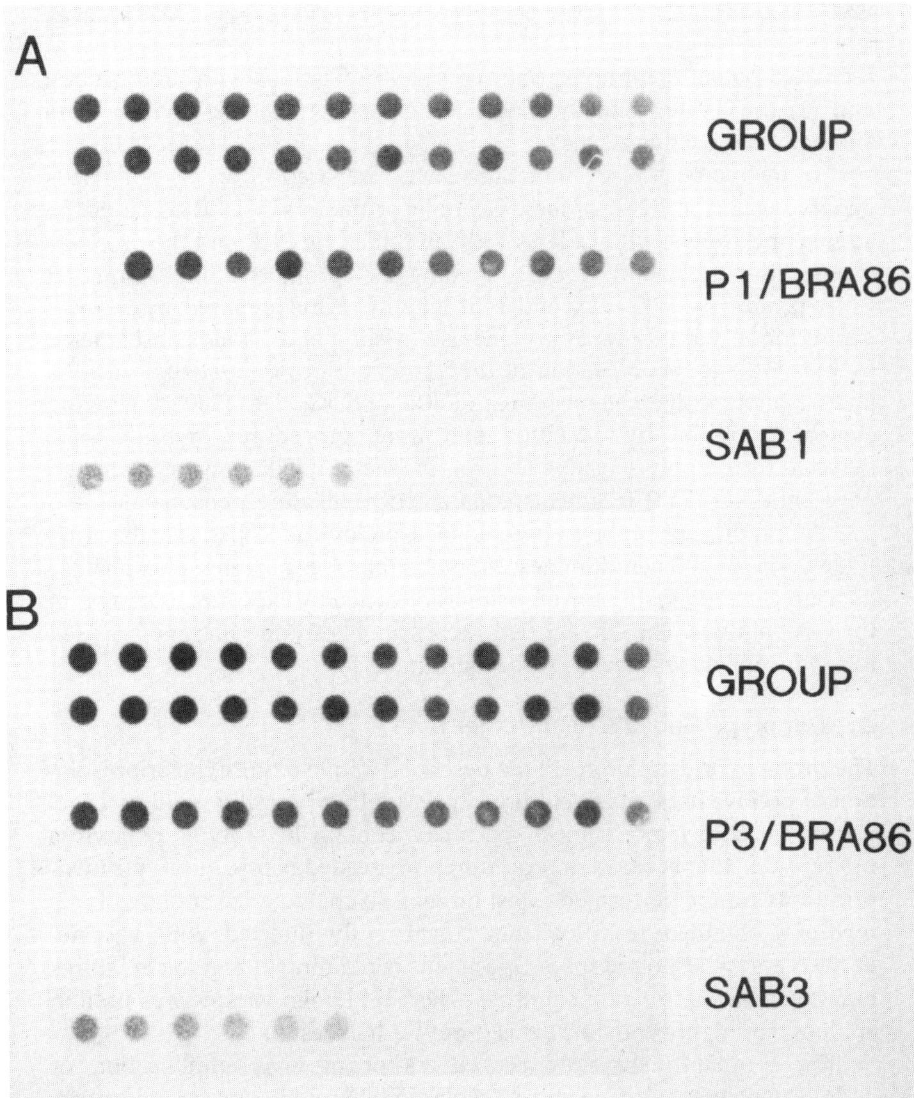

FIGURE 8 Autoradiogram of probe reactivities with 24 type 1 (panel A) and 24 type 3 (panel B) polioviruses. In each panel, suspensions of disrupted virions were blotted in three identical sets (two rows per set) and the blots hybridized with three different ^{32}P-labeled oligodeoxynucleotide probes (group, rows 1, 2, 7, 8; Brazil genotype-specific, rows 3, 4, 9, 10; Sabin-specific, rows 5, 6, 11, 12) were used, as described in the text. Samples were blotted from left to right as follows: *Panel A, type 1 isolates*. Wild isolates from Brazil (rows 1, 3, 5); Sabin 1-related isolates (rows 2, 4, 6 [left]); wild type 1 isolates from other regions (rows 2, 4, 6 [right]). *Panel B, type 3 isolates*. Wild isolates from Brazil (rows 7, 9, 11); Sabin 3-related isolates (rows 8, 10, 12 [left]); wild type 3 isolates from other regions (rows 8, 10, 12 [right]). (From da Silva et al., 1991.)

increased potential for nonspecific cross-hybridizations with short probes, and (4) the limited sites available for reporter molecules (which were generally radioactive atoms).

To overcome these limitations, we prepared sets of poliovirus genotype-specific RNA probes. Genomic sequences (Fig. 1) of the Sabin strains or different wild isolates were amplified by PCR and the products inserted into a plasmid vector containing a T7 promoter. Single-stranded RNA probes (90–100 nucleotides in length), were prepared by in vitro transcription with T7 RNA polymerase (Melton et al., 1984), and labeled by biosynthetic incorporation of uridylate residues derivatized with the steroid hapten, digoxigenin (DIG; Höltke and Kessler, 1989). Following standard dot-blot hybridization and wash procedures, hybrids were detected by a highly sensitive nonisotopic method. Filters were incubated with anti-DIG [Fab] fragments conjugated to alkaline phosphatase, and specific binding of probe to immobilized poliovirus RNAs visualized by hydrolysis of a chemiluminescent substrate for alkaline phosphatase (Schaap et al., 1989). Photon emission is recorded by exposure of x-ray film for 1–30 minutes. The DIG-labeled probes are highly specific, and are used to produce blots with very low backgrounds.

B. Genotype-Specific PCR Primer Sets

The probe hybridization methods described above require the prior isolation of polioviruses in cell culture, a process that typically requires 1 to 3 weeks. Because many clinical specimens contain heterotypic poliovirus mixtures, further separation procedures are needed before intratypic identifications can be performed. Most difficult to characterize are homotypic mixtures obtained from patients concurrently infected with vaccine-derived and wild polioviruses. Specimens containing homotypic mixtures have been encountered in countries where oral polio vaccine was used in epidemic or highly endemic areas (unpublished results).

The comparatively slow procedures of in vivo amplification of polioviruses in cell culture may be replaced by rapid in vitro amplification of viral RNA sequences by PCR. We have used the polymerase chain reaction (PCR) to obtain sensitive detection and identification of poliovirus RNA genomes. We designed primer pairs (Fig. 9) to permit identification of each Sabin poliovaccine strain by the electrophoretic mobilities of the amplified DNA products (Sabin 1: 97 bp; Sabin 2: 71 bp; Sabin 3: 44 bp; Fig. 10; Yang et al., 1991). The compositions of samples containing mixtures of vaccine strains could be readily determined by PCR. When the amplified products were visualized by ethidium bromide fluorescence, as few as 25 genomic copies in the original sample could be

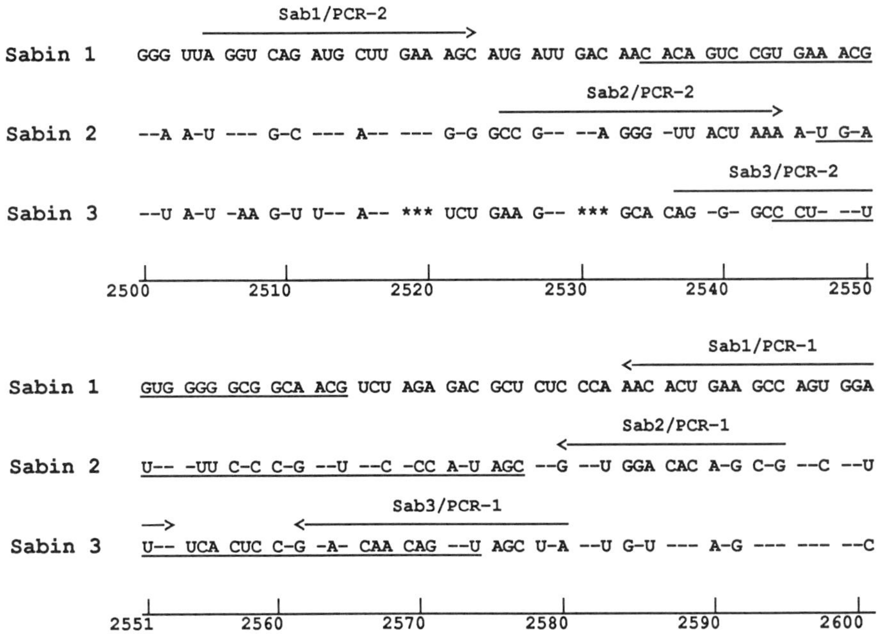

FIGURE 9 Location of Sabin strain genomic sequences complementary to (PCR-1 primers) or parallel with (PCR-2 primers) each PCR primer pair and oligodeoxynucleotide probe (antigenome polarity) set. Nucleotides encoding the amino terminal residues of VP1 (codons 1–32, types 1 and 2; codons 1–30, type 3) are aligned with the Sabin 1 reference sequence as originally shown by Toyoda et al. (1984). Dashes indicate sequence identities with Sabin 1, asterisks indicate nucleotide deletions. The predicted chain lengths of the amplified products are 97 bp (Sabin 1), 71 bp (Sabin 2), and 44 bp (Sabin 3). (From Yang et al., 1991.)

detected. When PCR was used in combination with strain-specific ^{32}P-labeled oligonucleotide probes, the limit of detection was ≤2.5 poliovirus genomes, which exceeded the sensitivity of poliovirus isolation in cell culture by at least 100-fold. PCR amplifications may be performed on virion RNAs extracted directly from clinical specimens, thus potentially eliminating the requirement for virus isolation in routine identifications while yielding reliable results within 8 h.

As described above, poliovirus isolates may be recognized as wild by their nonreactivity with the Sabin strain-specific PCR primer and probe sets (Yang et al., 1991). This approach, while reliable, does not take full advantage of the speed, sensitivity, and specificity potentially available

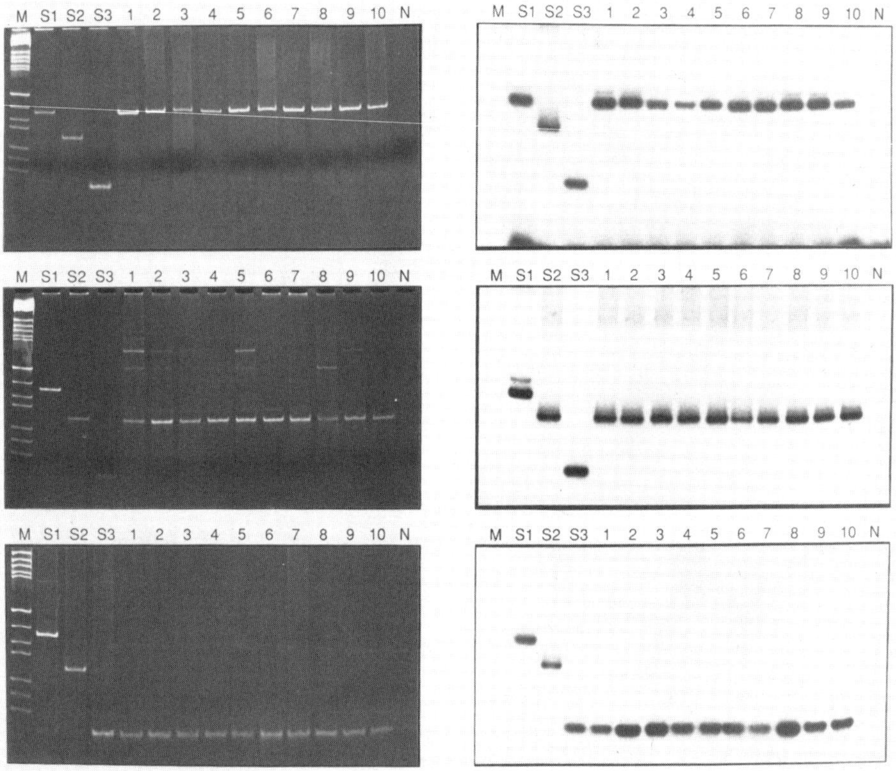

FIGURE 10 Specific amplification of the genomes of Sabin-related clinical isolates by PCR. DNA products were separated by electrophoresis on polyacrylamide gels and visualized by ethidium bromide fluorescence (left panels), or hybridized in solution to the corresponding ^{32}P-labeled Sabin strain probes before undergoing electrophoresis and the hybrids were detected by autoradiography (right panels). Each lane contains the products obtained from approximately 10^3 infected cells (left panels) or 5 infected cells (right panels). All Sabin-related isolates (type 1, top panels; type 2, middle panels; type 3, lower panels) were independently identified by genomic sequencing in the VP1/2A region. M, molecular weight markers; S1, S2, S3, reaction mixtures containing purified Sabin strain RNAs; N, reaction mixtures lacking RNA. (From Yang et al., 1991.)

from PCR analyses (Saiki et al., 1985, 1988). A clear improvement upon the above approach is to use PCR primer and probe sets that permit the direct detection of wild polioviruses. Such reagents would not only simplify analyses, but would also provide a clear, positive signal for the presence of wild poliovirus in the sample, even in specimens containing poliovirus or enterovirus mixtures. Therefore, we prepared PCR primer and probe sets specific for several wild poliovirus genotypes recently endemic to the Americas and elsewhere.

To illustrate this approach, we describe the properties of PCR primer sets permitting the selective amplification of the sequences of the wild type 3 poliovirus genotype recently associated with paralytic cases in Mexico and Guatemala. We first determined the VP1 nucleotide sequences of a type 3 virus representative of recent wild isolates from Mexico, PV3/9288/MEX89 (Fig. 11). The VP1 sequences of PV3/9288/MEX89 differed from those of Sabin 3 at 167 of 900 positions. From the sequence data, wild virus-specific primer pairs were designed to complement regions of high mismatch (>33%) with Sabin 3 templates. Primer binding sites were spaced along the genome so that the predicted amplification products (142 bp and 163 bp) could be easily resolved electrophoretically from the products generated with our Sabin strain-specific primers (Fig. 11). Two independent primer pairs were designed for each wild genotype: one set for routine screening and a second set for confirmation. RNAs of all wild type 3 poliovirus isolates from Mexico and Guatemala obtained over 13-year period (1977–1990) serve as efficient templates for amplification of the 142-bp and 163-bp products. Genomic templates derived from vaccine-related polioviruses and most heterologous wild polioviruses were inactive under equivalent reaction conditions. Amplifications generating a 114-bp product with a broadly reacting primer pair, matching highly conserved sequences in the 5′-noncoding region, provided a positive control for the presence in samples of poliovirus (or NPEV) RNAs. Selective amplification of wild Mexico–Guatemala type 3 poliovirus sequences was obtained with either primer set in reactions containing large stoichiometric excesses (up to 10^6-fold) of vaccine-related RNAs (Fig. 12). The use of wild genotype-specific PCR primer sets has facilitated identification of wild polioviruses present in both clinical and environmental samples.

VI. DETECTION OF SILENT POLIOVIRUS TRANSMISSION

To increase the sensitivity of virologic surveillance following investigations of sporadic cases of acute flaccid paralysis, the Pan American Health

```
                            9288/PCR-4 ----------------------->
001     G  I  E  D  L  I  S  E  V  A  Q  G  A  L  T  L  S  L  P  K  Q  Q  D  S  L
2477  GGUAUUGAAGAUUUGAUUUCUGAAGUUGCACAGGGCGCCCUAACUUUGUCACUCCCGAAGCAACAGGAUAGCUUA
2477  ---G-C--U--CC----C-----U--------A--A--AU-GG-CC-C--G--U--A-----G--AA-C--U---
001       V  D              D                    A                    N

026     P  D  T  K  A  S  G  P  A  H  S  K  E  V  P  A  L  T  A  V  E  T  G  A  T
2552  CCUGAUACUAAGGCCAGUGGCCCGGCGCAUUCCAAGGAGGUACCUGCACUCACUGCAGUCGAGACUGGAGCCACC
2552  --------C--A--------A-----A--------A--A--G--A-----A--C--U--U--A-----G------
026
          <--------------------- 9288/PCR-3
051     N  P  L  A  P  S  D  T  V  Q  T  R  H  V  V  Q  R  R  S  R  S  E  S  T  I
2627  AAUCCUCUGGCACCAUCCGACACAGUUCAAACGCGCCACGUAGUCCAACGACGCAGCAGGUCAGAGUCCACAAUA
2627  --C--CU-A-UU-----U--------C-----A--A-------------AG--------A--------A--G--C
051             V                                      Q

076     E  S  F  F  A  R  G  A  C  V  A  I  I  E  V  D  N  E  Q  P  T  T  R  A  Q
2702  GAAUCAUUCUUCGCACGCGGGGCGUGCGUCGCUAUUAUUGAGGUGGACAAUGAACAACCAACCACCCGGGCACAG
2702  --G--------U--------U--------------------A-----U--------G------------------
076

101     K  L  F  A  M  W  R  I  T  Y  K  D  T  V  Q  L  R  R  K  L  E  F  F  T  Y
2777  AAACUAUUUGCCAUGUGGCGCAUUACAUACAAAGAUACAGUGCAGUUGCGCCGUAAGUUGGAGUUUUUCACAUAC
2777  -----C-----U-CA-----------G--U-----C--------A--------C--A--A-----C-----U---
101                T

126     S  R  F  D  M  E  F  T  F  V  V  T  A  N  F  T  N  A  N  N  G  H  A  L  N
2852  UCUCGUUUUGACAUGGAAUUCACCUUCGUGGUAACCGCCAACUUCACCAACGCUAAUAAUGGGCAUGCACUCAAC
2852  --C-----C--------------------A--G--U--A------------A-C--------A--------A--U
126                                                       T

151     Q  V  Y  Q  I  M  Y  I  P  P  G  A  P  T  P  K  S  W  D  D  Y  T  W  Q  T
2927  CAGGUGUACCAGAUAAUGUACAUCCCCCCAGGGGCACCCACACCAAAGUCAUGGGACGACUACACUUGGCAAACA
2927  --A-----U-----U--------------G-----G--U--------A-----------U-----C-----G--G
151

176     S  S  N  P  S  I  F  Y  T  Y  G  A  A  P  A  R  I  S  V  P  Y  V  G  L  A
3002  UCUUCCAACCCGUCCAUAUUUUACACCUAUGGGGCUGCCCCGGCGCGAAUCUCAGUGCCAUACGUGGGGUUAGCC
3002  --C-----U-----------C-----U-----A--------A-----G-------------U-----C------
176

201     N  A  Y  S  H  F  Y  D  G  F  A  K  V  P  L  K  T  D  A  N  D  Q  I  G  D
3077  AAUGCUUACUCGCACUUUUACGACGGCUUCGCCAAGGUGCCAUUGAAGACAGAUGCCAAUGACCAGAUUGGUGAU
3077  -----C--U--U--U--C-----U-CU-----------A--GC------------AG--------A--C-----C
201                            A                             E
                           9288/PCR-2  ---------------------->
226     S  L  Y  S  A  M  T  V  D  D  F  G  V  L  A  V  R  V  V  N  D  H  N  P  T
3152  UCCUUGUACAGCGCCAUGACAGUUGAUGACUUUGGUGUAUUGGCAGUUCGUGUUGUCAAUGAUCACAACCCCACU
3152  --UC-A-----U--U-----G--G-----U--------GC-A---A-C--G-----U--C-----------U--C
226                                                I

251     K  V  T  S  K  V  R  I  Y  M  K  P  K  H  V  R  V  W  C  P  R  P  P  R  A
3227  AAAGUAACCUCCAAAGUCCGCAUUUACAUGAAACCCAAACACGUACGUGUCUGGUGCCCUAGACCGCCGCGCGCG
3227  --G--G--A-----G-----U--C--U-----------G-----G--C-----------------------U--A
251
                                    <--------------------- 9288/PCR-1
276     V  P  Y  Y  G  P  G  V  D  Y  R  N  N  L  D  P  L  S  E  K  G  L  T  T  Y
3302  GUACCUUAUUAUGGACCAGGGGUGGACUAUAGGAACAACUUGGACCCCUUAUCUGAGAAAGGUUUGACCACAUAU
3302  -----A--------G--G--A-----U--C-AAG-UG----AC-----C-G-----------------A--U---
276                                  K  D  D     H
```

FIGURE 11 Comparison of the VP1 sequences of Sabin type 3 (Leon 12 a$_1$b) and PV3/9288/MEX89. Nucleotide (line 2) and deduced amino acid (line 1) sequences of the Sabin 3 reference are shown; nucleotide (line 3) and amino acid (line 4) differences in PV3/9288/MEX89 are indicated. Sabin 3 nucleotide positions are numbered according to Stanway et al. (1984); those of PV3/9288/MEX89 are numbered similarly for comparability. VP1 amino acid residues are numbered 001–300. Sequences in bold letters identify amino acid residues that form neutralizing antigenic sites 1 (89–100), 2a (219–225), and 3a (286–290) (Minor et al., 1986b). Location of sequences matching wild genotype-specific PCR primer pairs (9288/PCR-1 + 9288/PCR-2; 9288/PCR-3 + 9288/PCR-4) are indicated by arrows. (From Yang et al., 1992.)

Organization recommended that stool samples be taken from every suspected case and five healthy community contacts under 5 years of age (Pan American Health Organization, 1991b). This strategy has been rewarded by the detection of wild polioviruses even when isolates could not be obtained from the case. In several studies, silent poliovirus transmission was detected in communities many weeks after the last case had occurred. All of these studies were supported by sequence characterizations of the poliovirus isolates, which confirmed that the virus isolates were of the local genotype.

Following these findings, a systematic study to detect silent poliovirus transmission was conducted in a high-risk community in Cartagena, Colombia (G. Tambini et al., personal communication). Continued silent transmission within Cartagena had been suspected because isolates from successive local cases occurring months apart had virtually identical VP1/2A sequences (unpublished results). Two different sampling strategies for detecting wild polioviruses were used: (1) characterization of viruses isolated from the stools of healthy children and (2) virologic and PCR analyses of community waste water. Both approaches confirmed the continued circulation of the indigenous wild type 1 polioviruses. Nearly 11% of the children sampled were infected with wild virus (J. Andrus et al., unpublished results), and approximately 20% of the environmental samples contained wild poliovirus (E. Marques et al., unpublished results). Wild poliovirus sequences were also detected directly by PCR of processed sewage samples (unpublished results).

The extent to which this approach can be generalized remains to be evaluated. Environmental studies were quite valuable in monitoring poliovirus transmission before the introduction of OPV (Melnick, 1947; Gravelle and Chin, 1961; Metcalf et al., 1988), and are still useful in countries where IPV is exclusively used for routine immunization (Pöyry et al., 1988). However, the use of OPV in most of the world has resulted in the overwhelming prevalence of OPV-derived polioviruses in most environmental specimens. The technical difficulties of detecting minute proportions of wild polioviruses in the environment (especially where OPV is distributed year-round) has reduced the potential value of environmental surveillance studies. The exceptional sensitivity and specificity of PCR for detecting wild poliovirus genomes in mixed samples (Fig. 12; Yang et al., 1992) may again permit the routine use of environmental surveillance. It may be possible, with the appropriate methodologic development, to establish a parallel surveillance system not dependent upon the appearance of paralytic cases. Ultimately, the inability to detect wild polioviruses in communities where they could be

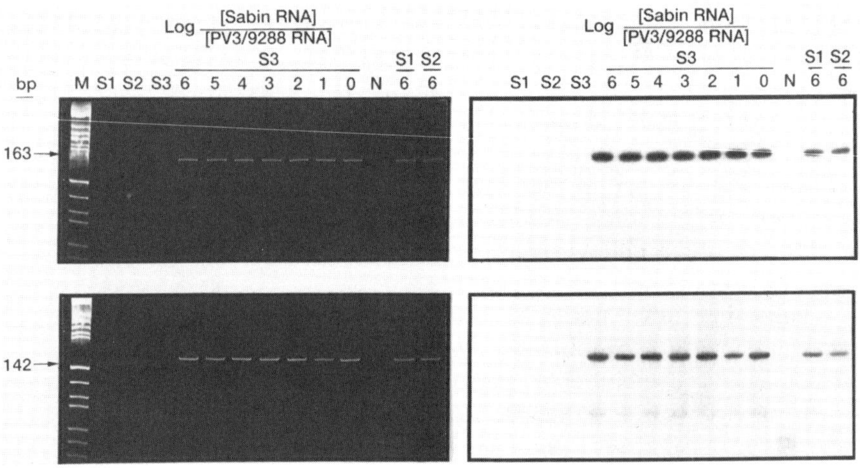

FIGURE 12 Selective detection of PV3/9288/MEX89 RNA in the presence of excess Sabin poliovaccine templates. Serial 10-fold dilutions of purified Sabin 3 RNA (1μg to 1 pg), or high template concentrations (1 μg) of Sabin 1 and 2 RNAs, were mixed with a constant amount of PV3/9288/MEX89 RNA (1 pg), and amplification reactions were performed using 9288/PCR-1 + 9288/PCR-2 (upper panels) and 9288/PCR-3 + 9288/PCR-4 (lower panels). The logarithm of the molar ratio of Sabin template to PV3/9288/MEX89 template is indicated above each sample lane. Products were resolved by polyacrylamide gel electrophoresis and visualized by ethidium bromide fluorescence (left panels) or autoradiography of ^{32}P-labeled products (right panels). (From Yang et al., 1992.)

readily detected previously provides supportive evidence that local chains of transmission have been broken.

VII. REMAINING SURVEILLANCE QUESTIONS

An integrated approach to poliomyelitis surveillance has deepened our understanding of the underlying dynamics of wild poliovirus transmission. The methods for detecting and identifying wild polioviruses are becoming increasingly faster, more sensitive, more precise, and more widely applicable. We have obtained partial answers to the set of basic epidemiologic questions that we initially considered. As answers to these first questions are found, we confront a new series of questions, again aimed at finding the most efficient means to break the chains of poliovirus transmission:

1. What are the limits of sensitivity for detecting wild polioviruses in the environment?
2. What are the quantitative effects of mass immunization campaigns on poliovirus circulation, and do these effects differ by serotype?
3. What is the minimum number of susceptibles in the community required to maintain transmission?
4. What is the relationship between infections in urban communities and adjacent rural areas?
5. What factors determine the rate and extent of transmission in areas having high population densities?
6. Is it possible to reconstruct the broad historical patterns of poliovirus transmission?

Exploration of these and related questions will require the best collaborative efforts of program managers, epidemiologists, virologists, and environmental scientists. The reward for these efforts will be a more direct path to the eradication of poliomyelitis.

VIII. CONCLUDING REMARKS

The long era of paralytic poliomyelitis is in twilight. The vigorous strategies applied thus far have had stunning success (de Quadros et al., 1991). We have already witnessed the disappearance of several major wild poliovirus lineages, and anticipate the extinction of many more in the near future. Nonetheless, formidable challenges lie ahead. Eradication activities are increasingly concentrated in regions with intense endemicity, high population densities, and reduced local infrastructure. However, our methods and tools are steadily improving to meet these challenges. We hope that a lasting legacy of the Poliomyelitis Eradication Initiative will be a stronger link between epidemiologic surveillance, laboratory studies, and programmatic action. We also look forward to the full establishment of a global network of diagnostic laboratories ready to apply the most powerful available tools to contribute to the worldwide triumph over poliomyelitis and other human diseases.

ACKNOWLEDGMENTS

We thank the virologists and epidemiologists throughout the world who contributed poliovirus samples for our studies, especially those from the Laboratory Network of the Americas: Jorge Boshell, Patricia Cáceres, Barbara Hull, Paula Padula, Victor Peña, Juan Ruiz Gómez, and Rosalba Salas. We also thank our CDC colleagues who have worked with us with outstanding skill and dedication. Kathy Crane, Mary Flemister, Beverlie Hamby, and George Marchetti prepared the poliovirus isolates. Brian Holloway, Edwin George, and Melissa Olson prepared the synthetic oligodeoxynucleotides used so extensively in our studies. Sharon Bloom (visiting from Stanford Medical School), Ana Maria Filippis (Fundação Oswaldo Cruz), Galina Lipskaya (visiting from Moscow State University), Michael McDonough, Rebeca Rico-Hesse (now at Yale University), Maria Sanz (visiting from Biokit, S.A., Barcelona), Su-Ju Yang, and Zheng Du-Ping (visiting from the Jiangxi Anti-Epidemic Station, China) contributed to our poliovirus sequence database. The vital assistance and collaboration of the Center for Prevention Services (CDC), the Pan American Health Organization, the World Health Organization, and the Task Force for Child Survival is gratefully acknowledged. Lina De was supported by the Poliomyelitis Eradication Initiative of the Expanded Program on Immunization, Pan American Health Organization, Washington. We thank Frederick Murphy (now at the University of California, Davis) for his leadership as Director, Center for Infectious Diseases, Centers for Disease Control.

REFERENCES

Balanant, J., Guillot, S., Candréa, A., Délpéyroux, F., and Crainic, R. (1991). *Virology 184*:645–654.

Benyesh-Melnick, M., Melnick, J. J., Rawls, W. E., Wimberly, I., Barrera-Oro, J., Ben-Porath, E., and Rennick, V. (1967). *Am. J. Epidemiol. 86*:112–136.

Bernal, A., García-Sáiz, A., Llácer, A., de Ory, F., Tello, O., and Nájera, R. (1987). *Am. J. Epidemiol. 126*:67–76.

Crainic, R., Coullin, P., Blondel, B., Cabau, N., Boué, A., and Horodniceanu, F. (1983). *Infect. Immun. 41*:1217–1225.

da Silva, E. E., Pallansch, M. A., Holloway, B. P., Cuoto Oliveira, M. J., Schatzmayr, H. G., and Kew, O. M. (1991). *Intervirology 32*:149–159.

de Quadros, C. A., Andrus, J. K., Olivé, J.-M., da Silveira, C. M., Eikhoff, R. M., Carrasco, P., Fitzsimmons, J. W., and Pinheiro, F. P. (1991). *Pediatr. Infect. Dis. J. 10*:222–229.

Domingo, E., Mateu, M. G., Martínez, M. A., Dopazo, J., Moya, A., and Sobrino, F. (1990). In *Applied Virology Research*, vol. 2, E. Kurstak, R. G. Marusyk, F. A. Murphy, and M. H. V. Van Regenmortel (Eds.), Plenum Press, New York, pp. 233–266.

Eigen, M., and Beibricher, C. K. (1988). In *RNA Genetics*, E. Domingo, J. J. Holland, and P. Ahlquist (Eds.), CRC Press, Boca Raton, FL.

Enterovirus Research Centre, Bombay (1990). Annual Report of Poliomyelitis Surveillance. Indian Council of Medical Research, New Delhi.

Evans, A. S. (1984). *Prog. Med. Virol. 29*:141–165.

Faden, H., Modlin, J. F., Thomas, M. L., McBean, A. M., Ferdon, M. B., and Ogra, P. L. (1990). *J. Infect. Dis. 162*:1291–1297.

Fenner, F., Henderson, D. A., Arita, I., Ježek, Z., and Ladnyi, I. D. (1988). *Smallpox and Its Eradication*, 1st ed. World Health Organization, Geneva.

Ferguson, M., Qui, Y.-H., Minor, P. D., Magrath, D. A., Spitz, M., and Schild, G. C. (1982). *Lancet 1*:122–124.

Figueroa, J. P., Ashley, D., King, D., and Hull, B. (1989). *J. Med. Virol. 29*:315–319.

Filman, D. J., Syed, R., Chow, M., Macadam, A. J., Minor, P. D., and Hogle, J. M. (1989). *EMBO J. 8*:1567–1579.

Fitch, W. M., and Margoliash, E. (1967). *Science 155*:279–284.

Gear, J. H. S. (1984). *Rev. Infect. Dis. 6*:S379–S384.

Glikmann, G., Pedersen, M., and Petersen, I. (1987). *J. Virol. Methods. 18*:25-36.

Gravelle, C. R., and Chin, T. D. Y. (1961). *J. Infect. Dis. 109*:205–209.

Grist, N., and Bell, E. (1984). *Rev. Infect. Dis. 6*:S385–S386.

Hayward, J. C., Gillespie, S. M., Kaplan, K. M., Packer, R., Pallansch, M., Plotkin, S., and Schonberger, L. B. (1989). *Pediatr. Infect. Dis. J. 8*:611–616.

Henderson, R. H., Keja, J., Hayden, G. A., Galazka, A., Clements, J., and Chan, C. (1988). *Bull. WHO 66*:535–543.

Hogle, J. M., Chow, M., and Filman, D. J. (1985). *Science 299*:1353–1365.

Holland, J. J., Domingo, E., de la Torre, J. C., and Steinhauer, D. A. (1990). *J. Virol. 64*:3960–3962.

Höltke, H. J., and Kessler, C. (1989). *Nucleic Acids Res. 18*:5843–5851.

Jansen, R. W., Siegl, G., and Lemon, S. N. (1990). *Proc. Natl. Acad. Sci. USA 87*: 2867–2871.

Kew, O. M., Nottay, B. K., Hatch, M. H., Nakano, J. H., and Obijeski, J. F. (1981). *J. Gen. Virol. 56*:337–347.

Kew, O. M., and Nottay, B. K. (1984). In *Modern Approaches to Vaccines*, R. Chanock and R. Lerner (Eds.). Cold Spring Harbor Laboratory, Cold Spring Harbor, New York, pp. 357–362.

Kew, O. M., Nottay, B. K., and Obijeski, J. F. (1984). In *Methods in Virology*, vol. 8, K. Maramorosch and H. Koprowski (Eds.). Academic Press, New York, pp. 41–84.

Kew, O. M., Nottay, B. K., Rico-Hesse, R. R., and Pallansch, M. A. (1990). In *Applied Virology Research*, vol. 2, E. Kurstak, R. G. Marusyk, F. A. Murphy, and M. H. V. Van Regenmortel (Eds.). Plenum Press, New York, pp. 199–221.

Kim-Farley, R. J., Bart, K. J., Schonberger, L. B., Orenstein, W. A., Nkowane, B. M., Hinman, A. R., Kew, O. M., Hatch, M. H., and Kaplan, J. E. (1984). *Lancet* 2:1315–1317.

Kinnunen, L., Huovilainen, A., Pöyry, T., and Hovi, T. (1990). *J. Gen. Virol. 71*: 317–324.

Kitamura, N., Semler, B., Rothberg, P. G., Larsen, G. R., Adler, C. J., Dorner, A. J., Emini, E. A., Hanecak, R., Lee, J. J., van der Werf, S., Anderson, C. W., and Wimmer, E. (1981). *Nature 291*:547–553.

Kwok, S., and Sninsky, J. J. (1989). In *PCR Technology, Principles and Applications for DNA Amplification*, H. A. Erlich (Ed.). Stockton Press, New York, pp. 235–244.

Lemon, S. B., and Robertson, S. E. (1991). *Prog. Med. Virol. 38*:42–55.
Melnick, J. L. (1947). *Am. J. Hyg. 45*:240–253.
Melnick, J. L. (1990). In *Virology*, 2nd ed., B. N. Fields, D. M. Knipe, R. M. Chanock, M. S. Hirsch, J. L. Melnick, T. P. Monath, and B. Roizman (Eds.). Raven Press, New York, pp. 549–605.
Melton, D. A., Krieg, P. A., Rebagliati, M. R., Maniatis, T., Zinn, K., and Green, M. R. (1984). *Nucleic Acids Res. 12*:7035–7056.
Metcalf, T. G., Jiang, X., Estes, M. K., and Melnick, J. L. (1988). *Prog. Med. Virol. 35*:186–214.
Minor, P. D., Schild, G. C., Ferguson, M., Mackay, A., Magrath, D. I., John, A., Yates, P. J., and Spitz, M. (1982). *J. Gen. Virol. 61*:167–176.
Minor, P. D., Ferguson, M., Evans, D. M. A., Almond, J. W., and Icenogle, J. P. (1986a). *J. Gen. Virol. 67*:1283–1291.
Minor, P. D., John, A., Ferguson, M., and Icenogle, J. P. (1986b). *J. Gen. Virol. 67*:693–706.
Morens, D. M., Pallansch, M. A., and Moore, M. (1990). In *Textbook of Human Virology*, 2nd ed., R. B. Belshe (Ed.). C. V. Mosby–Year Book, St. Louis, MO, pp. 427–497.
Nakano, J. H., Gelfand, H. M., and Cole, J. T. (1963). *Amer. J. Hyg. 78*:214–226.
Nakano, J. H., Hatch, M. H., Thieme, M. L., and Nottay, B. (1978). *Prog. Med. Virol. 24*:178–206.
Nkowane, B. M., Wassilak, S. G. F., Orenstein, W. A., Bart, K. J., Schonberger, L. B., Hinman, A. R., and Kew, O. M. (1987). *JAMA 257*:1335–1340.
Nomoto, A., Omata, T., Toyoda, H., Kuge, S., Horie, H., Kataoka, Y., Genba, Y., Nakano, Y., and Imura, N. (1982). *Proc. Natl. Acad. Sci. USA 79*:5793–5797.
Nottay, B. K., Kew, O. M., Hatch, M. H., Heyward, J. T., and Obijeski, J. F. (1981). *Virology 108*:405–423.
Osterhaus, A. D. M. E., van Wezel, A. L., Hazendonk, T. G., UytdeHaag, F. G. C. M., van Asten, J. A. A. M., and van Steenis, B. (1983). *Intervirology 20*:129–136.
Page, G. S., Mosser, A. G., Hogle, J. M., Filman, D. J., Rueckert, R. R., and Chow, M. (1988). *J. Virol. 62*:1781–1794.
Pallansch, M. A., Kew, O. M., Semler, B. L., Omilianowski, D. R., Anderson, C. W., Wimmer, E., and Rueckert, R. R. (1984). *J. Virol. 49*:873–880.
Pan American Health Organization (1985). *Eradication of Indigenous Transmission of the Wild Poliovirus from the Americas, Plan of Action*, Washington, D.C.
Pan American Health Organization (1991a). *EPI Newsletter 13*.
Pan American Health Organization (1991b). Proceedings of the Ninth Meeting of the EPI Technical Advisory Group on Vaccine-Preventable Diseases. Guatemala, 12–15 March, 1991.
Pan American Health Organization (1992). *Polio Surveillance in the Americas: Weekly Bulletin 7*(7), 1992.
Parks, W. P., Queiroga, L. T., and Melnick, J. L. (1967). *Am. J. Epidemiol. 85*:469–478.
Patriarca, P., Laender, F., Palmeira, G., Couto Oliveira, M. J., Lima Filho, I., de Souza Dantes, M. C., Tenorio Cordeiro, M., Risi, J. B., and Orenstein, W. A. (1988). *Lancet 1*:429–432.

Paul, J. R. (1971). *A History of Poliomyelitis.* Yale University Press, New Haven.
Pöyry, T., Kinnunen, L., Kapsenburg, J., Kew, O., and Hovi, T. (1990). *J. Gen. Virol. 71*:2535–2541.
Pöyry, T., Stenvik, M., and Hovi, T. (1988). *Appl. Environ. Microbiol. 54*:371–374.
Racaniello, V. R., and Baltimore, D. (1981). *Proc. Natl. Acad. Sci. USA 78*:4887–4891.
Reid, R. S. (1989). *Rev. Infect. Dis. 11*:S655–S658.
Reynolds, C., Page, G., Zhou, H., and Chow, M. (1990). *Virology 184*:391–396.
Rico-Hesse, R., Pallansch, M. A., Nottay, B. K., and Kew, O. M. (1987). *Virology 160*: 311–322.
Rombaut, B., Boeye, A., Ferguson, M., Minor, P. D., Mosser, A., and Rueckert, R. R. (1990). *Virology 174*:305–307.
Rueckert, R. R. (1990). In *Virology*, 2nd ed., B. N. Fields, D. M. Knipe, R. M. Chanock, M. S. Hirsch, J. L. Melnick, T. P. Monath, and B. Roizman (Eds.). Raven Press, New York, pp. 507–548.
Rueckert, R. R., and Wimmer, E. (1984). *J. Virol. 50*:957–959.
Sabin, A. B. (1985). *J. Infect. Dis. 151*:420–436.
Sabin, A. B., and Boulger, L. R. (1973). *J. Biol. Standard. 1*:115–118.
Sabin, A. B., Ramos-Alvarez, M., Alvarez-Amezquita, J., Pelon, W., Michaels, R. H., Spigland, I., Koch, M. A., Barnes, J. M., and Rhim, J. S. (1960). *JAMA 173*: 1521–1526.
Saiki, R. K., Scharf, S., Faloona, F., Mullis, K. B., Horn, G. T., Ehrlich, H. A., and Arnheim, N. (1985). *Science 230*:1350–1354.
Salk, J. E., Krech, U., Youngner, J. S., Bennett, B. L., Lewis, L. J., and Bazeley, P. L. (1954). *Am. J. Public Health 44*:563.
Salk, J., and Salk, D. (1977). *Science 195*:834–847.
Schaap, A. P., Akhavan, H., and Romano, L. J. (1989). *Clin. Chem. 35*:1863–1864.
Slater, P. E., Orenstein, W. A., Morag, A., Avni, A., Handsher, R., Green, M. S., Costin, C., Yarrow, A., Rishpon, S., Havkin, O., Ben-Zvi, T., Kew, O. M., Rey, M., Epstein, I., Swartz, T. A., and Melnick, J. L. (1990). *Lancet 335*:1192–1198.
Smith, D. B., and Inglis, S. C. (1987). *J. Gen. Virol. 68*:2729–2740.
Stanway, G., Hughes, P. J., Mountfort, R. C., Reeve, P., Minor, P. D., Schild, G. C., and Almond, J. W. (1984). *Proc. Natl. Acad. Sci. USA 81*:1539–1543.
Steinhauer, D. A., and Holland, J. J. (1987). *Annu. Rev. Microbiol. 41*:409–433.
Strebel, P. M., Sutter, R. W., Cochi, S. L., Biellik, R. J., Brink, E. W., Kew, O. M., Pallansch, M. A., Orenstein, W. A., and Hinman, A. R. (1992). *Clin. Infect. Dis. 14*:568–579.
Sutter, R. W., Patriarca, P. A., Brogan, S., Malankar, P. G., Pallansch, M. A., Kew, O. M., Bass, A. G., Cochi, S. L., Alexander, J., Hall, D. B., Sulieman, A. J. M., Al-Ghassany, A. A. K., and El-Bualy, M. S. (1991). *Lancet 338*:715–720.
Task Force for Child Survival. (1991). *World Immunization News 7*:19–24.
Toyoda, H., Kohara, M., Kataoka, Y., Suganuma, T., Omata, T., Imura, N., and Nomoto, A. (1984). *J. Mol. Biol. 174*:561–585.
Toyoda, H., Nicklin, M. J. H., Murray, M. G., Anderson, C. W., Dunn, J. J., Studier, F. W., and Wimmer, E. (1986). *Cell 45*:761–770.
van Wezel, A. L., and Hazendonk, A. G. (1979). *Intervirology 11*:2–8.

Varughese, P. V., Carter, A. O., Acres, S. E., and Furesz, J. (1989). *Can. J. Public Health* *80*:363–368.
Ward, C. D., Stokes, M. A. M., and Flanegan, J. B. (1988). *J. Virol.* *62*:558–562.
World Health Assembly (1988). *Global Eradication of Poliomyelitis by the Year 2000.* Resolution WHA41.28, Geneva.
World Health Organization (1989). *Manual for Immunization Programme Managers on Activities Related to Polio Eradication.* (WHO/EPI/89.1).
World Health Organization (1990). *Manual for the Virological Investigation of Poliomyelitis.* (WHO/EPI/CDS/POLIO/90.1).
World Health Organization (1991). *Weekly Epidemiol. Rec.* *65*:361–364; *66*:49–54, 70–71, 81–83.
Yang, C.-F., De, L., Holloway, B. P., Pallansch, M. A., and Kew, O. M. (1991). *Virus Res.* *20*:159–179.
Yang, C.-F., De, L., Yang, S.-J., Gómez, J. R., Cruz, J. R., Holloway, B. P., Pallansch, M. A., and Kew, O. M. (1992). *Virus Res.*, submitted.

10

POLIOMYELITIS ERADICATION

The Expanded Programme on Immunization of the World Health Organization

Nicholas A. Ward, Robert J. Kim-Farley, Julie B. Milstien, Harry F. Hull, and Carole Torel *World Health Organization, Geneva, Switzerland*

Ciro de Quadros *Pan American Health Organization, Washington, D.C.*

I. INTRODUCTION

The mission of the Expanded Programme on Immunization (EPI) is to reduce death and disability from six vaccine-preventable diseases (tuberculosis, diphtheria, tetanus, pertussis, measles, and poliomyelitis) by providing immunization services for all children and women of childbearing age in all parts of the world. The main thrust of the program has been to ensure that potent vaccines, stored and transported in an effective cold chain, are administered in full courses to children as early as possible in their first year of life, compatible with developing immunity. In addition, women of childbearing age should have received protective courses of immunization against tetanus to remove the threat of neonatal tetanus.

As immunization coverage levels improved through the 1980s, it became realistic to establish disease reduction targets for poliomyelitis, neonatal tetanus, and measles. Establishing these targets had the additional benefit of further promoting and developing the EPI, as well as intensifying specific control measures for each disease. Targets by the year 1995 were established for the elimination of neonatal tetanus and for the reduction by 90 and 95% of measles morbidity and mortality, respectively.

In May, 1988, the World Health Assembly (WHA) committed the World Health Organization (WHO) to the global eradication of poliomyelitis by the year 2000 (WHA, 1988). The WHA emphasized that eradication efforts should be pursued in ways that strengthen the development of the EPI, fostering its contribution, in turn, to the development of primary health care.

The WHA had as background the Declaration of Talloires (1988), which also cited the goal of poliomyelitis eradication. The Declaration was issued by the Task Force for Child Survival (comprised of WHO, UNICEF, the World Bank, United Nations Development Plan, and the Rockefeller Foundation) following a meeting in March 1988 in Talloires, France, attended by world leaders in health and development.

The experience gained in the Americas, which began its drive for hemispheric eradication of circulating wild poliovirus in 1985, was also used to develop the global poliomyelitis eradication initiative (Pan American Health Organization, 1985).

The progress of the EPI has provided grounds for optimism that an administrative structure and disease control strategy can be developed to allow poliomyelitis to be eradicated within the next decade. In 1974, when the EPI was started, it was estimated that fewer than 5% of children in developing countries were adequately immunized against the six common childhood diseases, including poliomyelitis. By the end of 1989, 74% of children worldwide had received a full course of poliomyelitis vaccine before age 12 months. This figure reached over 80% by the end of 1990 (Figs. 1 and 2).

It is hoped that the EPI target of 90% full immunization coverage, including all scheduled doses of poliomyelitis vaccines, can be achieved by the year 2000. By itself, this coverage would lead to a marked reduction in the incidence of the disease. When supplemented by additional policies to identify and eliminate residual, persisting chains of wild poliovirus transmission, there is every reason for optimism that poliomyelitis can be eradicated before the end of the decade.

The poliomyelitis eradication initiative aims for global eradication of the disease through a strengthened EPI. Its broad objectives are that no case of clinical poliomyelitis occurs associated with wild poliovirus, and no wild poliovirus can be identified worldwide through sampling of communities and environment.

II. STATUS OF POLIOMYELITIS: 1990

Following the development and use of effective poliomyelitis vaccines in the 1950s, the incidence of acute poliomyelitis rapidly declined in industrialized nations. Very few cases now occur in these countries and

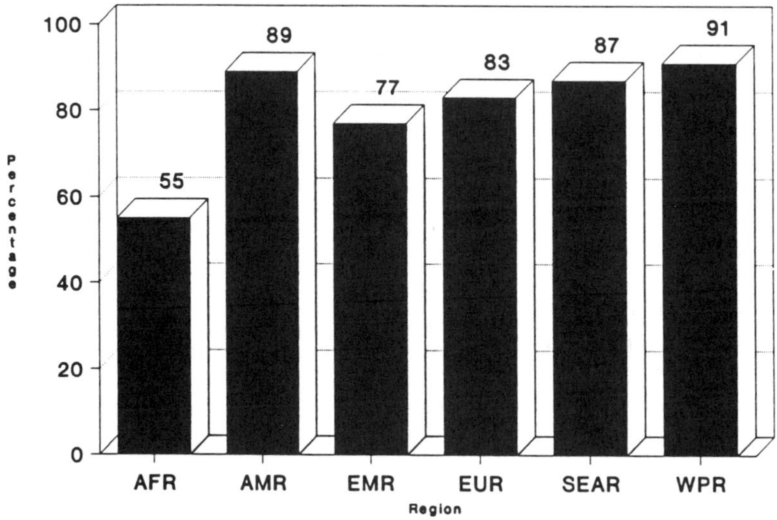

FIGURE 1 Immunization coverage with full courses of poliomyelitis vaccines in infants, by WHO Region, December, 1989.

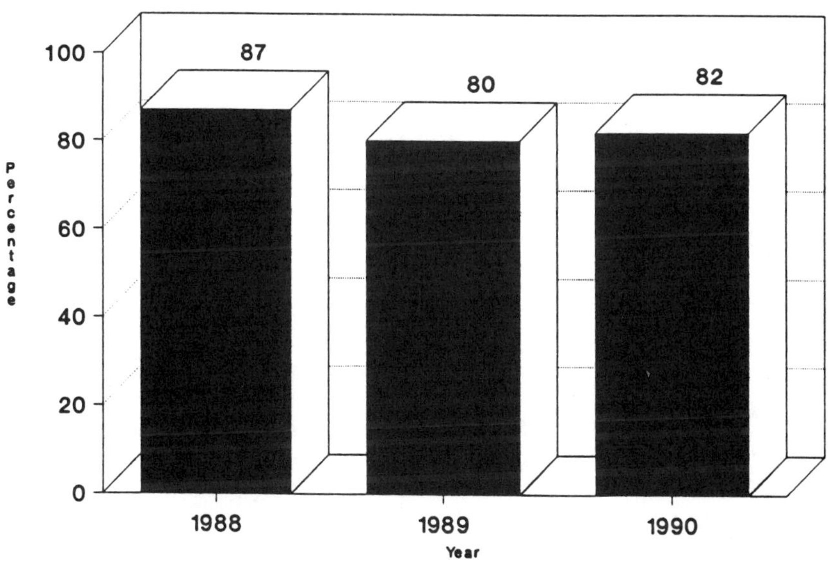

FIGURE 2 Global immunization coverage with full courses of poliomyelitis vaccines in infants, 1988–1990.

most can be attributed to importations, persistent transmission in minority groups, or are vaccine associated.

The pioneer work of Nicholas (1977) and Ofusu-Amaah (1977), who examined schoolchildren in Ghana for evidence of residual acute flaccid paralysis following polio, produced evidence that the disease was as widespread in the tropics and in developing countries as it had previously been in the temperate, industrialized world. This evidence was subsequently confirmed through many "lameness" surveys, which demonstrated that frequently fewer than 10% of cases were being officially reported (Table 1).

Greater awareness of the widespread prevalence of poliomyelitis coincided with marked increases in immunization coverage levels in children, facilitated by the development of the EPI. However, improved immunization coverage was not matched by corresponding improvements in surveillance. Consequently, although surveillance is much improved, officially reported cases can only be interpreted in most regions as showing

TABLE 1 Reported Incidence of Acute Poliomyelitis: Estimated Incidence Based on Lameness Surveys in 13 Countries and Reporting Completeness, 1978–1981

	Incidence of Poliomyelitis per 100,000 Population		
	Incidence Estimated from Lameness Surveys	Reported Incidence	Reporting Completeness (%)
Bangladesh	4	0.12	3
Burma	18	1.1	6
United Republic of Cameroon	24	1.2	5
Egypt	7	1.8	26
Ghana	31	2.5	7
India	18	2.1	12
Indonesia	13	0.1	1
Ivory Coast	34	1.2	4
Malawi	28	1.2	4
Nepal	5	0.3	6
Philippines	194	2.1	11
Thailand	7	1.7	24
Yemen	14	3.3	24

Source: From *Wkly. Epidemiol. Rec.* (1981).

trends in the incidence of poliomyelitis (sometimes confounded by variability in the completeness of reporting) and not as documenting absolute, reliable incidence (Fig. 3).

The distribution of cases of paralytic poliomyelitis in 1989, by WHO region is shown in Figure 4. In that year, 22,421 cases were officially reported, with 63% originating in Southeast Asia, 23% in the western Pacific, 10% in the Eastern Mediterranean, and 1% in each of the American and European regions. The African region, reporting only 4% of global cases, suffers more than any other region from incomplete reporting, both in terms of the percentage of cases officially reported and in the receipt of expected reports.

Figure 5 indicates trends in regional incidence rates for cases of acute poliomyelitis over a 16 year period from 1974 to 1989. These data suggest a steady decline in the incidence of the disease, especially since 1982 when infant immunization rates markedly increased through the acceleration of EPI activities.

Two factors are likely to produce real or apparent increases in the incidence of reported acute poliomyelitis as the eradication initiative

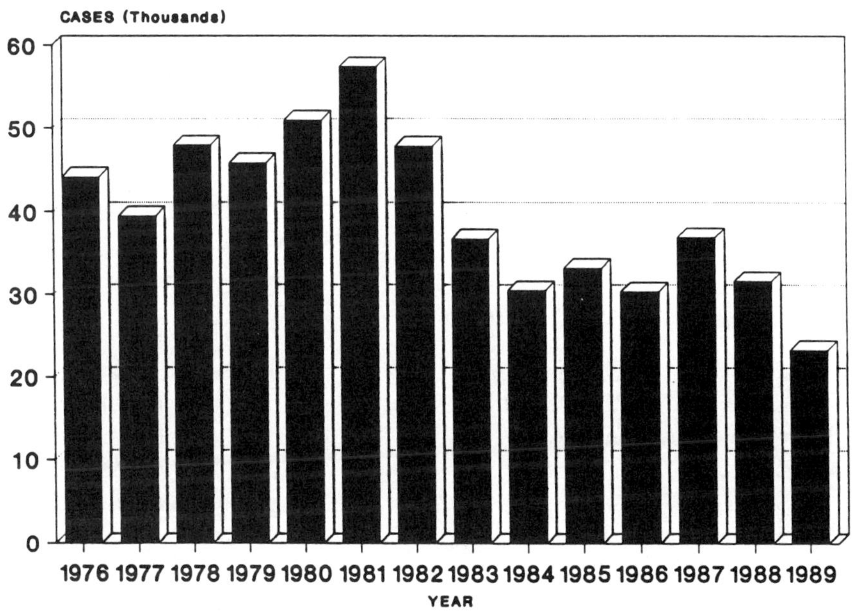

FIGURE 3 Reported global incidence of acute poliomyelitis, 1976–1989.

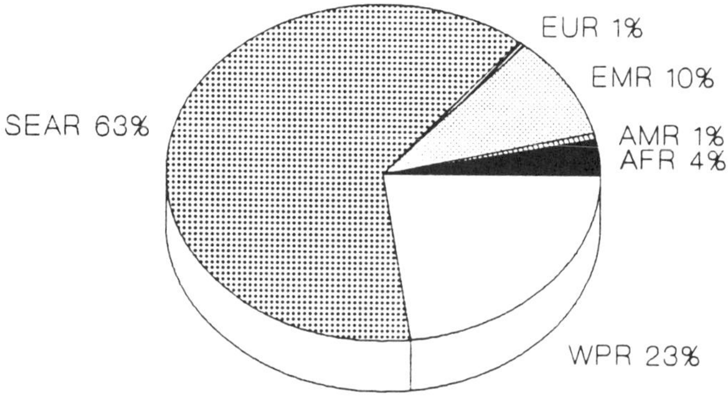

FIGURE 4 Distribution of reported poliomyelitis cases by WHO Region, 1989.

progresses. First, moderate immunization coverage levels carry the risk of temporary interruption of wild virus transmission, followed by a build-up of susceptibles and subsequent major epidemics if the virus is reintroduced. A number of countries, after a period of steadily declining numbers of cases, have suffered the disappointment of unexpected epidemics if the virus was not totally eradicated from the region. Second, improvements in surveillance, which is an increasingly high EPI priority, may lead to better reporting of cases and an apparent increase in incidence. Administrators and political leaders who have given strong support to the eradication initiative need to be aware that an increased incidence of the disease does not necessarily imply program failure.

III. ADMINISTRATIVE STRUCTURE FOR THE POLIOMYELITIS ERADICATION INITIATIVE

Since the WHA resolution to eradicate poliomyelitis stressed that it should be carried out within the context of EPI, the responsible officials within WHO are the regional advisers and, at the country level, the national EPI managers.

Within WHO, through the support of Rotary International and the Centers for Disease Control, Atlanta, a five-person team has been created within WHO/EPI headquarters to provide technical guidance to health staff in the regions and countries. In each region, except the Americas, an epidemiologist funded by Rotary International has been appointed to work primarily on the initiative.

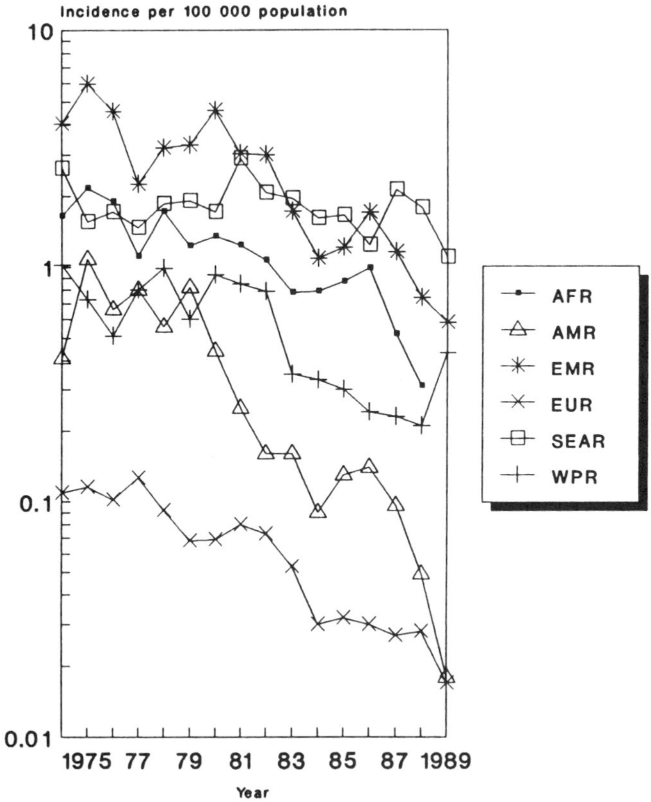

FIGURE 5 Reported incidence rates of poliomyelitis, by region, 1974–1989.

At the global level and in most regions, consultative or technical advisory groups were formed to advise on the development of strategies and policies most likely to achieve eradication of the disease. The first such global consultation took place in Geneva in September 1988, with a second meeting in 1989 and a third in 1990, at which, based on 2 years' experience, revised strategies for eradication activities were defined.

IV. INITIAL PLANNING FOR POLIOMYELITIS ERADICATION

At the start of the initiative, in 1988, managers were requested to assess the stage of achievement of EPI in their countries. Four stages of progress were defined.

1. *Stage D* The country had achieved immunization coverage of only 50% or less, or the coverage figure was unknown and there were more than 10 new cases of poliomyelitis each year, or the incidence was unknown. In this stage, priority was placed on increasing immunization coverage and developing sentinel surveillance.

2. *Stage C* Immunization coverage was over 50%, but there were still more than 10 new cases per year. The first priority remained increasing coverage, but greater emphasis was placed on developing surveillance.

3. *Stage B* Immunization coverage was over 50% and there were fewer than 10 new cases of acute poliomyelitis each year. At this stage, efforts were still to be placed on further increasing immunization coverage, aiming eventually for more than 90%, but surveillance was now of the highest importance, with full case investigation and laboratory confirmation of diagnosis.

4. *Stage A* Immunization coverage was over 80% and, in the presence of a reliable reporting system, no cases had been detected for over 3 years. Priority activities in this stage were to maintain immunization and surveillance and to investigate every case of acute flaccid paralysis.

This initial classification allowed EPI managers to assess priorities for action and develop policies appropriate for the epidemiologic status of poliomyelitis in their countries.

Seven areas for possible action were seen as being of particular importance:

1. *Immunization coverage,* aiming to achieve at least 80% coverage with a protective course of poliomyelitis vaccine within the first year of life, sustained for the age group 1–4 years, and in all geographic areas of the country.
2. *Surveillance* for suspected poliomyelitis cases, involving all areas, all reporting units with regular receipt of expected reports, including zero reporting, the use of a standard case definition, classification of isolated polioviruses, and full outbreak investigation and containment in countries reporting fewer than 50 cases per year.
3. *Vaccine quality control and laboratory services,* using only vaccine meeting WHO production requirements, developing the laboratory capacity to confirm clinical diagnoses with access to facilities able to perform virus characterization and vaccine potency testing. In addition, poliovirus surveillance, including environmental sampling, was to be developed.

4. *Training* of health service staff on strategies to achieve high coverage, developing surveillance, and using social mobilization and training of laboratory staff for virus isolation, strain differentiation, and vaccine quality control.
5. *Social mobilization*: sustaining a political and financial commitment as well as developing national communication plans.
6. *Strengthening rehabilitation* services, especially at the community level as the incidence of cases reaches low levels.
7. *Research and development* across a wide range of subjects, including aiming for improved laboratory diagnostic tests, epidemiologic studies on the transmission of both wild and vaccine virus strains, better control strategies, improved orally administered attenuated virus vaccines, the place of combinations of available vaccines.

In addition to these major areas for policy development, which were embodied in regional and national plans of action, one further principle for eradication was developed: eradication was to be particularly pursued by establishing and extending poliomyelitis-free geographical areas. At the same time, the incidence of poliomyelitis in other areas and countries would be reduced to a more manageable level by raising immunization coverage and establishing surveillance and outbreak response through a strengthened EPI.

Workshops were held in all regions; EPI managers and other responsible staff were briefed on the principles and policies of poliomyelitis eradication. In the course of these workshops, they developed and planned for specific activities aimed at achieving poliomyelitis eradication.

The seven areas for action have remained unchanged since policies for the eradication initiative were first developed in 1988. However, experience gained in various countries, especially in the Americas, has led to some rethinking of the principles on which successful eradication is most likely to be founded.

V. POLIOMYELITIS IN THE AMERICAS

In May, 1985, the Director of the Pan American Health Organization announced his organization's commitment to the goal of poliomyelitis eradication in the Western Hemisphere by 1990.

A key management tool of this commitment was the creation of an interagency coordinating committee, including representatives from all the major agencies involved in supporting the initiative. This committee had a key role not only in ensuring that adequate resources were available but also in being involved and informed on technical issues, policies, and progress. Similar groups were established in many countries to provide further interagency coordination and help to ensure mobilization of resources.

Countries were initially classified as either polio-infected, in which poliomyelitis cases had been reported within the previous 3 years; or poliomyelitis free, with no cases reported for 3 years, the latter being classified as high or low risk according to whether immunization coverage was over or under 80%.

In the poliomyelitis-infected countries, a policy of national vaccination days was developed: all available resources were mobilized to ensure that all children under 5 years of age received a dose of trivalent oral polio vaccine (OPV) on two occasions each year. This method was a potent weapon in supplementing routine immunization services and, coincidentally, led to marked increases in the uptake of all other EPI vaccines.

In view of the relatively small number of cases being reported in the region, it was possible to develop a policy in which each case could be treated as an emergency and investigated immediately. For operational purposes, cases were classified as suspected poliomyelitis if any child aged under 15 years developed acute paralysis, or if paralytic illness suspected as being polio occurred in a person of any age; probable poliomyelitis in any case of acute flaccid paralysis for which no other cause was immediately determined; and confirmed poliomyelitis when poliovirus was isolated, linkage with other cases could be demonstrated, paralysis persisted after 60 days, or the patient died or was lost to follow-up. Weekly reporting of numbers of suspected cases was instituted, with feedback to all countries if outbreaks occurred. Expert personnel were made available to all countries in which epidemiologic surveillance required strengthening. In the polio-free countries, a monetary reward was instituted for the reporting of subsequently confirmed cases.

An effective laboratory network was established with national laboratories and regional reference laboratories performing diagnostic tests using standardized reagents and methodologies.

The results achieved were immediate and dramatic. In the countries where polio was endemic, the policy of national vaccination days reduced poliomyelitis incidence to far lower levels than ever before recorded. Figure 6 shows the impact of these policies in Brazil.

By 1988, the initiative had consolidated its achievements and was backed by strong administrative and managerial support. Computerized information systems were installed in every country with feedback

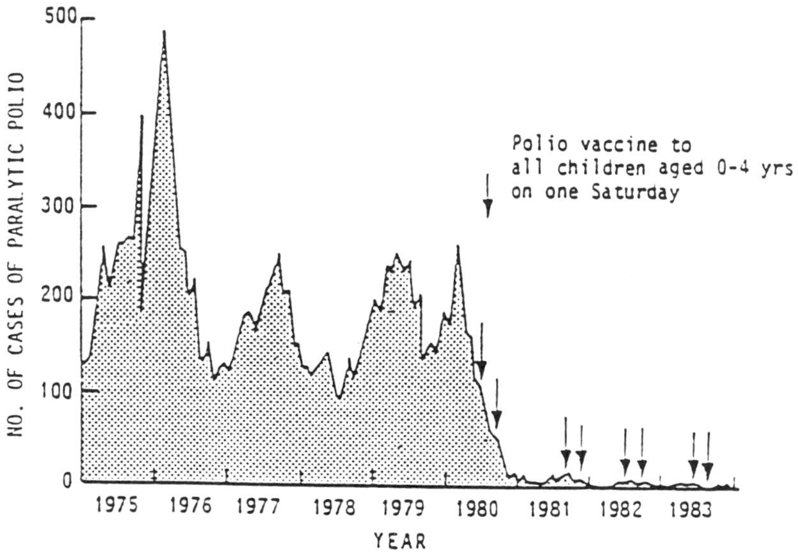

FIGURE 6 Reported cases of acute poliomyelitis, Brazil, 1975–1983, showing the impact of national vaccination days.

provided to health workers, initially through a newsletter and later supplemented by an information sheet on the status of case and laboratory investigation.

By the end of the year, the countries had moved to implement special "mop-up" operations aimed at increasing immunization coverage in districts and municipalities reporting either low coverage or the recent presence or persistence of poliomyelitis cases. These high-risk areas were identified by effective monitoring at subnational levels.

Where transmission of wild poliovirus persisted, as it did for limited periods in Brazil and Mexico, reasons could be identified. The cause usually related to vaccine failure, mostly reflecting unsatisfactory seroconversion to type 3, which was the responsible type in most late epidemics. Correction of the factors responsible, including increasing the vaccine content of type 3 virus, rapidly corrected the problems and stopped transmission.

Concomitant with the reduced transmission, EPI staff in WHO and the countries were able to perfect a system of surveillance for paralysis. They reclassified cases and narrowed the definition of proved cases to allow more accurate assessment of the real epidemiologic situation. Paralysis had an incidence of 1–2 cases per 100,000 children under 15 years of age in the absence of acute poliomyelitis caused by wild poliovirus, due to other causes such as Guillain-Barré syndrome, vaccine-associated paralysis, or traumatic and transverse myelitis. This finding provided a baseline against which surveillance performance could be assessed. Monitoring other indicators such as the promptness of reporting, case investigation, and the completeness of specimen collection and follow-up to detect residual paralysis proved effective in improving surveillance.

The initiative in the Americas proved to be well managed, effectively obtaining and using resources adequate for the purposes of poliomyelitis eradication and acceleration of EPI. Above all, however, policies were developed that were apparently appropriate in tackling eradication of the virus based on its epidemiology. The success is demonstrated in the Western Hemisphere in Figure 7.

The experience in the Americas confirmed that poliomyelitis could be eradicated over a continental area. It demonstrated that it was possible

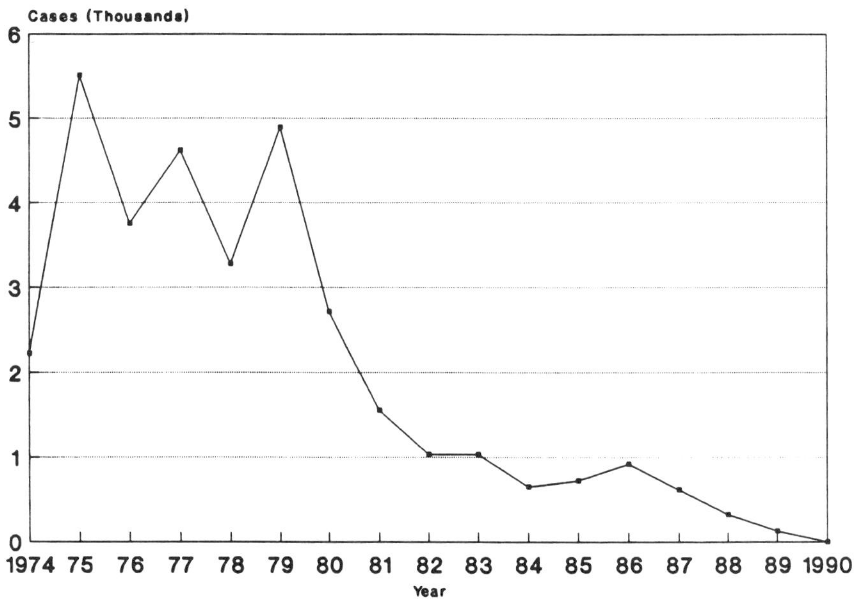

FIGURE 7 Reported cases of acute poliomyelitis in the Western Hemisphere, 1974–1990.

not only to stop transmission of the virus but also to establish surveillance and a laboratory network that could monitor and document progress. Most importantly, it demonstrated that supplementing delivery of all childhood vaccines through routine services, by the use of national and local vaccination days (i.e., the administration of OPV to all children of a defined age, usually those under 5 years, within a very short period of time), was highly effective in stopping persistent virus transmission.

This finding and success contrasted sharply with the increasingly frequent finding elsewhere in the world (Fig. 8) that, even with immunization coverage well over 80% apparently achieved with potent and well-stored vaccines, interruption of wild poliovirus transmission could not always be guaranteed.

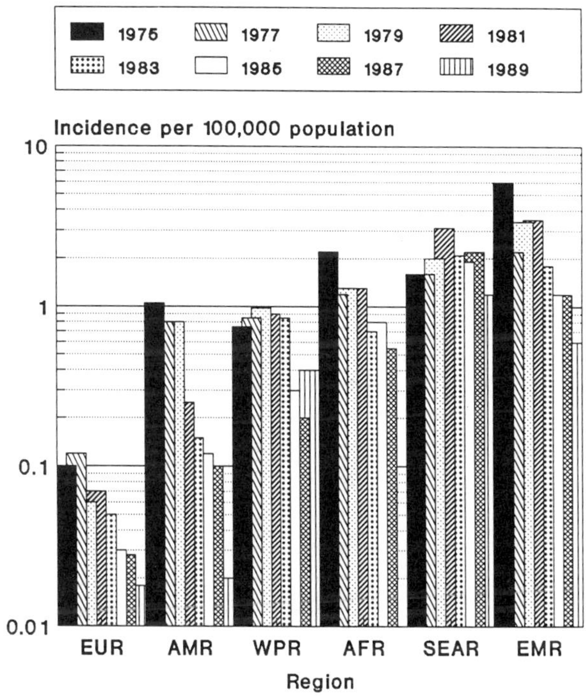

FIGURE 8 Reported incidence rates of poliomyelitis, by region. (Data reported to WHO as of July, 1990.)

VI. GLOBAL POLIOMYELITIS ERADICATION: PRESENT POLICIES

The Third Consultation on the Eradication of Poliomyelitis, meeting in Geneva in September, 1990, reviewed progress to date in all regions of the world and made recommendations that were later endorsed by the Global Advisory Group of the EPI. These recommendations, which supplemented the markedly successful EPI policies, now form the basis for global poliomyelitis eradication and are advocated by WHO to member states seeking to eradicate the disease.

A. Immunization Policies

The basis of poliomyelitis eradication rests firmly within the EPI and in its mandate to administer full courses of all scheduled vaccines to children, at an appropriate age, through the established infrastructure of fixed and outreach health services. The primary aim remains to achieve the highest possible level of immunization coverage, using potent vaccines that meet WHO production requirements and are subsequently stored and transported in an effective cold chain.

Immunization with presently available vaccines, whether administered through routine systems or through vaccination days, is highly effective in rapidly reducing the incidence of acute poliomyelitis. Interruption of wild virus transmission does not appear to occur immediately, however, even at high coverage levels, when only routine methods are used. Supplementary policies aimed at identifying high-risk areas and the administration of OPV within a short period of time to all possible susceptibles may be required. The key element of this policy revolves around displacing the wild virus from the community by saturating the community with high levels of coverage with vaccine virus in all possible susceptibles rather than only aiming to provide individual protection for each child.

It has long been realized that protection against poliomyelitis should be achieved before the time at which the child is at high risk of contracting the disease. To achieve this, WHO recommends the use of trivalent OPV as the vaccine of choice. There are no contraindications to its use. If the recipient has diarrhea at the time of immunization, the dose should still be given but not treated as one of the scheduled doses, and should be repeated 1 month later.

A recommended schedule for OPV, bacille Calmette-Guérin (BCG), measles, and diphtheria/pertussis/tetanus (DPT) vaccines has been promoted and widely implemented in many countries:

Contact	Age of child	Vaccines
1	At birth	OPV and BCG
2	6 weeks	OPV and DPT
3	10 weeks	OPV and DPT
4	14 weeks	OPV and DPT
5	9 months	Measles

The dose of OPV at birth is considered particularly important in urban areas and in countries where cases occur in the first year of life.

In vaccination days, the objective should be to give two or more doses per year to all children within a defined age, usually those up to the age of 5 years, within a short period of time, not usually longer than a week in any area. All available local resources (the media, teachers, religious and secular leaders) should be involved to ensure efficient and complete administration of the service and strong public support. Such vaccination days should use all EPI vaccines to raise immunization coverage for all target diseases.

Evidence in the Americas suggests that, like smallpox, poliomyelitis is a more focal disease than originally thought. Although, in view of the fact that 99% of cases are asymptomatic, it is not realistic to develop policies of local containment with tracing of contacts, it is desirable to develop activities around cases that will limit further spread. The policy of "mopping-up" addresses this issue. In this policy, high-risk areas are defined. In these areas, OPV is given house-to-house to all children within a defined age regardless of immunization status.

Experience has shown that these high-risk areas may involve 2–3% of the administrative units within a country. The area to be covered will vary according to the status of poliomyelitis within a country but could vary from a few thousand people, if there are many cases still occurring, to the whole country in the last stages of the initiative.

B. Surveillance

During the early stages of poliomyelitis eradication, while many cases are still occurring and before surveillance is efficient, the standard case definition of acute poliomyelitis has proved effective: "A case of poliomyelitis is defined as any patient with acute paralysis, including any child aged less than 15 years diagnosed to have the Guillain-Barré syndrome, for which no other cause can be identified."

As the number of cases declines to very low levels, it is possible that more specific definitions, excluding cases occurring at any age for which clear alternative diagnoses are evident, will become more practical.

WHO recommends that countries should develop surveillance as the critical strategy through which all cases of poliomyelitis are detected and the factors responsible for each case identified and analyzed. Such a strategy should allow for study of the epidemiology of the disease, forming the basis for sound and epidemiologically correct immunization policies. As examples of this, it is important to identify where cases are occurring, at which age, whether among specific groups within the community, whether there is a seasonal variation, and the location of cases occurring during the low season when local vaccination days may have a maximum impact.

It has been recommended that national programs establish case classification committees, consisting of pediatricians, neurologists, laboratory specialists, epidemiologists, and EPI staff, charged with classifying cases as poliomyelitis or not.

An additional responsibility of such a committee should be to classify cases after 60 days according to any viruses isolated (e.g., as wild virus, imported or endemic, vaccinelike virus, or unknown.

Reporting of cases should complement and strengthen routine communicable disease reporting systems. It should be mandatory to have both immediate reporting for action as soon as cases are identified, as well as regular reporting, weekly or monthly, to the national level and quarterly to the regional office of WHO on cases detected within the reporting period.

With the development of eradication activities, it is essential that case and outbreak investigation become rapid, competent, and comprehensive. Ensuring that this is achieved demands specific training and the designation of individuals to be responsible, possibly in addition to other existing duties, for investigation and control. Programs of training, reporting-form design, and logistic support are needed and time consuming, but investment in developing such a system should prove to be a major national investment for broader disease investigation and control.

Computer software is being developed, based on the experience gained in the Americas, which should help in promoting the collection of data, line listing of cases, analysis of epidemiologic information, and cross-referencing to avoid duplication.

Monitoring of surveillance is being developed through the use of progress indicators. WHO initially recommends that these indicators should address four factors:

1. Completeness of reporting at each level
2. Reporting sensitivity through identifying the percentage of cases detected within 1 week of onset of paralysis
3. The percentage of suspected cases that have been investigated and for which specimens have been collected
4. The identification of cases of paralysis compared with the expected figure of more than 1 case per 100,000 children under 15 years of age.

C. Outbreak Response

The level of outbreak response will vary according to the stage reached in the poliomyelitis eradication initiative. At the least, it should consist of an investigation and line listing of all cases, with specimens taken to confirm the diagnosis. The area around known cases constitutes a particularly high-risk zone and it should be submitted to intensive surveillance for further cases.

Immunization using trivalent OPV should be given to all children under 5 years of age within the appropriate at-risk area around the cases, ideally on a house-to-house basis. When zero or few cases are occurring, the area covered should be as wide as possible. At a minimum, the affected village and surrounding areas or the ward of an urban area should be covered.

D. Laboratory Network Development

A laboratory network to facilitate and standardize the diagnosis of poliomyelitis is being developed at three levels. At the first level, a limited number of specialized laboratories will provide reference services with advanced tests, training, research, and production of reagents. The second level is represented by regional reference laboratories, usually three or four in each WHO region, providing monitoring, training, some reagents, and reference services to the third level, the national laboratories that will assist diagnosis through virus isolation from fecal samples.

At this stage, the gold standard for diagnostic tests at the national level remains isolation through cell culture, although research and development are proceeding as a priority to develop simpler tests that do not depend on cell culture and provide results in a shorter time. At the regional level, intratypic differentiation will be available. More advanced testing, such as genomic sequencing, will be available when needed at the specialized laboratory level.

When the network is complete, it is anticipated that each country will have a channel of access to a laboratory able to conduct poliovirus isolation by well-trained staff using standardized techniques.

As progress is made towards eradication, it will become increasingly important to monitor the environment for the presence of wild polioviruses. Tests such as the polymerase chain reaction (PCR) are being investigated further to assess their role in such sampling, and research is being promoted to develop more effective environmental sampling techniques.

It is important that, as the number of suspected poliomyelitis cases decline, each case is fully investigated and fecal samples collected. These samples are transported to the laboratory in a refrigerated condition, made possible by the development of a "reverse cold chain" (i.e., cold boxes specifically designed for specimen transport similar to those used to carry poliomyelitis vaccine). Cold boxes, specimen containers, and collection kits that use containers and rectal "straws" have been developed and are being field tested. Stores of these kits and boxes will be available in each country.

E. Poliomyelitis Vaccines

Despite many recommendations by EPI advisory groups, only 5 of 17 producers of OPV are known to be producing vaccine in accord with WHO requirements, although three others produce nonpoliomyelitis vaccines that National Control Authorities certify for UNICEF supply.

The ideal formulation of OPV remains a subject for continuing research. It is now recommended, noting the data from the Americas suggesting improved epidemic control and in view of the heat stability of OPV, that the tender requirements for UNICEF supply should have a type 1, 2, and 3 formulation of 10:1:6. Because of the frequently disappointing type 3 seroconversion identified in many serologic studies, the possibility of further formulation studies is being explored.

In addition to such studies, a further research priority is to develop more thermostable OPV, possibly by the use of a better stabilizer. Equally important is the need to investigate alternative strategies of vaccine delivery (e.g., through vaccination days or through special activities during the low season of transmission). If such administration proves effective in displacing the wild virus, the relatively poor type 3 seroconversion may be of less significance than when vaccine is delivered through routine methods.

F. Training

As an integral part of EPI, poliomyelitis eradication benefits from the successful series of management training courses available to senior, midlevel, and peripheral health staff. In addition, two manuals have been produced: the *Manual for Managers of Immunization Programmes* and the *Manual for the Virological Investigation of Poliomyelitis*. These are standard works that will be updated regularly and should provide readily available reference for national EPI and laboratory staff.

Additional field guides have been produced for health staff concerned with the initiative in the Americas and in the eastern Mediterranean. Further guides appropriate for use in all countries where polio is endemic are needed and will be prepared, supplemented by training materials specific for surveillance and outbreak investigation and control. *Guidelines for the Prevention of Deformities in Polio,* a manual for staff on the development of community-based rehabilitation, has been developed.

In addition to those for training field staff, a number of courses and workshops have been held for laboratory staff, especially to standardize testing and procedures for vaccine quality control and virus isolation. These will be continued and will be conducted in all regions, so that staff at the regional reference laboratories will know the staff in all national laboratories in their area and will be able to monitor performance within the laboratory network.

G. Social Mobilization

Social mobilization, in which members of national and local communities are involved in developing and implementing immunization programs, has been one of the factors responsible for the success of EPI. Involvement has ranged from national leaders at the highest level, political and traditional leaders, and respected figures in the worlds of entertainment and sport, education, religion, and local government.

This technique, involving all those likely to influence decision-makers within the family, remains important as EPI further develops to a stage where disease reduction, investigation, and outbreak control become more important. The community will need to be aware of the need to sustain high coverage levels, assist in the follow-up of defaulters, report suspected cases, and help in the investigation and control of outbreaks. Experience to date suggests that not only will this prove possible, but that communities will also appreciate and themselves develop the capacity to participate in planning for their own services.

H. Research and Development

The eradication of poliomyelitis is a complex and difficult task. The success achieved to date has raised many questions that need to be answered if poliomyelitis eradication is to be achieved at the earliest possible date.

More knowledge is needed on the epidemiology of the disease, on the effectiveness of various eradication strategies, on ways to improve the oral poliomyelitis vaccine, on the development of simple and rapid diagnostic tests for poliovirus and the differentiation between wild and vaccine strains, and on ways of detecting the wild virus in the environment.

VII. CONCLUSIONS

The initiative to eradicate the scourge of poliomyelitis from the world by the year 2000 has made an impressive start with the remarkable progress achieved in the Americas, a region with a relatively strong health infrastructure and resource base. However, to achieve the global goal by adapting and applying the policies and strategies to achieve eradication in all the countries of the world is a challenging and formidable task that will require resource mobilization of the entire world community. Industrialized countries should become increasingly aware that support to the global eradication initiative is not only a noble humanitarian act but is also in their domestic interest. The cost of poliomyelitis vaccine (for example, some $114 million per year in the United States of America alone) is a recurrent cost that could ultimately be saved when the disease is eradicated and immunization can be discontinued, as was done in the case of smallpox vaccination. Let a world free of suffering, disability, and death due to poliomyelitis be the gift of this generation to those who follow.

REFERENCES

Declaration of Talloires, 1988.

Nicholas, D. D., Kratzer, J. H., Ofusu-Amaah, S. and Belcher, D. W. (1977). *Br. Med. J. 1*:1009–1012.

Ofusu-Amaah, S., Kratzer, J. H., and Nicholas, D. D. (1977). *Br. Med. J. 1*:1012–1013.

Pan American Health Organization. (1985). *Bull. PAHO 19*:213–215.

Wkly. Epidemiol. Rec. (1981). *56*:337–344.

World Health Assembly. (1988). Global eradication of poliomyelitis by the year 2000. Geneva, Resolution WHA 41.28.

11

Rabies Virus Infection

New Vaccines and Strategies in Immunization

James B. Campbell and Ying Zhang* *University of Toronto, Toronto, Ontario, Canada*

I. INTRODUCTION: FROM PASTEUR TO THE PRESENT DAY

The history of rabies vaccines is a long and distinguished one (Rosset, 1985; Théodoridès, 1986; Perrin et al., 1990). Although the discovery of the practicability of antirabies immunity was actually made by a young professor of the Veterinary College in Lyon, Pierre Victor Galtier, the work of Louis Pasteur in the 1880s determined the course of vaccine production for many decades following. In 1881, Galtier reported that he could protect sheep from later subcutaneous lethal challenge by the inoculation of rabid saliva directly into the jugular vein. However, Pasteur's realization that the central nervous system provided a more reliable and consistent source of the virus than saliva eventually resulted in the development of the first practical, nervous tissue vaccines (Table 1).

For the first half of the 20th century, rabies vaccines continued to be prepared from nervous tissue of some sort. Indeed, vaccines prepared from infected rabbit, sheep, or goat brain are still widely used today, especially in developing countries. The main advantage of these Semple-type vaccines is their low cost; their disadvantages include an unacceptably high incidence of neurologic complications due to brain-derived neuroallergenic components such as myelin (Hemachudha et al., 1987; Swaddiwudhipong et al., 1987; Javier et al., 1989), and of vaccine failures due to low immunogenic content. They present also the possibility of transmission of

**Present affiliation*: Dalian Medical College, Dalian, People's Republic of China.

TABLE 1 Vaccination Schedule of Joseph Meister, 1885

Inoculation Date	Inoculum	Rabbit Virulence of Inoculum
6 July, 8 p.m.	15 day cord	None
7 July, 9 a.m.	14 day cord	None
6 p.m.	12 day cord	None
8 July, 9 a.m.	11 day cord	None
6 p.m.	9 day cord	None
9 July, 11 a.m.	8 day cord	None
10 July, 11 a.m.	7 day cord	15 day incubation
11 July, 11 a.m.	6 day cord	15 day incubation
12 July, 11 a.m.	5 day cord	8 day incubation
13 July, 11 a.m.	4 day cord	8 day incubation
14 July, 11 a.m.	3 day cord	8 day incubation
15 July, 11 a.m.	2 day cord	7 day incubation
16 July, 11 a.m.	1 day cord	7 day incubation

Joseph Meister, a 9-year-old Alsatian boy, was Pasteur's first human patient. He had been bitten severely by an apparently rabid dog in the early morning of July 4, 1885. The vaccines were prepared from the spinal cords of rabbits dying of rabies. Source of the virus was a canine street virus that had been passaged repeatedly in rabbits, resulting in a virulent strain with a "fixed" incubation period of 7 days. Before use, the cords had been air-dried for varying lengths of time (1–15 days). Cords dried for 7 days or more were nonpathogenic in rabbits; those dried for shorter periods retained their virulence, killing test animals following incubation periods varying from 7 to 15 days, as detailed above. Each inoculum consisted of sterilized beef broth with a small piece of dried infected spinal cord mixed in it. Each dose consisted of "half a Pravaz syringe" (probably 3 cc; Marie, 1909) injected under the skin of the right abdomen. Meister survived both the rabies exposure and the vaccination procedure, and later became a gatekeeper at the Pasteur Institute. Data from Pasteur (1885).

"unconventional viruses," such as the Creutzfeldt-Jakob disease agent, via injection of contaminated sheep brain extracts (Arya, 1991).

The middle of the 20th century saw the adaptation of rabies virus to growth in nonnervous cell cultures, which provided the means for development of the present day vaccines. The best of these cell culture vaccines are only mildly, and even then rarely, reactogenic; they are safe and highly immunogenic, and have been developed for both human and veterinary use. Nevertheless, rabies remains a significant public health problem worldwide, and it is quite apparent that the present licensed vaccines do not provide the means to control the disease adequately in many parts of the world (Roumiantzeff, 1988; Vodopija, 1988; Warrell and Warrell, 1988). This is partly due to their cost and partly to the fact that the disease remains endemic in feral animals. In recent years, however, considerable progress has been made in developing new types of rabies vaccines and new vaccination strategies directed towards total eradication of the disease. This chapter describes these new approaches and considers their effectiveness in terms of achieving their ultimate aims. But to paraphrase Pasteur himself, if a cure is sought, it is important first to understand the course of the disease. Although impressive advances have been made in understanding the molecular biology of the virus, there is still much to be learned about its immunologic, pathogenetic and epizootiologic properties. A secondary purpose, therefore, is to provide a summary of the current state of knowledge of the virus and the infectious process itself.

II. THE VIRUS

A. Structure

Rabies virus is the prototype of the genus *Lyssavirus*, of the family Rhabdoviridae. It has the typical rhabdoviral bullet shape, with particles averaging 180 nm in length and with a diameter of about 75 nm (for reviews, see Wunner et al., 1988; Tordo and Poch, 1988; Wunner, 1991). The virions consist of a helical ribonucleoprotein (RNP) core surrounded by a lipid envelope derived from the host cell membrane. The exterior is uniformly covered by spikelike projections 9–10 nm long, glycoprotein in nature, which are embedded in the lipid membrane and probably anchored in the matrix protein located in the interior (Fig. 1).

The surface glycoprotein, or G protein, is the most important immunogenic component of the virion. It has hemagglutinating activity, and provides the receptor sites for attachment of the virion to host cells. The mature form contains 505 amino acids, with two or three potential glycosylation sites, depending on the strain. It is the only viral antigen capable of stimulating production of neutralizing antibodies as well as providing a target for virus-specific T-helper and cytotoxic T lymphocytes. By use of monoclonal antibodies, it has been determined that the largest number of virus-neutralizing epitopes occurs between amino acid positions 333 and 357. This region also contains a genotypic marker of pathogenicity (Dietzschold et al., 1983a; Tuffereau et al., 1989).

The RNP core consists of a single-stranded, negative-sense RNA molecule (the viral genome) of 4.6 kDa, complexed with three proteins: L, N, and NS. The L protein, a giant molecule that takes up about half the coding capacity of the genome, possesses most of the enzymic activities necessary for genomic transcription and replication. The N, or nucleocapsid, protein is the major internal protein and exists in close association with the viral RNA. In addition to protecting the genome from

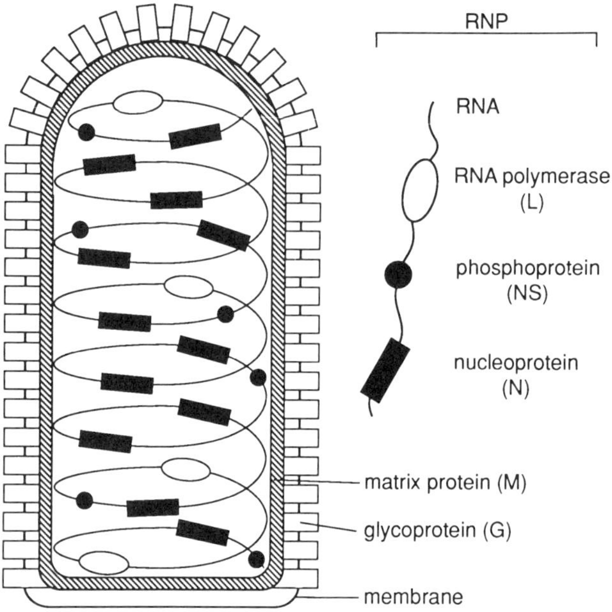

FIGURE 1 Schematic diagram of the rabies virion.

degradation it appears to have some role in regulating transcription. The NS component ("*N*onstructural": a misnomer) is a phosphoprotein, and is also associated with the viral RNA. Recent studies have shown that the RNP, as well as the G protein, can induce protective immunity, apparently by a complex interaction of various immune effector mechanisms, including B and T cells and cytokines such as interferon (Dietzschold and Rupprecht, 1989; Tollis et al., 1991).

The genomes of at least two strains of rabies virus have been sequenced in their entirety, as have large tracts of those of several other strains (Tordo et al., 1988; Conzelmann et al., 1990; Bourhy et al., 1989).

B. Antigenicity

Rabies virus isolates from all over the world can be neutralized with a single antiserum; indeed, many of the world's vaccines are prepared from derivatives of a pasteurian isolate. The virus, therefore, can be considered to be antigenically unique, although it is known that many different "variants" exist that can be differentiated on the basis of their reactivity with panels of monoclonal antibodies (Smith and Baer, 1988; Smith, 1989;

Rupprecht et al., 1991). Most of these viruses are variants of "classic" rabies; that is, the virus that has been studied since Pasteur's time. It is now apparent, however, that rabies-related viruses exist, which are sufficiently different to justify distinctive serogroupings within the genus *Lyssavirus*, but which show some degree of cross-reactivity with classic rabies. These include three African isolates: Lagos bat virus, Duvenhage, and Mokola (King and Crick, 1988; Fekadu et al., 1988; Bourhy et al., 1990; King et al., 1990). Recently, Duvenhage-like viruses have been recovered from European insectivorous bats (King et al., 1990). Commercially available rabies diagnostic reagents (monoclonal antibodies) have been used to identify cross-reactivity with several invertebrate viruses, including Obodhiang (isolated from *Mansonia uniformis* mosquitoes, Sudan), Kotonkan (from *Culicoides* spp., Nigeria), and Rochambeau (from *Coquillettidia albicosta* mosquitoes, New Guinea), and Adelaide River, a virus isolated from an asymptomatic bovine in the Northern Territory of Australia (Smith et al., 1989; Calisher et al., 1989).

The antigenic relationships between classic rabies and the rabies-related viruses have not been fully established (Calisher et al., 1989). The concept of a nucleocapsid-associated group-specific antigen may be an oversimplification (King and Crick, 1988), although immunization with RNP can confer cross-protective immunity against infection by heterologous lyssaviruses (Tollis et al., 1991).

C. Epizootiology

Rabies is found worldwide except in Australia, Antarctica, and some isolated islands and peninsular areas such as the British Isles, Japan, New Zealand, and Scandinavia. It is primarily a disease of dogs and related canids. In different parts of the world, different vector species predominate, sometimes to the extent that the majority of cases of rabies in a particular geographical region occur in a single species (Fig. 2). The reasons for the association of a particular animal species with the disease in any given area are unclear. It appears that the virus may develop specific tropisms for one or another animal species, rendering other species in the same geographical region less susceptible to that particular strain or "biotype" (Table 2; Blancou, 1986). Antigenic variants in different regions can be identified by panels of monoclonal antibodies, particularly those directed against the N protein. For example, the viruses affecting terrestrial animals in North America can be classified broadly into four major reactivity groups: one in arctic and red foxes (in the Arctic and southern Ontario/western Quebec, respectively); two in skunks (one in the north central United States and contiguous areas of Canada, the other

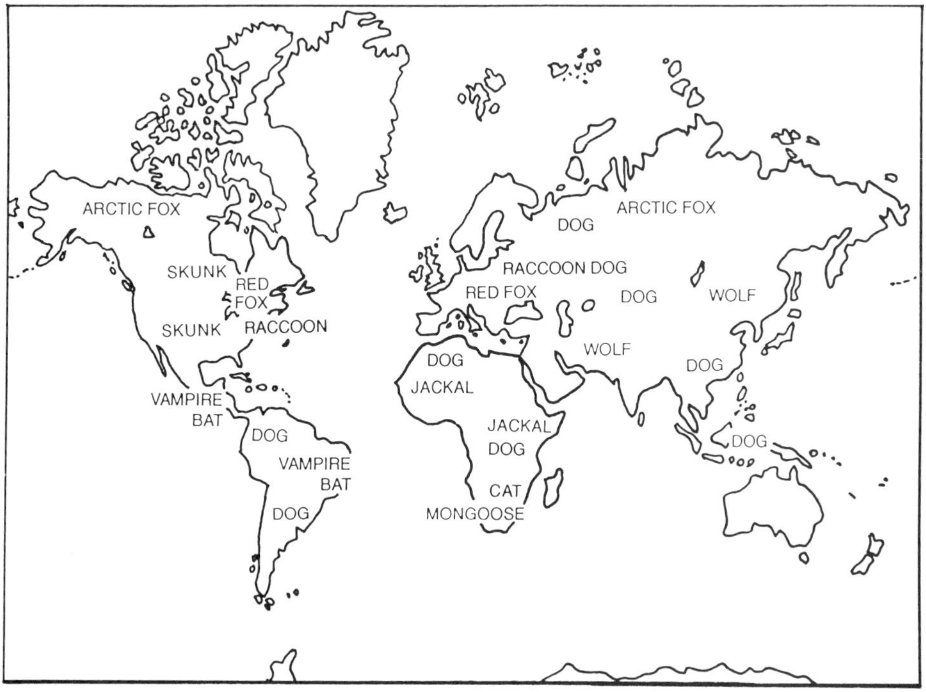

FIGURE 2 Worldwide distribution of rabies shows principal vector associations.

TABLE 2 Profiles of Two Rabies Biotypes

Animal Inoculated		Viral Biotype: Fox	Viral Biotype: Dog
Fox	S	●●●	○○○
	E	●●●	●○○
	A	○○○	●●○
Dog	S	○○○	●●●
	E	○○○	●●○
	A	●●●	○○○

○○○, low; ●○○, medium; ●●○, high; ●●●, very high.
S, level of susceptibility; E, propensity for excretion via the salivary glands; A, production of rabies-specific antibodies following a nonlethal infection. Data adapted from Blancou (1986).

in the south central states); and one in raccoons (with foci in the mid-Atlantic and southeast United States). Similar compartmentalization of rabies variants has been observed in other parts of the world (MacInnes, 1987; Smith and Baer, 1988; Smith et al., 1989).

Use of monoclonal antibody typing methods has provided important information on the origins and spread of epizootics. They have shown that strains of bat rabies are quite distinctive antigenically from those of terrestrial animals. This supports the theory that rabies in bats exists as enzootics largely independent of the cycles in terrestrial animals, and that bats, although widely distributed worldwide, are not important reservoirs for infection of other wildlife (Smith and Baer, 1988). This does not mean, however, that bat rabies can be ignored as being inconsequential. Three of the four cases of human rabies that have occurred in Canada since 1970 followed exposure to rabid bats. Duvenhage virus was first isolated from the brain of a 31-year-old South African who died 5 weeks after being bitten on the lip by an unknown bat, and there have been several human deaths associated with the European bat viruses (Lumio et al., 1986; King and Crick, 1988).

Figure 3 illustrates how the virus can be transmitted between species. The virus is maintained in wild animal reservoirs by direct animal-to-animal transmission within the same vector species. The current epizootic situation in southern Ontario provides an example of the kinds of interaction that may occur. In this geographical area, which is one of the most densely populated areas of Canada, both the red fox and the striped skunk are considered to be vector species. It is known that fox-to-fox and skunk-to-skunk transmissions occur, and fox-to-skunk (and vice versa) transmissions are at least virologically possible (MacDonald and Voigt, 1985). The extent to which interspecies transmission occurs, however, is uncertain. The saliva of a rabid fox generally contains a lower titer of infectious virus than that of a rabid skunk, and this may be a limiting factor in transmission of the disease from foxes to more resistant skunk (Smith and Baer, 1988). The virus appears, therefore, to be maintained more or less independently within the separate niches of these two species. However, a rabid fox (or skunk) may come in contact with, and infect, farm animals or pets. There is also the possibility that other wild animals may become infected by eating the carcasses of dead rabid animals (Ramsden and Johnston, 1975; Delpietro et al., 1990). In some cases, and especially if they are not carnivorous, the infected animals are simply "dead end" hosts: they do not transmit the virus to other animals. Nevertheless, if a pet cat or dog is infected, there is the potential for transmission to other contact animals, including humans. Humans may

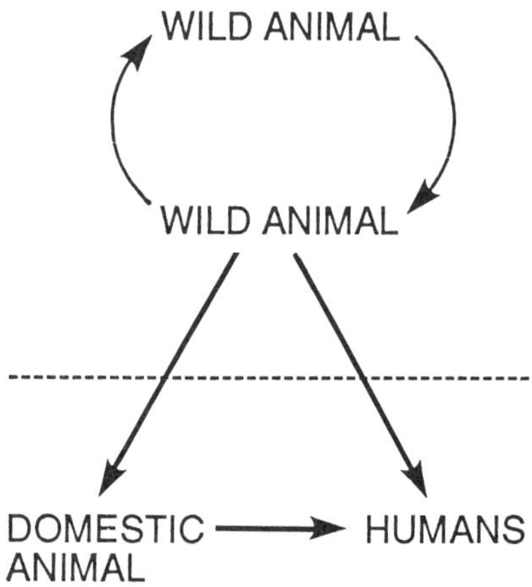

FIGURE 3 Transmission of rabies. The virus is maintained within wild animal reservoirs (mainly carnivorous species; see Fig. 2) but can spread to domestic animals (cattle, horses, dogs, cats, etc.), which can in turn infect human contacts. The broken line marks the boundary imposed by present vaccines: immunization of domestic animals especially can reduce human exposure. The schema has been reduced to its basic essentials; see text for further details.

also be exposed to the virus, and become infected, by direct contact with rabid wild animals (Sureau, 1990).

Table 3 summarizes the cases of laboratory-diagnosed animal rabies in North America during 1988. The actual incidence of rabies in wildlife is undoubtedly much higher than the laboratory figures indicate, especially in Mexico where the surveillance system is less well developed. The figures do, however, provide an indication of the relative levels of the disease in the various animal species. Most rabies cases in Mexico are in dogs, and the disease is maintained by dog-to-dog transmission of the virus. In 1988, there were also 74 human cases of rabies, 68 of which were the result of dog bites. In the United States and Canada, both of which have effective canine vaccination programs, the incidence of canine rabies is low, and cases in humans are practically nonexistent.

From the public health viewpoint, the disease has been identified as occurring in two epidemiologic forms: "urban" rabies, transmitted mainly by domestic and feral dogs in urban settlements; and "sylvatic" or "wildlife" rabies, with independent cycles in wildlife species. In fact, however, the distinction relates more to the biotype or monoclonal antibody

TABLE 3 Distribution of Rabies Cases in Animals, North America, 1988

	United States	Canada	Mexico
Wildlife (%)			
Skunk	37.9	29.3	
Raccoon	31.0	0.6	
Fox	3.9	47.3	
Bat	13.5	2.3	2
Other	2.1	0.9	2
Total cases (N)	3,826	1,837	665
Domestic (%)			
Cattle	3.6	9.6	
Dog	2.7	3.1	93
Cat	4.0	4.4	2
Other	1.3	2.4	1
Total cases (N)	898	447	12,627

In the United States, the south Atlantic, south central, north central, and mid-Atlantic states reported 81% of cases. In Canada, 80% of cases were in Ontario. Data from Varughese and Carter (1990).

reactivity profile of the virus strains than to their geographical situation. Rabid wildlife can exist within an urban environment; for example, skunks, foxes, and raccoons are commonly found throughout many North American cities. The strains of rabies infecting these urban animals are the same as those circulating in their country cousins. In terms of pathogenicity, however, the canine biotype is quite different from, for example, the fox biotype (see Table 2), and the viral cycles remain largely independent.

D. Pathogenesis

Entry into the Nervous System

One of the factors hindering progress in the development of antirabies strategies is that the pathogenetic mechanisms of the virus are far from being fully understood (for reviews, see Murphy, 1977, 1985; Rupprecht and Dietzschold, 1987; Charlton, 1988; Baer, 1991). It is apparent that the virus is transmitted primarily by the bite of a rabid animal, with deposition of virus-infected saliva in the wound. It is generally accepted that initial viral replication may occur in striated muscle cells in the vicinity of the bite, thereby facilitating invasion of exposed neuromuscular spindles and entry into the nervous system. The virus may also gain access to the nervous system via motor nerve endings, possibly following binding to the nicotinic acetylcholine receptor (AChR), to which it has a high affinity (Lentz, 1990; Baer and Lentz, 1991). Indeed, differences in susceptibility to infection among animal species may reflect their levels of AChR (Baer et al., 1990). The extent to which viral replication occurs prior to entry into the nervous system is uncertain, and may not even be necessary. For example, infected neurons have been detected in mice 18 hr after muscular injection of the CVS strain of virus (Coulon et al., 1989). In a recent study using a polymerase chain reaction assay, viral RNA was detected in the brainstem of mice as early as 24 hr after inoculation of infectious virus into the masseter muscle (Shankar et al., 1991).

Replication Within the CNS

Once within the nervous system, the virus is carried passively towards the CNS by retrograde axoplasmic flow (Iwasaki, 1991). Replication may occur en route in the cell bodies of the neurons, and budding from the dendritic plasma membranes probably provides the means for cell-to-cell transfer, such as across synaptic junctions. Additional amplification may occur in the neurons of the root ganglia. Once in the spinal cord, there is rapid progression of the virus to the brain. Viral replication in the hypothalamus results in neuronal dysfunction, producing hormonal imbalance, with consequent growth impairment, dehydration, and immunodepletion (Baczynski, 1989; Torres-Anjel et al., 1988). Infection of the limbic system produces personality changes such as aggressiveness and abnormal sexual behavior (Isaacson, 1989). As the disease progresses, the virus spreads throughout the brain, causing dysfunction of the higher centers, possibly through impairment of acetylcholine receptors. Nevertheless, even in the paralytic terminal stages of the disease, the brains of rabies-infected animals exhibit few degenerating neurons relative to the large number of infected ones.

Spread of the Virus

Even before there are signs of CNS involvement, the virus disseminates extraneurally, via the same axonal routes as before. Many tissues of the body are thereby infected: for example, skin biopsies and corneal impressions may reveal rabies antigen, even before death. From the standpoint of the perpetuation of the virus, however, the salivary gland is the most important target organ. Virus passes from peripheral nerves, in some as yet undetermined way, to the epithelial cells. Replication occurs in mucogenic cells, and virions are released in high titer into the glandular ducts and saliva by normal secretory flow. It is clear, therefore, that the virus in vivo replicates in both neural and nonneural tissues. Nevertheless, the neural networks appear to be necessary for widespread infection of glandular tissue: after inoculation of street virus directly into the submandibular salivary gland of skunks, antigen was not detected in the epithelial cells without its concurrent presence in the brain (Charlton et al., 1983).

Vector Species

The pathogenetic properties of the rabies virus are unique in a number of respects. The production of the virus in the saliva of infected animals provides a high-titer source for transmission, and virus-induced modifications of the limbic system, resulting in aggressive behavior, provide the means by which the virus *can* be transmitted. It is not surprising, therefore, that carnivores predominate among the terrestrial vector species and that these animals are the most susceptible to rabies infection.

Nonbite Transmission

Rabies can also be transmitted by nonbite routes, although the importance of these in nature is uncertain (Afshar, 1979). One unusual epizootic, among the greater kudu of southwest Africa, may fall into this category. The kudu, which are wild ruminants, appear to have been infected originally by a jackal virus. The disease was maintained in the herds from 1977 to 1983, seemingly by transfer of infected saliva during the feeding process. The infection has been transmitted experimentally to healthy kudu by the direct application of infected saliva to the oral cavity. In the natural state, the animals browse mainly on the leaves of thornbushes (*Acadia* spp.), the thorns of which produce lesions in the mouth, and this may facilitate the infection process (Hübschle, 1988).

Although not a common occurrence, transmission by aerosols is possible, as has been demonstrated experimentally and accidentally in bat-infested caves (Constantine et al., 1972). Infection by this route presumably occurs via the olfactory neuroepithelial cells, which extend into the olfactory bulb of the brain. Oral transmission by ingestion of infected tissues is also feasible. First reported by Galtier in 1881, it is now well established that oral administration of both street and fixed strains of virus can cause the disease, although high doses of virus are generally required (Bell and Moore, 1971; Lawson et al., 1989b). As with other routes, oral infection appears to require centripetal movement of the virus to the central nervous system before nonneural tissues are infected by centrifugal spread (Madhusudana and Tripathi, 1990).

Variations in Pathogenicity

There is a widely held belief that once clinical signs of the disease develop, the infection is almost invariably fatal. It is true that there are few well-documented cases of human survivors (Hattwick et al., 1972). There are numerous reports, however, of the recovery of lower animals from the disease with or without clinical signs, recovery with chronic disability, or with the development of a "carrier" state (Fekadu, 1991). In one study of dogs inoculated with virus strains from North American dogs, North American bats, or African dogs, up to 20% sickened and then recovered (Fekadu, 1988). There have also been reports of apparently healthy Ethiopian and Indian dogs that excreted rabies virus intermittently in their saliva for extended periods of time (Fekadu, 1988, 1991).

Strains of rabies virus isolated from naturally infected animals (Pasteur's "street" virus) have highly variable incubation periods. They may also exhibit different degrees of pathogenicity in different animal species (see section on Epizootiology, above). Laboratory passage of a street virus in another animal species (e.g., canine rabies virus in rabbits) results in shortening of the incubation period to a relatively fixed period (Pasteur's "fixed" virus). There is an increase in virulence of such fixed viruses for the new host, with a corresponding reduction in virulence for the original and other host species. Indeed, some fixed viruses cultured in vitro may become completely apathogenic in vivo, even when inoculated intracerebrally (e.g., Tuffereau et al., 1989). With those fixed viruses that are still pathogenic, there is generally a marked reduction in excretion of virus from the salivary glands compared with that resulting from street virus infections.

The occurrence of rabies-specific neutralizing antibodies in unvaccinated dogs and wild animals, clinically normal even when held captive for long periods, indicates that these animals have survived a natural infection (Gough and Niemeyer, 1975; Yasmuth et al., 1983; Wosu and Anyanwu, 1990). In some cases, the antibodies may have resulted from an infection with a heterologous rabies biotype (see Table 2), or from nonlethal infection with a cross-reacting rabies-related virus. They may also have resulted from infection with a naturally occurring variant of rabies virus with reduced pathogenicity, such as that reported in Nigerian dogs (Aghomo and Rupprecht, 1990).

III. THE IMMUNE RESPONSE

A. Natural Infection

In natural infection, antibodies appear only in the terminal stages of the disease, if at all (Kasempimolporn et al., 1991). This lack of response is probably related to the fact that there may be little, if any, replication of the viral inoculum at the site of entry. Consequently, the resulting antigenic mass may not be adequate to stimulate an early immune response. During the period of neuronal spread the virus is largely insulated from immunocompetent cells, so that only during the later stages of the infection is the virus susceptible to immunologic attack. At this stage, *any* response is probably too late to be effective, and death almost invariable follows, even in the presence of high levels of circulating antibody. Indeed, there is some evidence that the late immune response may contribute to the disease process (Hattwick and Gregg, 1975; Smith et al., 1982; Hemachudha, 1989). Paralysis following infection does not occur in immunosuppressed or athymic nude mice, which nevertheless eventually lose weight and die (Marcovistz et al., 1987).

B. Vaccination

The fact that effective rabies vaccines exist is clear evidence that the disease can be prevented if an appropriate immunologic response is stimulated. Nevertheless, there is still no clear picture as to the specific contributions of the various components of the immune system in the protective process (Turner, 1985; MacFarlan, 1988; Nathanson and Gonzalez-Scarano, 1991). In pre-exposure vaccination, there is frequently good correlation between antibody titer and the degree of protection conferred, but this is not the case when vaccine is administered after exposure (MacFarlan, 1988). For example, it has been found that passively transferred antibody per se fails to protect animals infected with rabies (Wiktor, 1978). Indeed, the role of postexposure vaccine-induced antibodies in protection remains poorly understood, although some experimental observations indicate the importance of a B-cell response (MacFarlan, 1988).

There is considerable evidence to implicate T cells in the protective mechanism(s) (Wiktor et al., 1977, 1985; Mifune et al., 1981). For example, Wiktor and co-workers found in mice that survival from rabies correlated with the induction of cytotoxic T lymphocytes (CTL) rather than with the other immunologic parameters examined (antibody and interferon responses). Mice infected with apathogenic viruses generated a strong antirabies CTL response, whereas those infected with pathogenic strains not only failed to do this, but also demonstrated suppressed responses to other antigens (Wiktor, 1978; Wiktor et al., 1985). In another type of experiment, an antirabies glycoprotein CTL clone transferred into rabies-infected syngeneic mice afforded protection to about 50% of the animals: protection was even greater in mice receiving both antirabies antibodies and CTL cells (Kawano et al., 1990). The question remains as to how T cells may contribute to protection. Two possibilities are by preventing spread of the infection by CTL-mediated killing of virus-infected cells; and by the release of soluble mediators such as γ-interferon (IFN) and interleukin-2 (IL-2).

The effectiveness of IFN in protecting against rabies, although still a controversial issue, has been demonstrated in a number of experimental studies (Turner, 1985; Tsiang, 1988). Nevertheless, studies on the efficacy of vaccine-induced IFN in human antirabies prophylaxis have yielded variable results (Turner, 1985). However, the work of Baer and colleagues (1979, 1989b) with mice and subhuman primates have indicated that post-exposure administration of vaccine together with IFN (or IFN inducer) afforded markedly better protection than vaccine alone. On the basis of a 10 year history of use in postexposure treatment, Vodopija and co-workers (1989a) have provided evidence for the capacity of IFN to inhibit rabies growth in humans.

Some recent observations have indicated that IL-2 plays a major role in antirabies immune responses (Perrin et al., 1991). In one study, exogenous recombinant human IL-2 protected about 50% of hamsters infected with lethal doses of virulent rabies virus and enhanced the protective activity of rabies vaccines in a pre-exposure potency test (Perrin et al., 1988). In another study, daily systemic administration of IL-2 in conjunction with inactivated rabies vaccine increased the potency of vaccination in outbred mice at least 25-fold. Enhanced protection was not correlated with an increase of neutralizing antibody, indicating that IL-2 acts to increase the cellular immune response (Nunberg et al., 1989).

The role of nonspecific cell-mediated soluble factors in protection against rabies has also been demonstrated in a series of studies in mice in which saponins (triterpenoid and steroidal glycosides) were used as oral immunostimulants (Campbell and Chavali, 1989). Given along with vaccine, saponins significantly increased T-helper and B-cell cooperation following vaccination, resulting in enhanced neutralizing antibody production and protection against lethal virus challenge. However, a significant proportion of animals fed saponins alone (i.e., no vaccine) survived intracerebral rabies challenge (Maharaj et al., 1986). In later studies, the saponins were found to induce CTL and natural killer cell activities, and to stimulate production of lymphokines (Chavali and Campbell, 1987a,b). These responses, therefore, may provide the basis for saponin-induced protection against rabies.

IV. PRESENT DAY VACCINES

A. Human Vaccines

Table 4 lists a number of tissue culture vaccines presently licensed for human postexposure use (see also Roumiantzeff et al., 1985; Crick and King, 1988; Vodopija and Clark, 1991). All are inactivated. The Wistar Institute's human diploid cell vaccine (HDCV), introduced in the mid-1970s, represented a major advance in terms of potency, safety, and reduction in reactogenicity, and it remains the standard against which new

TABLE 4 Inactivated Cell Culture Rabies Vaccines for Human Use

Cell Substrate	Virus Strain	Country of Production	References
Primary hamster kidney	Vnukovo-32 (SAD)	Soviet Union	Selimov et. al (1978)
Primary hamster kidney	Beijing	China	Lin (1990)
Primary fetal bovine kidney	Pasteur	France	Roumiantzeff et al. (1985)
Primary chicken embryo	Flury-LEP-C25	Germany	Barth et al. (1984, 1990)
Human diploid cell strain (WI-38)	Pitman-Moore (PM)	France, Germany	Wiktor et al. (1978), Wiktor (1985)
Human diploid cell strain (MRC-5)	Street-Alabama-Dufferin (SAD)	Canada	Lawrence et al. (1989)
Fetal rhesus lung diploid cell strain	Kissling	United States	Berlin et al. (1983), Berlin (1990)
African green monkey kidney cell line (Vero)	PM	France	Roumiantzeff et al. (1989)

vaccines are assessed. Its main disadvantage is its high cost, which puts it out of reach of all but the most affluent countries. The recommended postexposure regimen requires five to six doses: in the United States, in addition to human rabies immune globulin (RIG; 20 IU/kg) on day 0, 1 ml of vaccine is administered intramuscularly (IM) in the deltoid area on days 0, 3, 7, 14 and 28 (Centers for Disease Control, 1991). In Europe, a sixth dose is recommended on day 90 (the Essen scheme).

Introduction of new cell culture systems, virus strains, and more efficient production technologies have resulted in the development of less expensive, but equally effective, vaccines (Barth et al., 1990; Roumiantzeff et al., 1989). Much effort has been expended in attempts to reduce cost further by modifying dose schedules and route of administration. For example, the 2:1:1 regimen (two 1 ml IM doses on day 0, and one each on days 7 and 21) resulted in earlier antibody responses, with savings in both vaccine and time spent during clinic visits (Vodopija et al., 1986, 1989b; Sureau and Rollin, 1989). A 3:1 regimen, involving only two clinic visits, has been reported. In addition to producing a rapid antibody response, this triple dose on day 0 stimulated production of high interferon levels, lasting for more than 30 hr (Thraenhart et al., 1989). The higher immunogenicity of the intradermal (ID) route has also been exploited (Harverson and Wasi, 1984; Dreesen et al., 1984). As a result of these developments, cell culture vaccines are now within the means of some developing countries. In Thailand, purified Vero cell rabies vaccine (Mérieux), in a reduced ID regimen of two injections of 0.1 ml at 2 sites on days 0, 3, and 7, followed by two 0.1 ml boosters on days 30 and 90, plus the use of RIG, has provided a safe and affordable procedure (Wilde and Chutivongse, 1989). China, with a huge human population and a large canine rabies problem, has developed an inexpensive primary hamster kidney cell vaccine that now, with a production in excess of 50 million doses since 1980 (Lin, 1990), has completely replaced use of the Semple-type nervous tissue vaccines in this country.

Pre-exposure vaccination is presently limited to high-risk target populations, such as veterinarians, rabies laboratory workers, and health care personnel who may be exposed to rabies-infected patients. Recommended dose schedules involve either two doses administered on days 0 and 28, or three doses on days 0, 7, and 21–28. Administration boosters of 1 year later, with reinforcing doses every 1–3 years depending on the risk of exposure, maintains an acceptable level of protective immunity (Roumiantzeff et al., 1988; Nicholson, 1990).

Nervous tissue vaccines are considered too dangerous for pre-exposure immunization. Due to the expense of cell culture vaccines, preventive immunization is rare in developing countries, even in regions in which the risk of infection is high. However, with the advent of the more economical new vaccines, particularly if given by the ID route, this situation should eventually change.

B. Veterinary Vaccines

As with human rabies vaccines, domestic animal vaccines have evolved from the pasteurian nervous-tissue-derived preparations to those grown in cell culture. The vaccines available today can be classified into three groups: modified-live, inactivated nervous tissue origin, and inactivated cell culture origin (Bunn, 1988, 1991).

Modified-live vaccines for the control of dog rabies have a long history. A major advance was made in the 1940s when the Flury strain of rabies, isolated from, and named after, a young girl who died of rabies in 1939, was adapted to growth in embryonated chicken eggs. With increasing egg passage, the virus gradually lost its virulence for mammalian species. Two basic vaccines emerged: low egg passage (LEP) and high egg passage (HEP). When first licensed, the Flury LEP vaccine was considered safe for use in dogs more than 3 months old, but since it could cause rabies in younger puppies, and occasionally even in adult dogs, it has gradually been superseded by even safer vaccines. Despite the increased safety of the Flury HEP vaccine in cats, the occasional case of vaccine-induced rabies still occurred.

Another rabies virus with a long record in vaccine production is the Street-Alabama-Dufferin (SAD) strain. Originally a street virus isolated from a naturally infected dog in Alabama in 1935, it was adapted to growth in hamster kidney cell cultures by Fenje, in the Dufferin Division of the Connaught Laboratories, Toronto. The virus was further passaged in various cell systems to produce a number of vaccines. Among the most widely used of these are the ERA, grown in porcine kidney cells and named after its developers (*E*. Gaynor, A. *R*okitnicki, and M. K. *A*belseth), and the Vnukovo-32, developed in Russia by passage of the SAD virus, as its name indicates, at 32°C. Both vaccines have been recommended for use in dogs, cats, cattle, sheep, goats, and horses, and ERA vaccine has been widely used in South America to protect cattle against vampire bat rabies (Bunn, 1988; Arellano-Sota, 1988; Flores-Crespo and Arellano-Sota, 1991).

Despite the effectiveness of the modified-live vaccines, the fact that they have been associated with cases of vaccine-induced rabies (SAD as well as Flury) has led to their gradual withdrawal in North America and other countries. It is clear that the current trend is towards inactivated veterinary vaccines (NASPHV Committee, 1991). There are now many licensed vaccines that will provide a 3 year duration of immunity in dogs and cats following a single IM dose at 3 months and a second dose 1 year later. Some vaccines are also licensed for use in large domestic animals (cattle, sheep, and horses), with primary vaccination at 3 months followed by yearly boosters (NASPHV Committee, 1991).

V. NEW APPROACHES TO VACCINE DEVELOPMENT

There are practical limits to what can be done to improve the immunogenicity, and reduce the cost, of conventional rabies vaccines. There are also limitations imposed due to our incomplete understanding of the pathogenetic and immunogenetic properties of the virus. For example, what is the role of IFN in protection against rabies? Do antibodies protect, once the virus enters the nervous system? Although the rabies glycoprotein stimulates neutralizing antibodies, is it the only viral antigen necessary for provision of adequate protection under all circumstances? There are still no clear answers. Present pre- and postexposure vaccines are physically the same. Pre-exposure immunization, however, is for long-term protection; postexposure treatment is for a short-term emergency. Should separate vaccines be designed for these two widely differing purposes? One might surmise, for example, that vaccines stimulating high (but short-lived) IFN production would be of more value in postexposure protection than for pre-exposure immunization, in which a good cell-mediated response might be more appropriate. The fact that antirabies immunoglobulins are administered concurrently with the first vaccine dose in postexposure treatment indicates the considered importance of antibody in the early stages of infection, although passive administration of antibody reduces the immune response to the vaccine. Would a post-exposure vaccine designed to produce high IFN levels be more effective than the present vaccine/γ-globulin combination?

Even if we had the answers to these and other questions, the empirical methods used in the development of conventional vaccines would not provide ready solutions. New technologies, however, some involving high technologic "molecular" approaches, have provided a greater degree of flexibility (Table 5). This could result in the future production of rabies vaccines specially designed for their different uses.

A. Nonreplicating Vaccines

Inactivated whole-virus vaccines suffer from the inherent disadvantage of being produced from virulent material, and inadequate inactivation may have disastrous consequences. To circumvent this problem, attempts have

TABLE 5 Molecular Approaches to Rabies Vaccine Development

Nonreplicating vaccines	
	Anti-idiotypic antibodies
	Synthetic peptides
	Recombinant-derived proteins
Replicating ("live") vaccines	
	RNA-modified mutants
	Recombinant viruses

been made to develop subunit vaccines, free from nucleic acid and therefore unable to cause the disease under any circumstances. The following provides a summary of the most interesting approaches.

Liposomes

The ability of the rabies glycoprotein to induce neutralizing antibody is critically dependent on the integrity of the native secondary and tertiary structure. Extraction of the glycoprotein from the viral membrane by means of detergents generally results in a loss of immunogenicity. However, solubilized viral glycoprotein anchored to preformed unilamellar liposomes (synthetic phospholipid vesicles) regains its ability to induce protective antibodies and to stimulate a cell-mediated immunity (Oth et al., 1987; Sureau and Perrin, 1989). These "immunosomes" may therefore provide the basis for a nucleic acid–free, subunit vaccine. Also, since liposomes stimulate the production of IL-2 by primed splenocytes, there is the possibility of using them to potentiate rabies vaccines in vivo (Joffret et al., 1990).

Iscoms

One class of surfactants that permits retention of the immunogenic activity of the extracted glycoprotein is the saponins. As noted in an earlier section, these are triterpenoid and steroidal glycosides, the most common laboratory preparations being derived from the bark of a South American tree, *Quillaja saponaria* Molina. By incubating rabies virus with *Quillaja* saponin, Schneider et al. (1971) obtained a noninfectious, highly immunogenic viral subunit. Saponins have also been used as adjuvants in parenterally administered vaccines, including rabies, for veterinary use (Soulebot et al., 1985; Chavali and Campbell, 1987a).

Commercially available *Quillaja* saponin preparations frequently consist of complex and ill-defined mixtures of glycosides, contaminated with other components such as tannins. This has restricted their use in classic vaccines, since the adjuvant activity of different preparations can vary considerably, and many are highly hemolytic and therefore toxic when administered by the parenteral route. Nevertheless, there is increasing interest in their use as vaccines since they have been shown to interact with viral and other membrane glycoproteins to produce what have been named "iscoms" (*i*mmuno*s*timulating *com*plexes) (Morein et al., 1984). Iscoms are formed when detergent-solubilized glycoprotein is ultracentrifuged in sucrose gradients containing Quil A, a relatively refined fraction of *Quillaja* saponin. The detergent is replaced by the Quil A, and iscoms, which are multimicellar complexes of about 30–100 nm diameter, result. These complexes are nontoxic, highly immunogenic, and have been prepared using many different viral glycoproteins, including rabies (Morein et al., 1984; Morein and Simons, 1985; Höglund et al., 1989; Kersten, 1990). Using iscoms prepared with rabies glycoprotein, Berezin et al. (1987) have demonstrated a protective effect higher than that of subunit rabies vaccine adsorbed on aluminum hydroxide. Iscom vaccines may also have an advantage over inactivated vaccines in being able to induce antigen-specific major histocompatibility complex (MHC) class I restricted CTL responses (Takahashi et al., 1990).

Baculovirus Vectors

For large-scale vaccine production, preparation of immunogenic subunits from intact virus is costly due to limitations on the amount of antigen available. Expression of the appropriate genes to high levels in heterologous host systems has provided a possible solution. One of the most promising of these host systems is the baculovirus, an insect virus family whose members produce large amounts of proteinaceous crystalline materials, the polyhedra, which cover, and serve to protect, the intranuclear virion (Kang, 1988). The protein associated with these inclusion bodies is called the N-polyhedrin. Préhaud et al. (1989) inserted cloned rabies glycoprotein gene into the genome of the nuclear polyhedrosis virus of *Autographa californica* under control of the strong polyhedrin promoter, wherein it was expressed to high levels in an insect cell line. Intraperitoneal or IM injection of the expressed protein conferred protection on mice, and was associated with the production of high titers of neutralizing antibodies. Fu et al. (1991) have expressed the rabies viral nucleoprotein (N) gene in a similar system, and have shown the purified gene product to be efficacious as a vaccine. Although the N protein, either by itself or within the RNP complex, does not stimulate production of virus-neutralizing antibodies, it has been shown to induce a strong anti-ribonucleoprotein antibody response and to protect several animal species (mice, raccoons, and monkeys) against lethal challenge with rabies virus (Dietzschold et al., 1983b; Tollis et al., 1991; Fu et al., 1991). It has also been shown to prime animals for the induction of high antibody titers following a single dose of cell culture vaccine. The suggestion has been made that N proteins, produced and purified by biotechnology, could provide the basis for a low cost vaccine to prime entire human populations in parts of the world where rabies is endemic. Postexposure treatment might then require only a single whole-virus vaccine dose (Tollis et al., 1991; Fu et al., 1991).

Synthetic Peptides

Dietzschold and Ertl (1991) have summarized studies relating to the development of synthetic peptide vaccines. Such studies have provided valuable information on the antigenic determinants of the rabies G, N, and S proteins. Nevertheless, and although certain small synthetic peptides carrying epitopes for both B and T cells have provided inbred mice with protective immunity against lethal challenge, the feasibility of this approach for practical vaccine development is still uncertain.

Anti-Idiotypic Antibodies

Anti-idiotypic antibodies are antiantibodies: they have an antibody-binding site (or idiotype) structurally similar to the inducing epitope of the primary antigen (Dreesman and Kennedy, 1985). Anti-idiotypic antibodies, raised against antirabies monoclonal antibodies have protected mice against lethal rabies viral challenge (Reagan et al., 1985). Whether these laboratory observations can be developed into a practical vaccination strategy, however, remains to be determined.

B. Replicating Vaccines

As discussed above, conventional modified-live rabies vaccines have the inherent problem of residual virulence and may, on occasion, cause the disease itself in vaccinees. Part of the problem lies in the empirical way in which these vaccines have been developed; namely, repeated passage of a virulent virus in various in vivo or in vitro systems until an acceptable level of attenuation is reached, as determined by animal experimentation.

Arginine-333 Mutants

An alternative to this process of genetic roulette has been provided by the observation that mutations in two of the antigenic sites of the rabies glycoprotein can affect viral virulence, and that such mutants can be selected by their resistance to specific monoclonal antibodies. In particular, it has been found that strains virulent for adult mice by the IC or IM routes contained an arginine residue at position 333 of the mature viral glycoprotein (antigenic site III). Antigenic mutants in which arginine-333 was replaced by another amino acid such as leucine, isoleucine, methionine, cysteine, or serine were completely avirulent, whatever the dose or route of inoculation (Tuffereau et al., 1989). It would appear, therefore, that the replacement of arginine-333 in live vaccine strains by certain other amino acid residues could improve their safety without impairing their protective power.

Heterologous Recombinants

Advances in recombinant DNA technology over the last decade have made possible the construction of viable recombinant viruses capable of expressing one or more foreign genes in vivo. For use in the control of rabies, they can provide the advantages of a live vaccine without the drawback of possible vaccine-associated rabies. A number of rabies recombinants have been described, most expressing the glycoprotein gene, although interest is also turning to the N protein (Table 6). The next step may be the development of recombinants expressing both G and N proteins, and even IL-2 and/or IFN. In this way, future rabies vaccines might be "tailored" to exploit fully the host immunologic defense mechanisms.

Vaccinia virus is by far the most widely used expression vector for live recombinant vaccine development (Piccini and Paoletti, 1988; Moss, 1991). There are a number of very practical reasons. Being a poxvirus, it has a large DNA genome into which additional genes can be inserted without the packaging constraints of smaller viruses. It can be grown readily in a variety of cell systems. It is also a well-seasoned vaccine itself, having been used in the global smallpox eradication program. There remains, of course, the possibility of vaccinia-associated complications, although characterized strains of low virulence are already available, and even safer strains are being developed by molecular engineering (Rodriguez et al., 1989; Moss, 1991).

Although the vaccinia virus genome contains a number of regions that are nonessential for replication (at least in vitro), the most common molecular strategy for expression of foreign genes is by insertion into the viral thymidine kinase (TK) gene (Rupprecht and Kieny, 1988; Piccini and Paoletti, 1988). The cloned rabies glycoprotein gene, with suitable promoter and polyadenylation signal sequences, is inserted into a plasmid containing the vaccinia viral TK gene so that it is flanked by vaccinia TK-coding sequences. Permissive cells are then infected with wild-type (TK^+) vaccinia virus, and simultaneously transfected with the plasmid. Recombinational events between the replicating viral genome and the plasmid result in the production of vaccinia virus bearing the rabies gene. Since the rabies gene is inserted within the vaccinia TK gene, recombinant virus will have a TK^- phenotype. If the process is carried out in TK^- cells in medium containing hypoxanthine–aminopterin–thymidine (HAT) or 5-bromo-2′-deoxyuridine (which inhibits growth of TK^+ phenotypes), only TK^- virus can replicate. This provides a simple means for selection of recombinants.

Since the first successful development of a vaccinia-rabies glycoprotein (RG) recombinant in 1984, several other poxviruses have been used for the same purpose (Table 6). The rationale for using avipoxviruses (fowlpox and canarypox) is an interesting one. Although their natural productive host range is limited to birds, abortive infections can be initiated in vitro in cell lines derived from nonavian species (Taylor et al., 1988). In the recombinants, the rabies gene appears to be expressed, and the glycoprotein synthesized, processed, and presented on the cell surface, without infectious virus production. Following inoculation into a number of mammalian species, both avipox recombinants stimulated levels of protective immunity against lethal rabies virus challenge comparable to those produced by a vaccinia–RG recombinant (Taylor et al., 1988, 1991). They provide the possibility, therefore, of live vaccines that do not result in the production of infectious virus by the vaccinee.

Another virus family that is being used increasingly for expression of foreign genes is the Adenoviridae. These viruses can cause intestinal infections as well as acute upper respiratory disease, and can therefore be transmitted by the oral route. In fact, oral adenovirus vaccines have been available for many years, although restricted to military use for the protection of recruits against respiratory infections. These vaccines consist of nonattenuated strains (particularly types 4 and 7) that are taken orally in the form of enteric-coated tablets. In this way, infectious virus is released only in the intestine, but still stimulates the induction of systemic immunity that effectively protects against subsequent upper respiratory infection by the corresponding wild type viral strains (Chaloner-Larsson et al., 1986). This concept opens the possibility for development of recombinant vaccines that can be given orally, for protection against both systemic and intestinal infections.

TABLE 6 Live Recombinant Rabies Vaccines

Vector Virus	Rabies Gene	Host Animal	Route of Administration	Reference[a]
Vaccinia	G	Rabbit Mouse	ID tail scratch	Kieny et al. (1984)
Vaccinia	G	Mouse Dog	FP IM	Esposito et al. (1987)
Vaccinia	N	Mouse	ID	Sumner et al. (1991)
Raccoonpox	G	Raccoon	oral	Esposito et al. (1988)
Raccoonpox	N	Mouse	tail scratch	Lodmell et al. (1991)
Fowlpox	G	Mouse Dog, Cat	FP SC	Taylor et al. (1988)
Canarypox	G	Mouse Dog, Cat	FP SC	Taylor et al. (1991)
Human adeno-virus type 5	G	Mouse Dog	oral, IP SC, IN	Prevec et al. (1990)

[a]First construction of the recombinant(s).
FP, footpad; ID, intradermal; IM, intramuscular; IN, intranasal; IP, intraperitoneal; SC, subcutaneous.

As in vaccinia, several regions in the adenoviral genome are nonessential for viral replication in vitro. The best characterized of these is the E3 transcriptional unit, which codes for a number of proteins whose functions appear to be related to protection of the virus against host immune responses (Gooding and Wold, 1990). Mutants with this region almost completely deleted replicate in a number of cell systems as efficiently as wild-type strains. A human adenovirus type 5 recombinant expressing the rabies glycoprotein gene in the deleted E3 region has been described and tested in several animal species including mice, dogs, foxes, and skunks (Prevec et al., 1990; Charlton et al., 1991). It has stimulated high levels of protective antibody in all species tested; this was a somewhat unexpected observation since the recombinant did not appear to replicate to any extent. As with the avipoxvirus recombinants, there appears to have been abortive adenoviral replication in vivo but with expression of the rabies gene on the surface of infected cells.

VI. CONTROL OF RABIES

A. Urban Rabies

Because of the proximity of humans and lower animals, the existence of urban rabies poses the greatest human threat (Beran, 1991). Unfortunately, it is spreading in many developing countries, due to the increasing density and mobility of human and canine populations. In Canada, the United States and much of western Europe, mandatory vaccination of pets and eradication of strays virtually eliminated human rabies many years ago. The success of recent mass canine vaccination programs in several South American cities, including Buenos Aires (Argentina), Lima and Callao (Peru), and São Paulo (Brazil), has clearly demonstrated that elimination of canine rabies is one of the most effective ways of reducing human exposure and therefore infection (Belotto, 1988; Chomel et al., 1988; Larghi et al., 1988; Bögel and Meslin, 1990; PAHO, 1990). Before initiation of such a program, Buenos Aires reported more than 4,000 cases of rabies per year (1976). Nine years after implementation of the program, this figure had been reduced to zero (Larghi et al., 1988). Because of ethical, economic, and administrative problems, however, it is not easy for many developing countries to undertake such mass immunization programs (Lin, 1990). In such countries, including China, human postexposure treatment continues to be the most practicable method for preventing human rabies.

Figure 3 emphasizes the point that domestic animals and humans *can* be protected by vaccination, but this will remain a necessity as long as the virus remains circulating in its wildlife vectors.

B. Wildlife Rabies

Until recently, the only practical means of controlling epizootics of rabies in wildlife was by reducing the population density of the affected animal species. Methods such as shooting, poisoning, and gassing of dens have met with limited success but, with some notable exceptions (Rosatte et al., 1986), they usually provide only short-term solutions. Due to the rapid population turnover of vector species such as foxes and raccoons, potentially infected animals soon move in to fill the ecologic "vacuum" created by population reduction, and the disease cycle repeats itself. In addition to being ethically questionable, population reduction methods also suffer from the disadvantages of being highly labor-intensive, expensive, and generally inefficient (Wandeler, 1988).

The concept of vaccinating susceptible free-ranging wildlife has provided a more attractive alternative. If a sufficiently high proportion of rabies vectors (e.g., 70%, to use a widely quoted figure) in a given ecosystem can be rendered immune to the disease, the virus is not able to spread effectively and the disease dies out. Following up on observations that foxes can be immunized against rabies by the oral route with live vaccine (Black and Lawson, 1970, 1973; Baer et al., 1971; Mayr et al., 1972), extensive field studies in a growing number of countries have now provided evidence that control of rabies in wildlife by immunization is not only practicable but also economically feasible (Fig. 4; Table 7) (Wandeler, 1988, 1991; MacInnes, 1988; Pastoret et al., 1988; Schneider and Cox, 1989; *Wkly. Epidemiol. Rec.* 1989; Wilhelm and Schneider, 1990).

Immunization of target wildlife animals in their natural habitat requires that the vaccine be presented to them not only in an immunogenically active form but also in one that is sufficiently attractive to induce the animal to find and eat it. The first field trials (in Switzerland) used chicken heads, into which were inserted small plastic/aluminum blisterpacks containing liquid vaccine. These were prepared in large quantities and distributed manually in Alpine valleys upstream of advancing rabies epizootics. Foxes (the main wildlife rabies vector in western Europe) readily found these baits and, during the process of eating them, punctured the blister packs, thereby releasing sufficient vaccine into the buccal cavity to permit immunization. Switzerland is now practically rabies-free (Wandeler et al., 1988; Wandeler, 1988, 1991), which attests to the high effectiveness of these vaccine baits. Nevertheless, their manufacture is labor-intensive and does not lend itself to automation, which is a drawback when large quantities have to be produced. Most field studies in other countries have therefore used baits containing ingredients such as paraffin wax, beef fat, and either fish meal or chicken essence. These are poured in molds in heated liquid form, and the vaccine-containing blister packs are inserted before the wax-fat mixture solidifies (Bachmann et al., 1990).

For a vaccine to be considered completely acceptable for use in the immunization of free-changing wildlife, it should meet a number of requirements. First and foremost, it must be safe, not only in the target species but also in any other animal species (including human) that may come in contact with it. It must not revert to higher pathogenicity. Of course, it must be able to immunize target animals effectively by the oral route. There are more practical considerations such as stability, and the ease and cost of manufacture.

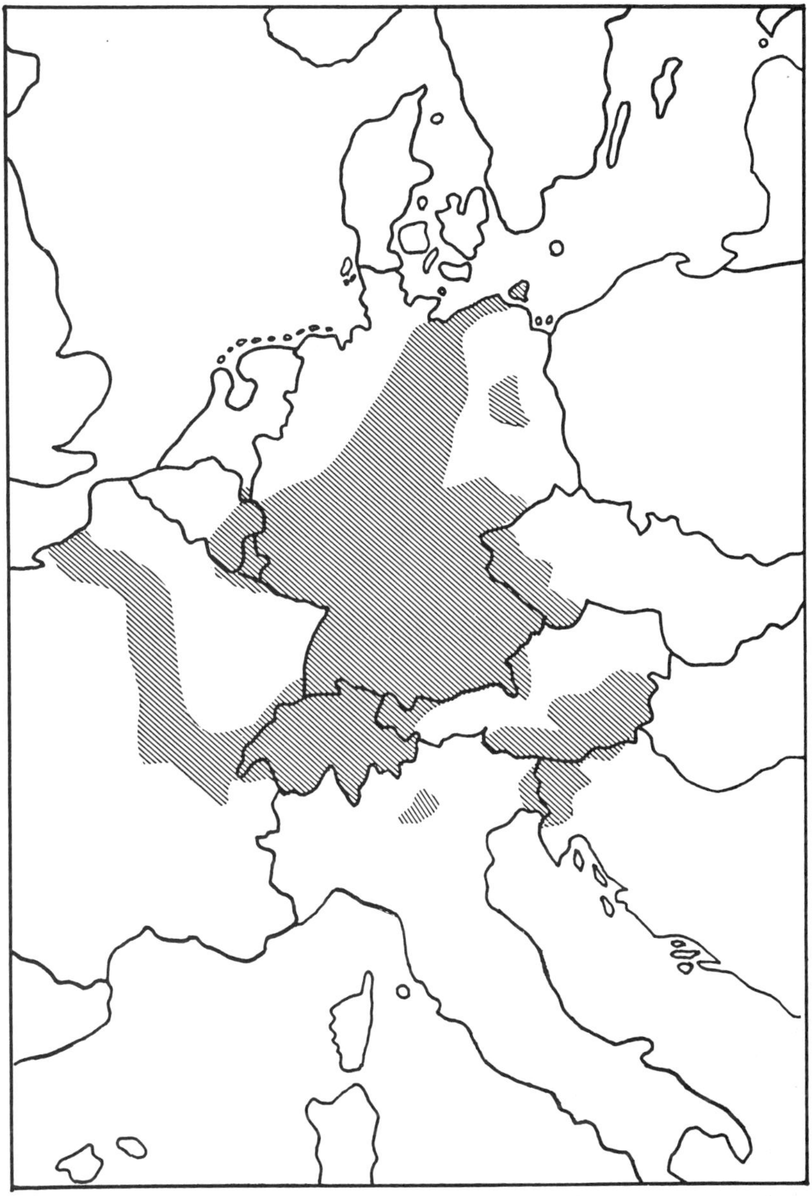

FIGURE 4 Areas of oral fox vaccination in Europe, 1978–1990. Hatched regions have been vaccine-baited at least once. Baits have also been distributed in Finland, from the Gulf of Finland along the southeastern border with the Soviet Union. (*Source*: *Rabies Bull. Eur.* 14/4, 1990.)

TABLE 7 Milestones in the Oral Immunization of Wildlife Against Rabies

1970	Demonstration that foxes can be immunized orally (Black and Lawson, 1970, 1973; Baer et al., 1971; Baer, 1985)
1978	First field trial, Switzerland (SAD-Bern vaccine) (Wandeler, 1988; Wandeler et al., 1988)
1983	Start of field trials in Germany (SAD-B19 vaccine) Schneider and Cox, 1989; Wilhelm and Schneider, 1990)
1985	Automation of vaccine bait production. Extension of SAD-B19 field trials to Italy, Austria, Luxembourg, Belgium, and France (later to other European countries) (Wilhelm and Schneider, 1990)
1987	First North American field trial, Ontario, Canada (ERA vaccine) MacInnes, 1988)
1988	First field trial, vaccinia RG recombinant vaccine, Belgium (Pastoret et al., 1988; Desmettre et al., 1990; Brochier et al., 1990, 1991)
1988	Start of vaccinia RG vaccine field trials in France (Desmettre et al., 1990)
1990	First field trial in the United States (vaccinia-RG vaccine) (Fox, 1990)

When wildlife vaccination was first contemplated in the 1970s, there were no completely safe live vaccines. The SAD strain was known to have residual pathogenicity for certain rodent species, as well as to cause the occasional case of rabies in adult animals. Safety considerations prompted some research groups to investigate the possible use of inactivated vaccine, and it was shown that a number of animal species *would* seroconvert following administration of killed antigen orally or by direct instillation into the duodenum (Atanasiu et al., 1982; Campbell et al., 1984; Lawson et al., 1989a). Nevertheless, this form of vaccination remains impracticable for immunization of wildlife. One drawback is that very large concentrations of viral antigen are required: perhaps baculovirus vaccines may overcome eventually this problem.

Most European trials have used live SAD-derived vaccines, particularly the B19 strain, which was selected for heat stability and good growth characteristics in BHK-21 cells. Concerns about safety appear to have been unfounded: following deposition of more than 8 million vaccine baits over an area in Europe covering at least 100,000 square miles, extensive studies have shown little evidence of vaccine-associated rabies (Wilhelm and Schneider, 1990). Use of an ERA/BHK-21 vaccine in Canadian trials has also given no evidence of causing the disease in any species (MacInnes, personal communication). This notwithstanding, the use of a completely avirulent, arginine-333-substituted vaccine, SAG1 (*SAD-avirulent-Gif*; Le Blois et al., 1990), in recent French field trials is a positive step forward.

One of the limitations of conventional live rabies vaccines for wildlife use is that, although effective by the oral route in foxes, they fail to immunize certain other important vector species such as skunks (Tolson et al., 1990; Rupprecht et al., 1990). Because of their wider host range, the rabies recombinant vaccines may prove to be more effective, and field trials with the vaccinia-RG are under way in Belgium, France, and the United States (Pastoret et al., 1988; Brochier et al., 1990; Desmettre et al., 1990; Fox, 1990). The human adenovirus rabies recombinant (Prevec et al., 1990) is possibly even more effective in skunks than the vaccinia-RG (Charlton et al., 1991), and it is currently under consideration in Canada as a potential wildlife vaccine.

Adenovirus-vectored vaccines may have intrinsic advantages as oral vaccines. For example, canine adenovirus type 1 (infectious canine hepatitis virus) is a natural pathogen of carnivores, with a worldwide distribution (Appel, 1987). Canine adenovirus type 2 is a serologically related virus, the causative agent of "kennel cough" in dogs (Appel, 1987). Both are transmitted in their natural host species by the respiratory or oral route, and there are vaccine strains of both types. Both are completely nonpathogenic for humans. In theory, a canine adenovirus-vectored vaccine should provide an ideal means for the control of canine and wildlife rabies, and research towards its development is in progress (Baer et al., 1989a; Dragulev et al., 1991).

Another, admittedly more fanciful, possibility is the use of adenovirus-based vaccines for the control of rabies in bats. Since most bats are insectivorous, they are unlikely to be attracted to the type of vaccine bait presently used for terrestrial animals. Bats, however, are highly social animals with habits that include mutual grooming, and this characteristic has been used in the control of vampire bat rabies. Mist-netted vampire bats are coated with anticoagulant and released so that they can lethally contaminate roost members (Linhart et al., 1972; Flores-Crespo and Arellano-Sota, 1991). Using this approach, if captured insectivorous bats were to be coated with an infectious vaccine (such as an adenovirus expressing the rabies glycoprotein gene) and then released, the consequence might be autoimmunization that could result in the elimination of rabies from the whole colony. If the recombinant virus were to be transmitted via fecal excretions, the mass immunization process would be correspondingly more efficient. This is highly speculative, however, and requires a nonpathogenic vector virus that will infect bats (unknown as yet), and that such a vaccine could be produced in a form nonpathogenic for any other species. It might not provide the most suitable strategy for control of the vampire bat problem, since a stable vampire population feeding on cattle would still cause problems such as blood loss and disease resulting from infection of bite wounds. With regard to hematophagous bats, therefore, future antirabies strategies are likely to consists of more efficient vector population reduction measures together with more extensive use of the effective vaccines presently available for cattle (Arellano-Sota, 1988). Trials with a vaccinia rabies glycoprotein recombinant in cattle provide optimism that the new generation of rabies vaccines will be effective (Koprowski, 1988).

C. Urban Wildlife

Control of rabies in wild animals living in urban areas presents another problem. Since there is no clear assurance that the present conventional modified live rabies vaccine bait formulations are safe enough to permit possible handling by uninformed humans, their large-scale use has been restricted mainly to rural areas, away from human habitation. As noted above, conventional vaccines are also practically ineffective in skunks, which are urban dwellers over most of North America. Recombinant vaccines may provide a solution. Since these have not yet been approved for use in Canada, however, an alternative method is being tested for the control of skunk and raccoon rabies in urban areas of southern Ontario. This involves live-trapping animals, vaccinating them IM with commercial inactivated vaccine, and releasing them (Rosatte et al., 1990). Experiments so far have indicated that this approach is effective with animals that can be easily trapped, such as skunks and raccoons, although the costs are considerably higher than for oral immunization using vaccine baits (Rosatte et al., 1987; MacInnes, 1987, 1988).

VII. CONCLUSIONS

The end of the first century of rabies vaccination saw the development of safe and effective vaccines for human pre- and postexposure treatment, and for pre-exposure protection of the more common domestic animals, especially dogs. Human cases of rabies are rare in the parts of the world in which these vaccines have been used systematically. Yet worldwide, human deaths from rabies still number yearly in the tens of thousands. These occur mainly in the developing countries of Asia, most of which concentrate their limited resources for rabies control on human post-exposure treatment. Bögel and Meslin (1990) have presented a compelling argument for the establishment of national programs for the elimination of canine rabies, which would include mass vaccination campaigns or continuing vaccination schemes, together with management of the dog population. Their calculations indicate that the yearly implementation of a combined national human postexposure treatment/canine rabies control program would be less costly within 5 years than a human postexposure treatment program alone. Fishbein et al. (1991) have presented similar statistics relating to the cost-effectiveness of canine rabies elimination in the Philippines.

Although considerable logistical problems stand in the way of the development of these programs in many countries, the recent advances in rabies vaccine production will undoubtedly facilitate the process. International technology transfer programs are being instituted so that developing countries can themselves produce more effective, but still inexpensive, vaccines (Halstead, 1988). It is therefore reasonable to anticipate further progress in the global control of canine rabies, with a concomitant reduction in the number of human cases in the coming years.

The start of the second century of rabies vaccination has heralded new concepts in vaccines and the establishment of previously unthinkable goals in rabies control. The continuing expansion of national and international programs for the immunization of free-ranging wildlife indicates that the ultimate bastions of the virus are under increasingly strong attack. It is too early to determine if wildlife rabies *can* be controlled by such methods, but the new live recombinant vaccines should provide powerful weapons. Although their proposed use is still under the careful scrutiny of national and international regulatory agencies, recombinant vaccines may eventually replace conventional human and veterinary vaccines as safer (both to produce and to use), more easily administered (orally), and less costly. Indeed, by virtue of their theoretical ability to spread horizontally in contact animals, they may even provide the means for the total eradication of the virus. This is still a far-distant goal, but there is increasing reason to believe that it may not be an unattainable one.

ACKNOWLEDGMENTS

We are grateful to Drs. M. Aubert, W. Franke, A. King, C. D. MacInnes, F.-X. Meslin, P.-P. Pastoret, C. E. Rupprecht, L. G. Schneider, Zhu Jiahong and Mme. A. Perrot for providing critical appraisals and/or relevant materials. The authors' work described herein has been supported by the National Science and Engineering Research Council of Canada, Tsumura & Co., Japan, and the Ontario Ministry of Natural Resources.

REFERENCES

Afshar, A. (1979). *Br. Vet. J. 135*:142–148.

Aghomo, H. O., and Rupprecht, C. E. (1990). *Vet. Microbiol.* 22:17–22.

Appel, M. J. (1987). In *Virus Infections of Carnivores*, M. J. Appel (Ed.). Elsevier, Amsterdam, pp. 29–51.

Arrelano-Sota, C. (1988). *Rev. Infect. Dis. 10* Suppl. *4*:S707–S709.

Arya, S. C. (1991). *Vaccine 9*:70.

Atanasiu, P., Metianu, T., and Bolanos, A. (1982). *Comp. Immunol. Microbiol. Infect. Dis. 5*:187–191.

Bachmann, P., Bramwell, R. N., Fraser, S. J., Gilmore, D. A., Johnston, D. H., Lawson, K. F., MacInnes, C. D., Matejka, F. O., Miles, H. E., Pedde, M. A., and Voigt, D. R. (1990). *J. Wildlife Dis. 26*:486–501.

Baczynski, Z. (1989). In *Progress in Rabies Control*, O. Thraenhart, H. Koprowski, K. Bögel, and P. Sureau (Eds.). Wells Medical, Royal Tunbridge Wells, pp. 48–53.

Baer, G. M. (1991). (Ed.), *The Natural History of Rabies*, 2nd ed. CRC Press, Boca Raton.

Baer, G. M. (1985). In *World's Debt to Pasteur*, H. Koprowski and S. A. Plotkin (Eds.). Alan R. Liss, New York, pp. 235–247.

Baer, G. M., Abelseth, M. K., and Debbie, J. G. (1971). *Am. J. Epidemiol. 93*:487–490.

Baer, G. M., and Lentz, T. L. (1991). In *The Natural History of Rabies*, 2nd ed., G. M. Baer (Ed.). CRC Press, Boca Raton, pp. 105–120.

Baer, G. M., Moore, S. A., and Levy, H. B. (1979). *Bull. W.H.O. 57*:807–813.

Baer, G. M., Brooks, R. C., and Foggin, C. M. (1989a). *Am. J. Vet. Res. 50*:836–837.

Baer, G. M., Shaddock, J. H., Levy, H., and Johnston, P. (1989b). In *Progress in Rabies Control*, O. Thraenhart, H. Koprowski, K. Bögel, and P. Sureau (Eds.). Wells Medical, Royal Tunbridge Wells, pp. 245–250.

Baer, G. M., Shaddock, J. H., Quirion, R., Dam, T. V., and Lentz, T. L. (1990). *Lancet 335*:664–665.

Barth, R., Gruschkau, H., Bijok, U., Hilfenhaus, J., Hinz, J., Milke, L., Moser, H., Jaeger, O., Ronneberger, H., and Weinmann, E. (1984). *J. Biol. Stand. 12*:29–46.

Barth, R., Franke, V., Müller, H., and Weinmann, E. (1990). *Vaccine 8*:41–48.

Bell, J. F., and Moore, G. J. (1971). *Am. J. Epidemiol. 93*:176–182.

Belotto, A. J. (1988). *Rev. Infect. Dis. 10* Suppl. *4*:S693–S696.

Beran, G. W. (1991). In *The Natural History of Rabies*, 2nd ed., G. M. Baer (Ed.). CRC Press, Boca Raton, pp. 427–443.

Berezin, V. E., Zaides, V. E., Grigoriev, V. B., Klimenko, S. M., and Zhdanov, V. M. (1987). *Vopr. Virusol. 32*:312–317.

Berlin, B. S., Mitchell, J. R., Burgoyne, G. H., Brown, W. E., and Goswick, C. (1983). *JAMA 249*:2663–2665.

Berlin, B. S. (1990). *Am. J. Public Health 80*:476–477.

Black, J. G., and Lawson, K. F. (1970). *Can. J. Comp. Med. 34*:309–311.
Black, J. G., and Lawson, K. F. (1973). *Can. Vet. J. 14*:206–211.
Blancou, J. (1986). In *Proc. 9th Int. Congr. Infect. Parasit. Dis.*, vol. 1, W. Margret, W. Lang, and E. Gabler-Sandberger (Eds.). MMV Medizin Verlag, Munich, pp. 134–137.
Bögel, K., and Meslin, F.-X. (1990). *Bull. W.H.O. 68*:281–291.
Bourhy, H., Tordo, N., Lafon, M., and Sureau, P. (1989). *J. Gen. Virol. 70*:2063–2074.
Bourhy, H., Sureau, P., and Tordo, N. (1990). *Vet. Microbiol. 23*:115–128.
Brochier, B., Thomas, I., Leveau, T., Pastoret, P.-P., Languet, B., Chappuis, G., Desmettre, P., Blancou, J., and Artois, M. (1990). *Vaccine 8*:101–104.
Brochier, B., Costy, F., Hallet, L., Duhaut, R., Peharpre, D., Afiademanyo, K., Bauduin, B., and Pastoret, P.-P. (1991). *Ann. Méd. Vét. 135*:191–201.
Bunn, T. O. (1988). In *Rabies*, J. B. Campbell and K. M. Charlton (Eds.). Kluwer Academic Publishing, Boston, pp. 323–333.
Bunn, T. O. (1991). In *The Natural History of Rabies*, 2nd ed., G. M. Baer (Ed.). CRC Press, Boca Raton, pp. 415–425.
Calisher, C. H., Karabatsos, N., Zeller, H., Digoutte, J.-P., Tesh, R. B., Shope, R. E., Travassos da Rosa, A. P. A., and St. George, T. D. (1989). *Intervirology 30*: 241–257.
Campbell, J. B., Maharaj, I., and Roith, J. (1984). In *Rabies in the Tropics*, E. Kuwert, C. Mérieux, K. Bögel, and H. Koprowski (Eds.). Springer-Verlag, Berlin, pp. 285–293.
Campbell, J. B., and Chavali, S. R. (1989). In *Progress in Rabies Control*, O. Thraenhart, H. Koprowski, K. Bögel, and P. Sureau (Eds.). Wells Medical, Royal Tunbridge Wells, pp. 263–273.
Centers for Disease Control. (1991). *M.M.W.R. 40*:1–19.
Chaloner-Larsson, G., Contreras, G., Furesz, J., Boucher, D. W., Krepps, D., Humphreys, G. R., and Mohanna, S. M. (1986). *Can. J. Public Health 77*:367–370.
Charlton, K. M. (1988). In *Rabies*, J. B. Campbell and K. M. Charlton (Eds.). Kluwer Academic Publishing, Boston, pp. 101–150.
Charlton, K. M., Casey, G. A., and Campbell, J. B. (1983). *Can. J. Comp. Med. 47*:363–369.
Charlton, K. M., Artois, M., Prevec, L., Campbell, J. B., Casey, G. A., Wandeler, A. I., and Armstrong, J. (1991). *Arch. Virol.*, in press.
Chavali, S. R., and Campbell, J. B. (1987a). *Immunobiology 174*:347–359.
Chavali, S. R., and Campbell, J. B. (1987b). *Int. Arch. Allergy Appl. Immunol. 84*: 129–134.
Chomel, B., Chappuis, G., Bullon, F., Cardenas, E., David de Beublain, T., Lombard, M., and Giambruno, E. (1988). *Rev. Infect. Dis. 10* Suppl. 4:S697–S702.
Constantine, D. G., Emmons, R. W., and Woddie, J. D. (1972). *Science 175*:1255–1256.
Conzelmann, K. K., Cox, J. H., Schneider, L. G., and Thiel, H. J. (1990). *Virology 175*:485–489.
Coulon, P., Derbin, C., Kučera, P., Lafay, F., Préhaud, C., and Flamand, A. (1989). *J. Virol. 63*:3550–3554.
Crick, J., and Brown, F. (1978). *Dev. Biol. Stand. 40*:255–264.

Crick, J., and King, A. (1988). In *Rabies*, J. B. Campbell and K. M. Charlton (Eds.). Kluwer Academic Publishing, Boston, pp. 47–66.

Delpietro, H., Segre, L., Marchevsky, N., and Berisso, M. (1990). *Medicina B. Aires* *50*:356–360.

Desmettre, P., Languet, B., Chappuis, G., Brochier, B., Thomas, I., Lecocq, J.-P., Kieny, M.-P., Blancou, J., Aubert, M., Artois, M., and Pastoret, P.-P. (1990). *Vet. Microbiol.* *23*:227–236.

Dietzschold, B., and Ertl, H. C. J. (1991). *Crit. Rev. Immunol.* *10*:427–439.

Dietzschold, B., and Rupprecht, C. E. (1989). In *Progress in Rabies Control*, O. Thraenhart, H. Koprowski, K. Bögel, and P. Sureau (Eds.). Wells Medical, Royal Tunbridge Wells, pp. 199–206.

Dietzschold, B., Wunner, W. H., Wiktor, T. J., Lopes, A. D., Lafon, M., Smith, C., and Koprowski, H. (1983a). *Proc. Natl. Acad. Sci. U.S.A.* *80*:70–74.

Dietzschold, B., Wang, H., Rupprecht, C. E., Celis, E., Tollis, M., Ertl, H., Heber-Katz, E., and Koprowski, H. (1983b). *Proc. Natl. Acad. Sci. U.S.A.* *84*:9165–9169.

Dragulev, B. P., Sira, S., AbouHaidar, M. G., and Campbell, J. B. (1991). *Virology* *183*:298–305.

Dreesen, D. W., Brown, W. J., Kemp, D. T., Brown, J., Reid, F. L., and Baer, G. M. (1984). *Vaccine* 2:185–188.

Dreesman, G. R., and Kennedy, R. C. (1985). *J. Infect. Dis.* *151*:761–775.

Esposito, J. J. (1989). *Res. Virol.* *40*:480–482.

Esposito, J. J., Brechling, K., Baer, G. M., and Moss, B. (1987). *Virus Genes* *1*:7–21.

Esposito, J. J., Knight, J. C., Shaddock, J. H., Novembre, F. J., and Baer, G. M. (1988). *Virology* *165*:313–316.

Fekadu, M. (1988). *Rev. Infect. Dis.* *10* Suppl. 4:S678–S683.

Fekadu, M. (1991). In *The Natural History of Rabies*, 2nd ed. G. M. Baer (Ed.). CRC Press, Boca Raton, pp. 191–198.

Fekadu, M., Shaddock, J. H., Sanderlin, D. W., and Smith, J. S. (1988). *Vaccine* *6*:533–539.

Fishbein, D. B., Miranda, N. J., Merrill, P., Camba, R. A., Meltzer, M., Carlos, E. T., Bautista, C. F., Sopungco, P. V., Mangahas, L. C., Hernandes, L. M., Leoncio, M. M., Mercado, D., Gregorio, S., Salva, E., Dobbins, J. G., and Winkler, W. G. (1991). *Vaccine* *9*:581–587.

Flores-Crespo, R., and Arellano-Sota, C. (1991). In *The Natural History of Rabies*, 2nd ed. G. M. Baer (Ed.). CRC Press, Boca Raton, pp. 461–476.

Fox, J. L. (1990). *A.S.M. News* *56*:579–583.

Fu, Z. F., Dietzschold, B., Schumacher, C. L., Wunner, W. H., Ertl, H. C. J., and Koprowski, H. (1991). *Proc. Natl. Acad. Sci. U.S.A.* *88*:2001–2005.

Galtier, P. V. (1881). *C. R. Acad. Sci.* *93*:284–285.

Gooding, L. R., and Wold, W. S. M. (1990). *Crit. Rev. Immunol.* *10*:53–71.

Gough, P. M., and Niemeyer, C. (1975). *J. Wildlife Dis.* *11*:170–176.

Halstead, S. B. (1988). *Rev. Infect. Dis.* *10* Suppl. 4:S764–S765.

Harverson, G., and Wasi, C. (1984). *Lancet* 2:313–315.

Hattwick, M. A. W., and Gregg, M. B. (1975). In *The Natural History of Rabies*, vol. 2, G. M. Baer (Ed.). Academic Press, New York, pp. 281–304.

Hattwick, M. A. W., Weiss, T. T., Stechschulte, C. J., Baaer, G. M., and Gregg, M. B. (1972). *Ann. Intern. Med. 76*:931–942.
Hemachudha, T. (1989). In *Progress in Rabies Control*, O. Thraenhart, H. Koprowski, K. Bögel, and P. Sureau (Eds.). Wells Medical, Royal Tunbridge Wells, pp. 54–64.
Hemachudha, T., Phanuphak, P., Johnson, R. T., Griffin, D. E., Ratanavongsiri, J., and Siriprasomsup, W. (1987). *Neurology 37*:550–556.
Höglund, S., Dalsgaard, K., Lövgren, K., Sundquist, B., Osterhaus, A. D. M. E., and Morein, B. (1989). *Subcell. Biochem. 15*:39–68.
Hübschle, O. J. B. (1988). *Rev. Infect. Dis. 10* Suppl. 4:S629–S633.
Isaacson, R. L. (1989). In *Progress in Rabies Control*, O. Thraenhart, H. Koprowski, K. Bögel, and P. Sureau (Eds.). Wells Medical, Royal Tunbridge Wells, pp. 17–23.
Iwasaki, Y. (1991). In *The Natural History of Rabies*, 2nd ed., G. M. Baer (Ed.). CRC Press, Boca Raton, pp. 121–132.
Javier, R. S., Kunishita, T., Koike, F., and Tabira, T. (1989). *J. Neurol. Sci. 93*: 221–230.
Joffret, M.-L., Morgeaux, S., Leclerc, C., Oth, D., Zanetti, C., Sureau, P., and Perrin, P. (1990). *Vaccine 8*:385–389.
Kang, C. Y. (1988). *Adv. Virus Res. 35*:177–192.
Kasempimolporn, S., Hemadchudha, T., Khawplod, P., and Manatsathit, S. (1991). *Clin. Exp. Immunol. 84*:195–199.
Kawano, H., Mifune, K., Ohuchi, M., Mannen, K., Cho, S., Hiramatsu, K., and Shichijo, A. (1990). *J. Gen. Virol. 71*:281–287.
Kersten, G. (1990). Doctoral thesis, University of Utrecht, The Netherlands.
Kieny, M. P., Lathe, R., Drillien, R., Spehner, D., Skory, S., Schmitt, D., Wiktor, T., Koprowski, H., and Lecocq, J. P. (1984). *Nature 312*:163–166.
King, A., and Crick, J. (1988). In *Rabies*, J. B. Campbell, and K. M. Charlton (Eds.). Kluwer Academic Publishing, Boston, pp. 177–199.
King, A., Davies, P., and Lawrie, A. (1990). *Vet. Microbiol. 23*:165–174.
Koprowski, H. (1988). *Rev. Infect. Dis. 10* Suppl. 4:S810–S813.
Larghi, O. P., Arrosi, J. C., Nakajata-A. J., and Villa-Nova, A. (1988). In *Rabies*, J. B. Campbell, and K. M. Charlton (Eds.). Kluwer Academic Publishing, Boston, pp. 407–422.
Lawrence, G. D., Kanarek, A. D., and Wachmann, B. (1989). In *Progress in Rabies Control*, O. Thraenhart, H. Koprowski, K. Bögel, and P. Sureau (Eds.). Wells Medical, Royal Tunbridge Wells, pp. 221–227.
Lawson, K. F., Johnston, D. H., Patterson, J. M., Hertler, R., Campbell, J. B., and Rhodes, A. J. (1989a). *Can. J. Vet. Res. 53*:56–61.
Lawson, K. F., Hertler, R., Charlton, K. M., Campbell, J. B., and Rhodes, A. J. (1989b). *Can. J. Vet. Res. 53*:438–444.
LeBlois, H., Tuffereau, C., Blancou, J., Artois, M., Aubert, A., and Flamand, A. (1990). *Vet. Microbiol. 23*:259–266.
Lentz, T. L. (1990). *J. Mol. Recog. 3*:82–88.
Lin, F. T. (1990). *Bull. W.H.O. 68*:449–454.

Linhart, S. B., Flores Crespo, R., and Mitchell, G. C. (1972). *Bull. PAHO 6*: 31–38.
Lodmell, D. L., Sumner, J. W., Esposito, J. J., Bellini, W., and Ewalt, L. C. (1991). *J. Virol. 65*:3400–3405.
Lumio, J., Hilbom, M., Roine, R., Ketonen, L., Haltia, M., Valle, M., Neuvonen, E., and Lahdevirta, J. (1986). *Lancet 1*:378.
Macdonald, D. W., and Voigt, D. R. (1985). In *Population Dynamics of Rabies in Wildlife*, P. J. Bacon (Ed.). Academic Press, London, pp. 71–108.
MacFarlan, R. I. (1988). In *Rabies*, J. B. Campbell and K. M. Charlton (Eds.). Kluwer Academic Publishing, Boston, pp. 163–176.
MacInnes, C. D. (1987). In *Wild Furbearer Management and Conservation in North America*, M. Novak, J. A. Baker, M. E. Obbard, and B. Malloch (Eds.). Ontario Trappers Association, Ontario, pp. 910–929.
MacInnes, C. D. (1988). In *Rabies*, J. B. Campbell and K. M. Charlton (Eds.). Kluwer Academic Publishing, Boston, pp. 381–405.
Madhusudana, S. N., and Tripathi, K. K. (1990). *Ind. J. Med. Res. 28*:497–499.
Maharaj, I., Froh, K. J., and Campbell, J. B. (1986). *Can. J. Microbiol. 32*:414–420.
Marie, A. (1909). *L'étude expérimentale de la rage*. Octave Doin et fils, Paris.
Markovistz, R., Germano, P. M., Riviere, Y., Tsiang, H., and Hovanessian, A. G. (1987). *J. Interferon Res. 7*:17–27.
Mayr, A., Kraft, H., Jaeger, O., and Haacke, H. (1972). *Zentralbl. Veterinärmed. [B] 19*:615–625.
Mifune, K., Takeuchi, E., Napiorkowski, P., Yamada, A., and Sakamoto, K. (1981). *Microbiol. Immunol. 25*:895–904.
Morein, B., and Simons, K. (1985). *Vaccine 3*:83–93.
Morein, B., Sundquist, B., Höglund, S., Dalsgaard, K., and Osterhaus, A. (1984). *Nature 308*:457–460.
Moss, B. (1991). *Science 252*:1662–1667.
Murphy, F. A. (1977). *Arch. Virol. 54*:279–297.
Murphy, F. A. (1985). In *World's Debt to Pasteur*, H. Koprowski and S. A. Plotkin (Eds.). Alan R. Liss, New York, pp. 153–169.
NASPHV Committee. (1991). Compendium of animal rabies control. *J. Am. Vet. Med. Assoc. 198*:37–41.
Nathanson, N., and Gonzalez-Scarano, F. (1991). In *The Natural History of Rabies*, 2nd ed. G. M. Baer (Ed.). CRC Press, Boca Raton, pp. 145–161.
Nicholson, K. G. (1990). *Lancet 335*:1201–1205.
Nunberg, J. H., Doyle, M. V., York, S. M., and York, C. J. (1989). *Proc. Natl. Acad. Sci. U.S.A. 86*:4240–4243.
Oth, D., Mercier, G., Perrin, P., Joffret, M. L., Sureau, P., and Thibodeau, L. (1987). *Cell. Immunol. 108*:220–226.
PAHO. (1990). *Report of the Director: Quadrennial 1986–1989, Annual 1989*. PAHO, Washington, D.C. ISBN 92 75 17234X.
Pasteur, L. (1885). *C. R. Acad. Sci. 101*:765–774.
Pastoret, P.-P., Brochier, B., Thomas, I., and Blancou, J. (Eds.) (1988a). *Vaccination to Control Rabies in Foxes*. EUR 1439. Office for Official Publications of the European Community, Luxembourg.

Pastoret, P.-P., Brochier, B., Languet, B., Thomas, I., Paquot, A., Bauduin, B., Kieny, M. P., Lecocq, J. P., De Bruyn, J., Costy, F., Antoine, H., and Desmettre, P. (1988b). *Vet. Rec. 123*:481–483.

Perrin, P., Joffret, M.-L., Leclerc, C., Oth, D., Sureau, P., and Thibodeau, L. (1988). *Immunobiology 177*:199–209.

Perrin, P., Lafon, M., and Sureau, P. (1990). *Adv. Biotechnol. Proc. 14*:325–345.

Perrin, P., Joffret, M.-L., Zanetti, C., Bourhy, H., Gontier, C., Fritzell, C., Leclerc, C., and Sureau, P. (1991). *Vaccine 9*:549–558.

Piccini, A., and Paoletti, E. (1988). *Adv. Virus Res. 34*:43–64.

Préhaud, C., Takehara, K., Flamand, A., and Bishop, D. H. (1989). *Virology 173*: 390–399.

Prevec, L., Campbell, J. B., Christie, B. S., Belbeck, L., and Graham, F. L. (1990). *J. Infect. Dis. 161*:27–30.

Ramsden, R. O., and Johnston, D. H. (1975). *J. Wildlife Dis. 11*:318–324.

Reagan, K. J., Wunner, W. H., and Koprowski, H. (1985). In *High-Technology Route to Virus Vaccines*, G. R. Dreesman, J. D. Bronson, and R. C. Kennedy (Eds.). A.S.M., Washington, pp. 117–124.

Rodriguez, D., Rodriguez, J. R., Rodriguez, J. F., Trauber, D., and Esteban, M. (1989). *Proc. Natl. Acad. Sci. U.S.A. 86*:1287–1291.

Rosatte, R. C., Pybus, M. J., and Gunson, J. R. (1986). *J. Wildlife Dis. 22*:459–467.

Rosatte, R. C., Kelly-Ward, P. M., and MacInnes, C. D. (1987). In *Integrating Man and Nature in the Metropolitan Environment*, L. W. Adams and D. L. Leedy (Eds.). National Institute for Urban Wildlife, Columbia, MD, pp. 161–167.

Rosatte, R. C., Howard, D. R., Campbell, J. B., and MacInnes, C. D. (1990). *J. Wildlife Dis. 26*:225–230.

Rosset, R. (1985) (Ed.). *Pasteur et la Rage*, Informations Techniques des Services Vétérinaires, Ministère de l'Agriculture, Paris.

Roumiantzeff, M. (1988). *S.E. Asian J. Trop. Med. Public Health 19*:549–561.

Roumiantzeff, M., Ajjan, N., Montagnon, B., and Vincent-Falquet, J. C. (1985). *Ann. Inst. Pasteur/Virol. 136E*:413–424.

Roumiantzeff, M., Ajjan, N., and Vincent-Falquet, J. C. (1988). *J. Infect. Dis. 10* Suppl. 4:S751–S757.

Roumiantzeff, M., Montagnon, B., and Vincent-Falquet, J. C. (1989). In *Progress in Rabies Control*, O. Thraenhart, H. Koprowski, K. Bögel, and P. Sureau (Eds.). Wells Medical, Royal Tunbridge Wells, pp. 483–492.

Rupprecht, C. E., and Dietzschold, B. (1987). *Lab. Invest. 57*:603–606.

Rupprecht, C. E., and Kieny, M.-P. (1988). In *Rabies*, J. B. Campbell and K. M. Charlton (Eds.). Kluwer Academic Publishing, Boston, pp. 335–364.

Rupprecht, C. E., Charlton, K. M., Artois, M., Casey, G. A., Webster, W. A., Campbell, J. B., Lawson, K. F., and Schneider, L. G. (1990). *J. Wildlife Dis. 26*:99–102.

Rupprecht, C. E., Dietzschold, B., Wunner, W. H., and Koprowski, H. (1991). In *The Natural History of Rabies*, 2nd ed., G. M. Baer (Ed.). CRC Press, Boca Raton, pp. 69–100.

Schneider, L. G., and Cox, J. H. (1989). In *Progress in Rabies Control*, O. Thraenhart, H. Koprowski, K. Bögel, and P. Sureau (Eds.). Wells Medical, Royal Tunbridge Wells, pp. 159–168.
Schneider, L. G., Horzinek, M., and Novický, R. (1971). *Arch. Ges. Virusforsch.* *34*:360–370.
Selimov, M., Aksenova, T., Klyueva, E., Gribencha, L., and Lebedeva, I. (1978). *Dev. Biol. Stand.* *40*:57–62.
Shankar, V., Dietzschold, B., and Koprowski, H. (1991). *J. Virol.* *65*:2736–2738.
Smith, J. S. (1989). *Adv. Virus Res.* *36*:215–253.
Smith, J. S., and Baer, G. M. (1988). In *Rabies*, J. B. Campbell and K. M. Charlton (Eds.). Kluwer Academic Publishing, Boston, pp. 267–299.
Smith, J. S., McClelland, C. L., Reid, F. L., and Baer, G. M. (1982). *Infect. Immun.* *35*:213–221.
Smith, J. S., Sanderlin, D. W., and Yager, P. A. (1989). In *Progress in Rabies Control*, O. Thraenhart, H. Koprowski, K. Bögel, and P. Sureau (Eds.). Wells Medical, Royal Tunbridge Wells, pp. 115–125.
Soulebot, J. P., Précausta, P., Brun, A., Blancou, J. M., Pépin, M., Chappuis, G., and Petermann, H. G. (1985). In *Rabies in the Tropics*, E. Kuwert, C. Mérieux, K. Bögel, and H. Koprowski (Eds.). Springer-Verlag, Berlin, pp. 274–284.
Sumner, J. W., Fekadu, M., Shaddock, J. H., Esposito, J. J., and Bellini, W. J. (1991). *Virology* *183*:703–710.
Sureau, P. (1990). *Comp. Immunol. Microbiol. Infect. Dis.* *13*:107–110.
Sureau, P., and Perrin, P. (1989). *Eur. J. Epidemiol.* *5*:275–278.
Sureau, P., and Rollin, P. (1989). In *Progress in Rabies Control*, O. Thraenhart, H. Koprowski, K. Bögel, and P. Sureau (Eds.). Wells Medical, Royal Tunbridge Wells, pp. 548–549.
Swaddiwudhipong, W., Prayoonwiwat, N., Kunasol, P., and Choomkasien, P. (1987). *S.E. Asian J. Trop. Med. Public Health* *18*:526–531.
Takahashi, H., Takeshita, T., Morein, B., Putney, S., Germain, R. N., and Berzofsky, J. A. (1990). *Nature* *344*:873–875.
Taylor, J., Weinberg, R., Languet, B., Desmettre, P., and Paoletti, E. (1988). *Vaccine* *6*:497–503.
Taylor, J., Trimarchi, C., Weinberg, R., Languet, B., Guillemin, F., Desmettre, P., and Paoletti, E. (1991). *Vaccine* *9*:190–193.
Théodoridès, J. (1986). *Histoire de la Rage*. Masson, Paris.
Thraenhart, O., Marcus, I., Scheiermann, N., Baer, J., Hilfenhaus, J., Jäger, O., and Ramakrishnan, K. (1989). In *Progress in Rabies Control*, O. Thraenhart, H. Koprowski, K. Bögel, and P. Sureau (Eds.). Wells Medical, Royal Tunbridge Wells, pp. 536–547.
Tollis, M., Dietzschold, B., Volia, C. B., and Koprowski, H. (1991). *Vaccine* *9*:134–136.
Tolson, N. D., Charlton, K. M., Stewart, R. B., Webster, W. A., MacKenzie, K., Campbell, J. B., and Lawson, K. F. (1990). *Can. J. Vet. Res.* *54*:178–183.
Tordo, N., and Poch, O. (1988). In *Rabies*, J. B. Campbell and K. M. Charlton. (Eds.). Kluwer Academic Publishing, Boston, pp. 25–45.

Tordo, N., Poch, O., Ermine, A., Keith, G., and Rougeon, F. (1988). *Virology 165*: 565–576.

Torres-Anjel, M. J., Volz, D., Torres, M. J. R., Turk, M., and Tshikuka, J. G. (1988). *Rev. Infect. Dis. 10* Suppl. 4:S710–S725.

Tsiang, H. (1988). In *Rabies*, J. B. Campbell and K. M. Charlton (Eds.). Kluwer Academic Publishing, Boston, pp. 67–100.

Tuffereau, C., Leblois, H., Benejean, J., Coulon, P., Lafay, F., and Flamand, A. (1989). *Virology 172*:206–212.

Turner, G. (1985). *Ann. Inst. Pasteur/Virol. 136E*:453–460.

Varughese, P. V., and Carter, A. O. (1990). *Canada Dis. Wkly, Rep. 16-28*:131–136.

Vodopija, I. (1988). *Rev. Infect. Dis. 10* Suppl. 4:S758–S763.

Vodopija, I., Sureau, P., Lafon, M., Ljubičić, M., Baklaić, Z., Svjetličić, M., and Smerdel, S. (1986). *Vaccine 4*:245–248.

Vodopija, I., and Clark, H. F. (1991). In *The Natural History of Rabies*, 2nd ed., G. M. Baer (Ed.). CRC Press, Boca Raton, pp. 571–595.

Vodopija, I., Smerdel, S., Ljubičić, M., Baklaić, Z., Svjetličić, M., and Lojkić. (1989a). In *Progress in Rabies Control*, O. Thraenhart, H. Koprowski, K. Bögel, and P. Sureau (Eds.). Wells Medical, Royal Tunbridge Wells, pp. 243–244.

Vodopija, I., Ljubičić, M., Baklaić, Z., Svjetličić, M., and Smerdel, S. (1989b). In *Progress in Rabies Control*, O. Thraenhart, H. Koprowski, K. Bögel, and P. Sureau (Eds.). Wells Medical, Royal Tunbridge Wells, pp. 523–528.

Wandeler, A. I. (1988). In *Rabies*, J. B. Campbell and K. M. Charlton (Eds.). Kluwer Academic Publishing, Boston, pp. 365–380.

Wandeler, A. I., Capt, S., Kappeler, A., and Hauser, R. (1988). *Rev. Infect. Dis. 10* Suppl. 4:S649–653.

Wandeler, A. I. (1991). In *The Natural History of Rabies*, 2nd ed., G. M. Baer (Ed.). CRC Press, Boca Raton, pp. 485–503.

Warrell, D. A., and Warrell, M. J. (1988). *Rev. Infect. Dis.* 10 Suppl. 4:S726–S731.

Wiktor, T. J. (1978). *Dev. Biol. Stand. 40*:255–264.

Wiktor, T. J. (1985). In *World's Debt to Pasteur*, H. Koprowski and S. A. Plotkin (Eds.). Alan R. Liss, New York, pp. 141–151.

Wiktor, T. J., Doherty, P. C., and Koprowski, H. (1977). *Proc. Natl. Acad. Sci. U.S.A. 74*:334–338.

Wiktor, T. J., Plotkin, S. A., and Koprowski, H. (1978). *Dev. Biol. Stand. 40*:3–9.

Wiktor, T. J., MacFarlan, R. I., and Koprowski, H. (1985). In *Rabies in the Tropics*, E. Kuwert, C. Mérieux, K. Bögel, and H. Koprowski (Eds.). Springer-Verlag, Berlin, pp. 21–29.

Wilde, H., and Chutivongse, S. (1989). In *Progress in Rabies Control*, O. Thraenhart, H. Koprowski, K. Bögel, and P. Sureau (Eds.). Wells Medical, Royal Tunbridge Wells, pp. 529–535.

Wilhelm, U., and Schneider, L. G. (1990). *Bull. W.H.O. 68*:87–92.

Wkly. Epidemiol. Rec. (1989). *25*:189–192.

Wkly. Epidemiol. Rec. (1990). *15*:114–115.

Wosu, L. O., and Anyanwu, H. N. (1990). *Zentralbl. Veterinärmed. B 37*:47–52.

Wunner, W. H. (1991). In *The Natural History of Rabies,* 2nd ed., G. M. Baer (Ed.). CRC Press, Boca Raton, pp. 31–67.

Wunner, W. H., Larson, J. K., Dietzschold, B., and Smith, C. L. (1988). *Rev. Infect. Dis. 10* Suppl. *4*:S771–S784.

Yasmuth, C., Nelson, K. E., Laima, T., Supawdee, J., and Thaiyanant, P. (1983). *J. Med. Assoc. Thai. 66*:169–175.

Part V

Japanese Encephalitis and Dengue

12

JAPANESE ENCEPHALITIS
Virus, Infection, and Control

Akira Igarashi *Institute of Tropical Medicine, Nagasaki University, Nagasaki City, Japan*

I. JAPANESE ENCEPHALITIS VIRUS

A. Taxonomy

Japanese encephalitis (JE) virus, causative agent of a serious acute infectious human disease, belongs to the family Flaviviridae (Westaway et al., 1985), which comprises approximately 60 members (Calisher et al., 1989). Most of the flaviviruses, including JE virus, were formerly classified as group B arboviruses according to their transmission cycle in nature and antigenic cross-reactivity (Clarke and Casals, 1965). Several flaviviruses or group B arboviruses have been documented as human or veterinary pathogens (Shope, 1980; Monath, 1986). By results of classic serologic tests of hemagglutination–inhibition (HI), complement-fixation (CF), or neutralization (N), JE virus was closely related to Murray Valley encephalitis, West Nile, and St. Louis encephalitis viruses, constituting a subgroup or complex (Clarke and Casals, 1958; DeMadrid and Porterfield, 1974).

B. Virion Morphology and Physicochemical Properties

Electron microscopic examination of thin sections of infected cells/tissues (Ota, 1965; Yasuzumi and Tsubo, 1965; Oyanagi et al., 1969) or negatively stained purified preparation (Kitano et al., 1974) revealed enveloped particles 38–53 nm in diameter, similar to other flaviviruses (Fig. 1).

Sedimentation coefficient of the infections virion was estimated as 200S with density of 1.23 g/ml in sucrose-D_2O (Shapiro et al., 1971). Besides complete virion, slowly sedimenting hemagglutinin (SHA) and soluble

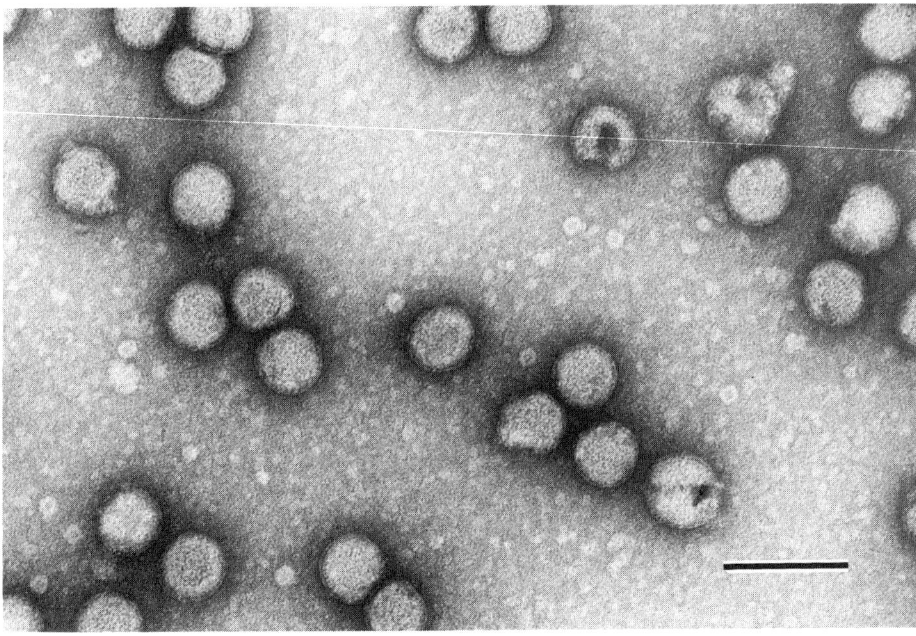

FIGURE 1 Morphology of JE virion. Purified preparation of mouse brain-derived and formalin-inactivated JE vaccine concentrate (scale: 100 nm). Figure kindly provided by Mr. S. Yoshida, Kanonji Institute, Research Foundation for Microbial Diseases of Osaka University, by courtesy of Professor K. Fukai, Director.

compartment-fixing antigen (SCF) were recognized in the infected mouse brain homogenate supernatant or infected cell culture fluid (Igarashi et al., 1963a; Kitaoka and Nishimura, 1965; Shapiro et al., 1971; Shameem et al., 1989).

C. Virion Structural Proteins

Like other flaviviruses, three structural proteins have been identified for JE virus: membrane protein V1 (or M, molecular weight [MW], 8 kD), core protein V2 (or C, Mw, 14 kD) and envelope glycoprotein V3 (or E, Mw, 54 kD) (Shapiro et al., 1971; Kitano et al., 1974). Of these structural proteins, the E protein on the virion surface has been considered to play the most important role in the initial step of virus–cell interaction. Neutralizing (N) antibodies were produced in mice by immunization with purified E protein (Takegami et al., 1982). Passively immunized mice with detectable neutralizing antibodies at 1:10 serum dilution was protected from lethal challenge of JE virus (Oya, 1988). Analysis by monoclonal antibodies (MCA) identified multiple epitopes on the E protein with various cross-reactivity and biological properties (Kimura-Kuroda and Yasui, 1983, 1986, 1988; Cecilia et al., 1988). Among different groups of MCA reported by Kimura-Kuroda and Yasui, their group 8 MCA was JE virus-specific and protective in a mouse model system (Table 1).

D. Genomic RNA

The genome of JE virus is a single-stranded RNA of approximately 45 S and infectious (Nakamura, 1961; Igarashi et al., 1963b, 1964), therefore positive-sense. Analysis of the complete nucleotide sequence of a wild strain JaOArS982 showed that the genome consisted of 10,976 nucleotides (nt): 95 nt in the 5′-noncoding region, 10,296 nt in a long open reading frame (ORF), and 585 nt in the 3′-noncoding region (Sumiyoshi et al., 1986, 1987). The ORF could code a polyprotein of 3,432 amino acids and its 5′ one-fourth consists of the structural protein genes in the order of C-PreM (precursor of M)-E, and the remaining part of the ORF is the nonstructural protein genes (Fig. 2). The 3′-end of JE virus genomic RNA did not contain poly(A) tract but was considered to form stem and loop secondary structure (Takegami et al., 1986). This genomic organization is essentially the same as other flaviviruses represented by yellow fever virus (Rice et al.,

TABLE 1 Groups of MCA Specific to JE Virus E Protein

Epitope Group	Biological Activity[a] HI	N	PA	Cross-Reactivity
1	++	–	+	Flaviviruses
2	—	–	+	Subgroup
3	–	+	++	JE-specific[b]
4	–	+	–	Subgroup
5	–	+	+	Subgroup
6	–	–	+	Subgroup
7	++	++	++	Subgroup
8	–	+++	+++	JE-specific
9	–	–	+	Flaviviruses

[a]HI, hemagglutination-inhibition; N, neutralization; PA, protection by passive immunization.
[b]Also strain-specific.
Source: Modified by permission from Yasui (1987), summarized from Kimura-Kuroda and Yasui (1983, 1986, 1988).

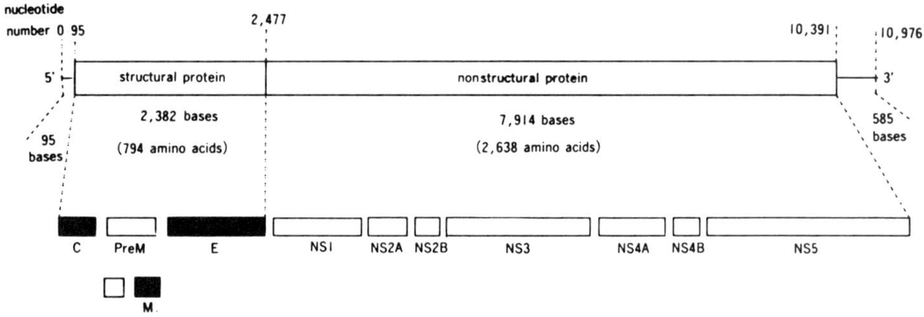

FIGURE 2 Genomic organization of JE virus RNA. (Reproduced from Igarashi [1988] by permission.)

1985). Partial or complete nt sequences of several other JE virus strains were analyzed and the results were consistent with the overall genomic organization mentioned above, although several nt substitutions were present (McAda et al., 1987; Hashimoto et al., 1988; Nitayaphan et al., 1990; Aihara et al., 1991).

E. Virus Infection to Host Cells

Virus–Host Cell Interaction

The initial step of JE virus attachment to host cell membrane was considered to take place by interaction between virion E protein and cell receptor(s). Isolation of biologically active JE virus receptor from host cells or tissues showed that the active components contained lipids, saccharides, and peptides (Mori and Nozima, 1965; Nozima et al., 1968; Yasui et al., 1971). However, their structure and function were not analyzed further. Electron microscopic observation of virus-infected mosquito C6/36 cells indicated that the entry mode of JE virus is different from that of Semliki Forest (SF) virus, an alphavirus of the family Togaviridae (Hase et al., 1989). At physiological pH, SF virus particles were observed mainly within plasma membrane invaginations and cytoplasmic vesicles, indicating receptor-mediated endocytosis. On the other hand, JE virus particles remained exclusively at the cell surface, indicating virus penetration and disintegration at or near the adsorption site. From these observations, the authors postulated that the fusion protein of SF virus is inactive at physiological pH and needs to be activated by acidic endosomal pH, while that of JE is active to dissolve plasma membrane at physiological pH.

Viral RNA Synthesis

Viral RNA synthesis appeared to take place in close proximity to or association with nuclear membrane, as shown by radiolabeling followed by autoradiographic observation (Takeda et al., 1965, 1977) and cell fractionation (Takeda et al., 1978). Assay of viral RNA polymerase in JE virus-infected cells showed that the enzyme activity was closely associated with membrane or nuclear fraction (Takegami and Hotta, 1989, 1990). These findings may be related to the report that the replication of JE virus did not take place in cells enucleated before the infection, but did occur at reduced level in the cells enucleated 4 hr or later after the infection (Kos et al., 1975).

Virus-specific RNA species synthesized in JE virus-infected cells was analyzed by sucrose gradient sedimentation of radiolabeled specimens (Nishimura and Tsukeda, 1971). The label was first incorporated into 10–15S component, which was soluble in 2M NaCl, and then moved to RNase-resistant 26S component. These components were suggested as intermediates before 43S virion RNA and 20S double-stranded RNA were synthesized. These intermediate-type RNA were obtained from outer membrane fractions of nuclear envelope, while 42S virion RNA was identified from large vesicles membranes and plasma membranes (Takeda et al., 1978). With the use of strand-specific probes, Takegami and Hotta (1990) indicated that (+) strand of viral RNA accumulated mostly in membrane fraction, while (–) strand accumulated mostly in supernatant fraction.

Viral Protein Synthesis

Intracellular viral protein synthesis was analyzed by radiolabeling of the infected cells treated with actinomycin D, cycloheximide or puromycin to reduce the background of cellular protein synthesis (Shapiro et al., 1973). The synthesis of structural as well as nonstructural viral proteins appeared to take place in the cytoplasm and their syntheses were affected in different degree by these metabolic inhibitors. The smallest structural protein (M) was not associated with the intracellular form of JE virion, which contained instead its glycosylated precursor, PreM. Processing of PreM to M appeared to take place in the Golgi apparatus (Shapiro et al., 1971). Two virus-specific nonstructural proteins, NS3 and NS5, were found in association with a membrane fraction rich in viral RNA polymerase activity (Takegami and Hotta, 1989).

Secretion of Viral Glycoprotein

Studies of the virus-specified glycoproteins in the infected cells indicated two forms of the nonstructural protein NS1, which was formerly designated as SCF antigen. These two forms of NS1, were considered to be generated by different posttranslational cleavage of the polyprotein. All three glycosylated virus-specific proteins (E and two forms of NS1) were secreted slowly into the culture medium of the infected mammalian Vero cells as a particulate form. In the infected mosquito cells, only the E protein was excreted and two forms of the NS1 protein were retained inside the cells (Mason et al., 1987; Mason, 1989). In the transient expression system of recombinant vaccinia virus-infected BHK21 cells, the NS1 gene was expressed, processed, glycosylated, and secreted into the culture medium without participation of other viral genes (Fan and Mason, 1990).

Morphogenesis

Morphologically mature JE virion was observed inside cytoplasmic vacuoles or lumen of smooth endoplasmic reticulum (Ota, 1965; Yasuzumi and Tsubo, 1965; Oyanagi et al., 1969). This observation suggested virion maturation in association with membrane of these cytoplasmic organelles; however, a convincing picture of the "budding process" of the precursor "core" structure was not obtained.

II. JE VIRUS INFECTION

A. Transmission Cycle

Epidemic Cycle of Transmission

As a typical arbovirus, JE virus is maintained in nature by alternative growth in vertebrate hosts and arthropod vectors. The most important vector species is *Culex tritaeniorhynchus* and related mosquitoes that breed in watered rice fields (Mitamura et al., 1938; Buescher et al., 1959). Among vertebrate hosts susceptible to JE virus, swine has been documented as the most important "amplifier" because of its significant viremia following JE virus infection, large numbers of population, high turnover rate, and preferential feeding by the vectors (Scherer et al., 1959b; Konno et al., 1966; Oya, 1967). Except stillbirth and/or abortion that occurs among pregnant swine infected with JE virus, swine did not exhibit any apparent diseases (Sugawara et al., 1973). Although cows are much less sensitive to JE virus, they are an effective attractants of the vector and thus could modulate JE virus transmission (Carey et al., 1968). Besides swine, some avian species such as black herons and egrets have been described as important amplifier vertebrates in nature (Scherer et al., 1959a). In India, several avian and multiple mosquito species were considered to be involved in JE virus transmission (National Institute of Virology, 1989). Equine species are quite sensitive to JE virus and exhibit apparent encephalitis with significant fatality rates (Hoshi and Ito, 1951). Fatal JE among horses has been a serious economic and social problem in China. Because of their relatively smaller number of population, horses as amplifiers of JE virus transmission in nature would not be as important as swine or avian species.

Humans are relatively insensitive to JE virus and no appreciable transmission of JE virus from infected humans to other humans or vector mosquitoes has been documented. Therefore, humans were considered deadend hosts in the transmission cycle of JE virus, although they could be infected by bite of infective vector mosquitoes (Fig. 3). Only one of several hundred infected humans manifests apparent encephalitis. The majority of disease remains as inapparent infection that could be detectable by antibody survey (Southam, 1956; Halstead and Grosz, 1962; Grossman et al., 1973c).

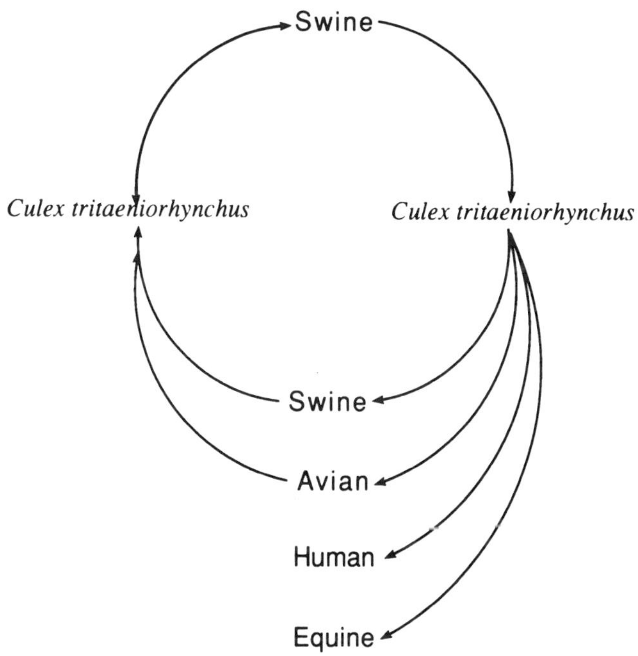

FIGURE 3 Epidemic transmission cycle of JE virus.

Epidemiologic Survey

In Japan, JE virus dissemination in nature has been monitored by antibody survey of slaughtered swine blood and virus isolation from field-caught female *C. tritaeniorhynchus*. The swine antibody survey has been performed countrywide as a program of the Ministry of Health and Welfare of Japan. The specimens were examined for anti-JE antibodies by the HI test combined with 2-mercaptoethanol (2ME) treatment. A HI titer decrease equal to or greater than eightfold by 2ME treatment was regarded as showing the predominance of IgM class antibodies, indicating recent infection. When 2ME-sensitive HI antibody was demonstrated or the antibody-positive swine proportion reached 50% or greater, the relevant area was considered to be contaminated with JE virus. This survey method would be valid in temperate climates like that of Japan, but would require further consideration in the areas where JE virus transmission could take place for longer periods of the year.

Another surveillance method of virus isolation was not performed as routinely as swine antibody survey, but provided more direct evidence for the existence of JE virus in nature. Field-collected female *C. tritaeniorhynchus* pools were processed for virus isolation by inoculation into the brain of suckling mice, which are the most sensitive animal host for JE virus (Shope and Sather, 1979). The virus isolates were identified by serologic methods, with final identification by the neutralization test. Indirect fluorescent antibody staining of the infected brain specimen could offer a quick estimate of the virus isolates. The virus isolation procedure was improved by the introduction of virus-sensitive *Aedes albopictus* clone C6/36 cells (Igarashi, 1978). This method had similar or even better sensitivity in isolating JE virus from field-collected *C. tritaeniorhynchus* females (Igarashi et al., 1981a), and could detect mutant arboviruses and other unknown viruses that could not be detected by mouse brain inoculation (Igarashi et al., 1981b). Other mosquito cell lines were also used for isolation of JE virus from field specimens (Hsu et al., 1978; Leake et al., 1986).

B. Geographic Distribution of JE and JE Virus

Although the name JE results from the first isolation of its causative agent in Japan around 1935, JE and JE virus are known to exist in wide areas of the far eastern Soviet Union, Korea, China, and several countries in Southeast Asia and South Asia (Fig. 4; Miles, 1960; Umenai et al., 1985). Most of these countries in the Asia monsoon areas have the climatic condition of sufficiently high temperature during summer and precipitation during rainy season, allowing for rice cultivation in watered paddy

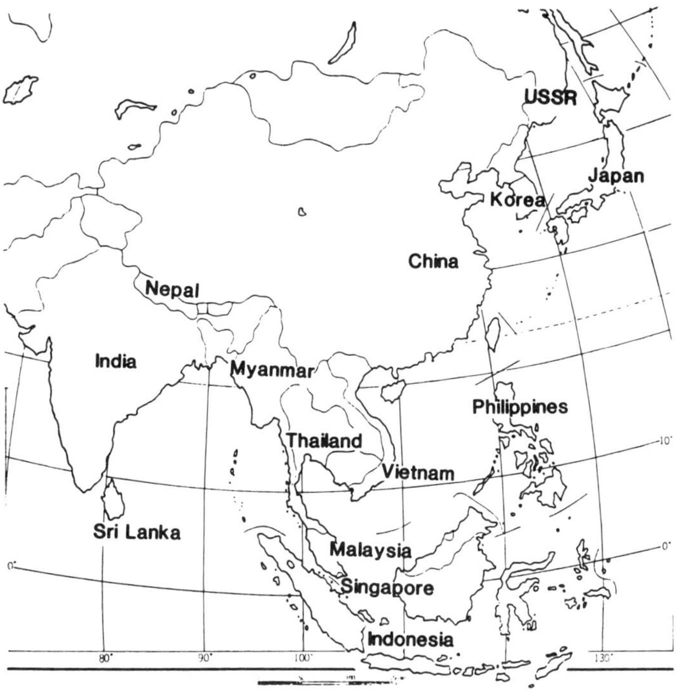

FIGURE 4 Geographic distribution of JE.

fields. Swine raising is quite common in this area, except for Moslem areas. These socioagricultural background could facilitate the circulation of JE virus in nature by providing ample breeding site for the vectors and abundant amplifier vertebrates, leading to outbreaks of human JE.

C. Annual Trend of Human JE in Several Asian Countries

Japan

Large outbreaks of human JE were recorded until 1966, with more than 1,000 cases and 30–50% case fatality rate. Then the number of cases showed a dramatic decrease and only fewer than 100 cases have been reported annually after 1972 (Fig. 5, top panel; Ministry of Health and Welfare, Japan, 1988). Two factors have been documented as influencing this dramatic change: decreased vector population and mass vaccination of humans. The decrease of the vectors was not the result of JE control

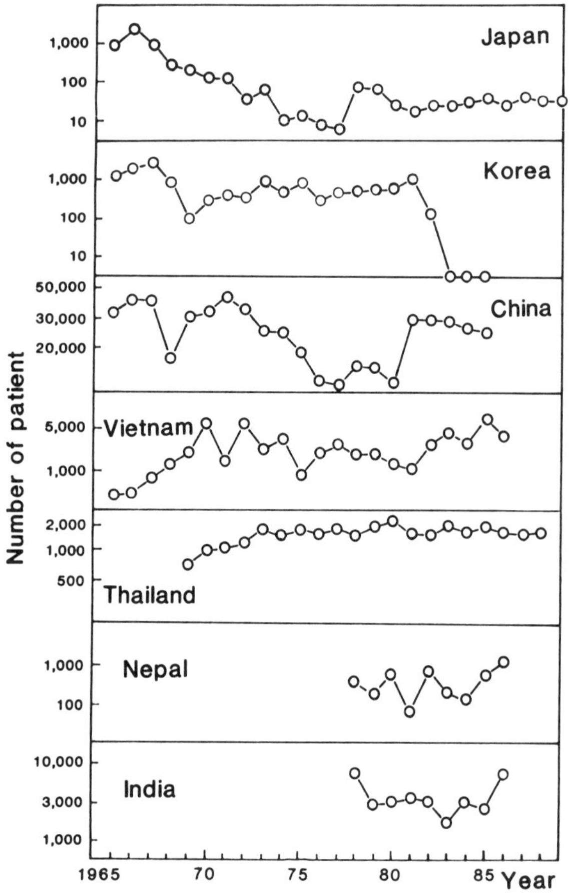

FIGURE 5 Annual trend of JE incidence in Asia. (Modified from Igarashi [1991] by permission. Summarized from the Ministry of Health and Welfare, Japan [1988], Cho [1988], Thongcharoen [1988], Igarashi [1986], Joshi [1986, 1987], and Shegal [1989].)

program but of the widespread spraying in pesticides in rice fields by the farmers to protect rice crops. However, *C. tritaeniorhynchus* collected in the field after the 1980s were found to be highly resistant to pesticides, especially organophosphorus (Table 2; Kamimura and Maruyama, 1983; Takahashi and Yasutomi, 1987). This resistance was observed for all *C. tritaeniorhynchus* captured in various parts of Japan (Yasutomi and Takahashi, 1987). As a result, the *C. tritaeniorhynchus* population in the

TABLE 2 Insecticidal Resistance of Fourth Instar Larvae of Two Strains of *Culex tritaeniorhynchus*: Sensitive Toyama and Resistant Taiwan

	Organophosphorus				
Strain	Temephos	Malathion	Fenitrothion	Diazone	Fenthion
Toyama	>100	24.0	21.2	4.75	32.1
Taiwan	0.0008	0.0004	0.0008	0.015	0.0014
Ratio	>125,000	6,000	26,500	317	22,929

	Carbamate		
Strain	Propoxur	Carbaryl	Pyrethroid: Permethrin
Toyama	29.8	14.2	0.0028
Taiwan	0.095	0.268	0.0024
Ratio	314	53	1.2

Figures for Toyama and Taiwan represent LC_{50} (ppm).
Source: Reproduced from Takahashi and Yasutomi (1987) by permission.

Toyama prefecture of Japan was found to be increasing after the 1980s (Watanabe, 1988). However, the number of human JE cases in Japan has stayed at a low level, probably because of the sustained vaccination of young children in epidemic areas (approximately 80% of 3–15-year-old children have been vaccinated every year) and the dissociation between the swine–*Culex* cycle and human dwellings.

Republic of Korea

The number of human JE cases decreased significantly after 1981 and no human JE cases have officially been recognized after 1983. This decrease was reported as the result of mass vaccination in that country (Fig. 5, second panel; Cho, 1988).

China

China, however, has been recording more than 10,000 to sometimes 20,000 human JE every year despite extensive use of hamster kidney cell-derived inactivated vaccine (Fig. 5, third panel; Thongcharoeng, 1989). Except for the desert Xintian area and mountainous Tibet and Chin Hai provinces, all areas of the country have become epidemic areas.

Vietnam

In 1965, the first outbreak of acute encephalitic syndrome (AES) was recognized in North Vietnam, and JE virus was isolated from patients, mosquitoes, swine, and wild birds. Then the disease spread out and more than 1,000 cases were recorded every year (Fig. 5, fourth panel). The disease is present both in the north and the south; however, the epidemic season in the subtropical north is June to August with a peak in July, while the disease has been reported all year round in the tropical south, with slight increase in July. Children under 9 years old were most frequently affected. The HI test was positive with JE antigen in approximately 30% of AES cases (Igarashi, 1986).

Thailand

In 1969, the first outbreak of viral encephalitis was reported in the Chiang Main area of northern Thailand and surveillance confirmed the presence of JE and JE virus (Yamada et al., 1971; Grossmann et al., 1973a,b,c, 1974; Gould et al., 1974; Johnsen et al., 1974). Then the epidemic area spread and the number of patients increased to more than 2,000 in 1979 (Fig. 5, fifth panel; Thongcharoeng, 1985). Further studies in northern Thailand showed a continuation of JE virus and its infection in this area together with dengue virus infection (Igarashi et al., 1983). Epidemics were found in the rainy season from June to August with a peak in July in the north, while no definite seasonal variation was observed in the south. Although the morbidity rate of viral encephalitis is relatively low in southern Thailand, extensive transmission of JE virus among swine has been demonstrated (Burke et al., 1986). Children under 14 years old were most frequently affected, and the HI test showed positive reaction with JE antigen in approximately 30% of cases of viral encephalitis.

India and Nepal

In India, a large epidemic of JE occurred in 1978 affecting several thousand patients. Since then the outbreaks have included more than 1,000 cases every year (Fig. 5, bottom panel; Shegal, 1989). In the same year in 1978, a JE epidemic occurred in the southern Terai belt in Nepal, along the Indian border. The disease has been occurring every year with fluctuating number of cases and 30–50% case fatality rate (Fig. 5, second panel from the bottom; Joshi, 1986, 1987).

D. Possible Reason for Increased Outbreaks in Asia

The most remarkable and apparent change in developing Asian countries has been a "population explosion" since World War II. This increase has often been ascribed to the progress of medical care and improved public health and sanitation, and it is generally accepted that the population growth is mutually dependent on economic growth. However, population growth definitely requires increased food production (i.e., rice production in the case of the Asian monsoon area). Although the introduction of high-yielding rice varieties by the "green revolution" should have provided a certain amount of increased food supply, in Sri Lanka at least, JE epidemics were reported in the areas where rice fields were newly developed (Vitarana et al., 1988). A similar situation was said to have been observed in India and Nepal. It is easy to imagine that newly developed rice fields have offered ample breeding sites for JE vector mosquitoes, while increased swine raising to obtain proteinaceous food would have provided increased amplifier hosts. Thus, the economic, particularly agricultural, development to compensate for the population explosion may have provided increased JE virus transmission, leading to outbreaks of human JE.

E. Experimental Infection

Host Factors

Among several susceptible experimental animals, mice have been studied most extensively as a model of JE virus infection in a whole animal. It has been recognized that the lethal effect of JE virus infection in mice is dependent on both host and viral factors as well as the inoculation route and virus dose. Young mice are more susceptible than old mice and the difference in susceptibility is more pronounced when the virus was inoculated by peripheral route than intracerebrally (Lennette and Koprowski, 1949; Grossberg adn Scherer, 1966; Huang, 1982). Recently, Ogata et al. (1991) demonstrated that JE virus neurotropism in rat is dependent on the degree of neuronal maturity. While a difference in the susceptibility to JE virus among mouse strains has also been recognized, this was recently reported to be controlled by a single dominant gene (Miura et al., 1990).

Viral Factors

Differences among JE virus strains in relation to neurovirulence in mice have been described (Huang, 1957; Nakamura and Nakamura, 1963; Oya et al., 1963). Neurovirulence of the virus was related to peripheral multiplication of the virus and its heat stability (Huang, 1957; Huang and Wong, 1963). Nt sequence analysis on MCA-escaped mutants showed that particular amino acid replacements on the E protein resulted in the loss of mouse neurovirulence (Cecilia and Gould, 1991). Comparative nt sequence analysis on the virulent parental and attenuated progeny paired strains identified multiple nt and amino acid replacements (Nitayaphan et al., 1990; Aihara et al., 1991). Comparison with a published sequence of other strains of JE virus suggested several mutations specific to the attenuation; however, a definite characterization of the virulence gene would require further studies to construct infectious DNA clones and site-directed mutagenesis.

Neuroinvasion

The sequence of the events taking place in vivo during invasion of neurotropic virus has been discussed by Monath (1990), and is summarized in Figure 6 for JE virus. In the case of peripheral virus inoculation, neuroinvasion would be determined by the viremia level and prevented by the integrity of the blood–brain barrier. The level of viremia would depend on virus multiplication in extraneural tissues and would be counteracted by the clearance in the reticuloendothelial (RES) system and neutralization by humoral antibodies. However, the primary focus of JE virus replication in extraneural tissue has not well been studied, nor has the role of RES. While artificial procedures to break the blood–brain barrier, such as intracerebral inoculation of balanced salt solution

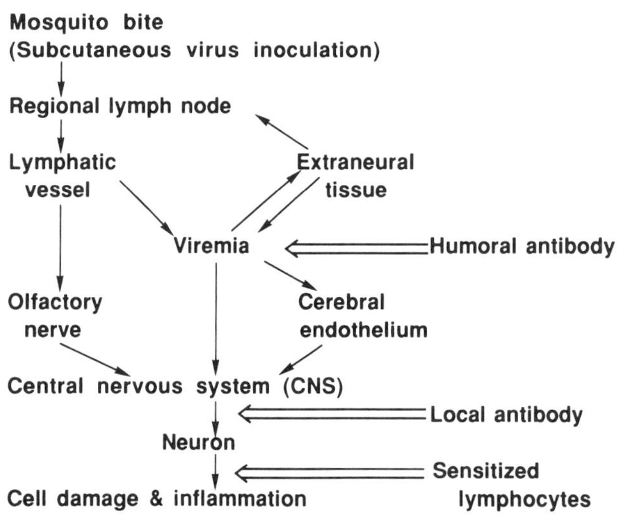

FIGURE 6 Sequence of JE virus infection in experimental animals. (Modified from Yasui [1987] and Monath [1990] by permission.)

simultaneously with peripheral inoculation of JE virus, was shown to increase its neurovirulence. The latter method was used in the vaccine potency test in China (Shope, 1987). Passive transfer of immune sera was shown to protect mice from lethal challenge of JE virus (Oya, 1964). Assay of serum antibody titers in these passively immunized mice showed that detectable neutralizing antibodies at 1:10 serum dilution were able to protect mice against 10^4 LD_{50} challenge virus, which was the maximum amount of the virus inoculated by a single bite of infective *C. tritaenio-rhynchus* (Takahashi, 1976; Oya, 1988). These observations provided a scientific base for the potency test on JE vaccine in Japan by neutralizing antibody production in vaccine-immunized mice.

Once the virus gets into the central nervous system (CNS), it can efficiently replicate in the neurons. Local antibody production against JE virus in the CNS was reported to be related to better prognosis in humans (Burke et al., 1985b). On the other hand, cellular immunity as represented by cytotoxic T lymphocytes was believed to accelerate overt symptoms of neuronal involvement by damaging virus-infected cells and inducing inflammatory reactions.

F. Clinical Aspects

Japanese encephalitis has been recognized as a serious acute disease, with a triad of high fever, headache, and impaired consciousness. Other frequently observed signs and symptoms are chills, vomiting, malaise, myalgia, photophobia, nuchal rigidity, pareses, and tremors. On laboratory examination, cerebrospinal fluid (CSF) shows lymphocytic pleocytosis and moderately elevated protein levels but normal sugar levels, while the blood cell count usually shows moderate leukocytosis (Dickerson et al., 1952; Ketel and Ognibene, 1971). There is no specific treatment for JE except supportive care. Because of its high case fatality rate (25–50%) and grave sequelae, with neurologic and/or psychiatric disorders occurring among approximately half of the patients who survive, JE has been regarded as a serious medical and public health problem in epidemic areas (Monath, 1988).

G. Virologic Diagnosis

Virus Isolation

Virologic diagnosis of JE consists of virus isolation and serologic examination (Shope and Sather, 1979). A classic method of virus isolation was performed using suckling mouse brain inoculation as explained above. Isolation by C6/36 cell culture inoculation appears to be superior to mouse brain inoculation in terms of its sensitivity and simplicity. Since the virus could be isolated most efficiently from brain specimens of patients who died from JE, diagnosis by virus isolation was often possible postmortem. While JE virus was sometimes isolated from the CSF of patients in the acute phase of disease, presence of the virus in the CSF was considered a sign of poor prognosis (Burke et al., 1985b).

Even without isolation of infectious virus, indirect fluorescent antibody staining of brain tissue from fatal cases to demonstrate viral antigen could offer diagnostic evidence for JE (Kimoto et al., 1968).

Serologic Diagnosis

Classic serologic diagnosis of JE depended on the demonstration of a significant antibody rise between acute and convalescent paired sera or significantly high antibody titers by the HI or CF test, as shown by the diagnostic guidelines in Japan (Table 3). These diagnostic criteria would be valid in Japan, where JE virus is practically the only prevalent flavivirus, but would not be suitable in areas where multiple flaviviruses are circulating. For example, frequent dengue virus infection in Southeast Asia made the result of the HI test complicated to interpret, sometimes providing the diagnosis only of flavivirus infection. Since IgM-class antibody exists transiently and is more specific to recently infecting virus

TABLE 3 Guideline for Serodiagnosis of JE in Japan

		Paired Sera		Single Serum:	2ME Treatment:
Test	Diagnosis[a]	Titer Rise	Maximum Titer	Maximum Titer	Titer Decrease
HI	++	≥ 4	≥ 1:320	≥ 1:640	—
	+	≥ 4	1:160	1:320	eightfold
	+−	≥ 4	1:40–1:80	1:160	fourfold
	−			< 1:10	—
CF	++	≥ 4	≥ 1:16	≥ 1:32	
	+	≥ 4	1:8	1:16	
	+−	<1:4–1:4			
	−			1:8	
				< 1:4	

[a]++ probably JE, + possibly JE, +− dubious, −negative. Specimens that do not fit into any of the above categories are uninterpretable.

Source: Modified from the diagnostic guideline by JE study group in Japan (1967).

(Westaway, 1969a,b), sucrose gradient centrifugation of patient's sera followed the HI test on IgM fraction was used to detect JE-specific antibodies (Edelman and Pariyanonda, 1973). In Japan, demonstration of 2ME-sensitive HI antibodies was recognized as diagnostic of predominant IgM class antibodies. IgM antibody detection was simplified by radioimmunoassay and ELISA (Burke and Nisalak, 1982; Burke et al., 1985a; Bundo and Igarashi, 1985). Demonstration of anti-JE IgM antibodies in CSF is particularly diagnostic of CNS involvement. Although serum IgM antibodies could be produced also by inapparent systemic infection, its assay was used in a serologic survey (Burke et al., 1985c).

III. JE CONTROL MEASURES

A. Mosquito Control

Based on the natural transmission cycle of JE virus (Fig. 3), three strategies have been considered for the control of human JE epidemics: vector control, swine immunization, and immunization of humans.

Attempts have been made to control JE vector mosquitoes by spraying chemical insecticides, which apparently reduced vector density but their effect was relatively transient (Self et al., 1973a,b; Mitchell et al., 1974). It has generally been accepted that wide spraying of pesticides in rice fields that led to the dramatic decrease of vector density in Japan was carried out by farmers to protect their rice crops, rather than as part of a JE vector control project. Practical application of insecticides to control JE virus transmission was not generally considered cost-effective because of the large area of vector breeding sites in watered rice fields.

B. Swine Immunization

Practical Applications

Immunization of swine to control JE virus transmission in nature was brought into operation in several restricted areas in Japan. An apparent reduction of JE in human patients was reported in Iki Island in Nagasaki prefecture, where swine immunization was performed in 1967 (Fig. 7). Although the data could be criticized for the absence of a control area, no fatal human cases of JE were reported after swine immunization here (Nagasaki Prefectural Institute, 1972). Similar successful results were said to be observed in Kumamoto prefecture after 1985, before which the prefecture had recorded the most human cases of JE in Japan. In a controlled field study in Osaka prefecture, Ueba et al. (1972) reported modification of JE virus transmission by swine vaccination using live-attenuated

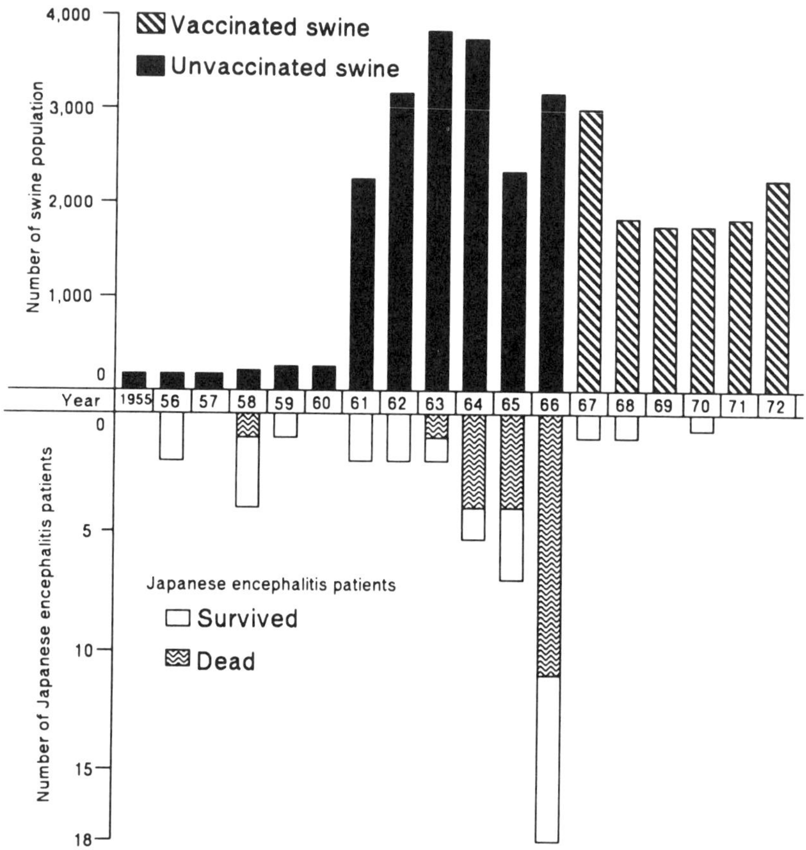

FIGURE 7 Swine immunization and patients with JE in Iki Island, Nagasaki prefecture, Japan. (Modified from Nagasaki Prefectural Institute of Public Health [1972] by permission.)

ML-17 strain JE virus. This strain was developed for the particular purpose of swine immunization and possessed several different biological characteristics from its parental virulent strain, such as reduced mouse virulence, absence of swine viremia, and limited growth in vector mosquitoes (Yoshida et al., 1981).

Problems

The following problems of swine immunization have been recognized. First, most of the swine population raised in their farms are slaughtered after 6–8 months and such a high turnover rate requires immunization of newly born piglets every year before the JE epidemic season. Second, live-attenuated JE vaccine for swine immunization will not be "taken" by piglets that possess maternal antibodies until about 6 months. This restricts the window period for swine immunization to a narrow range. Therefore, swine immunization was performed only in a limited area in Japan. In tropical areas where JE virus transmission could take place all year, it would be more difficult to determine the proper timing for swine immunization.

C. Human Immunization

Mouse Brain–Derived Inactivated Vaccine Developed in Japan

Improvement of Human JE Vaccine in Japan. Human immunization by inactivated JE vaccine derived from infected mouse brains has been studied by the U.S. military personnel (Sabin, 1947; Sabin et al., 1943). Classic achievements in this type of vaccine were summarized by Hammon et al. (1971). Improvement in the national standard for formalin-inactivated JE vaccine in Japan is a history of purification to remove brain materials from the final vaccine preparation to avoid possible allergic encephalopathy (Table 4). The first national standard for JE vaccine in 1954 was formalin-inactivated in 5% supernatant of infected mouse brain homogenate, with total solid materials making up less than 20 mg/ml. The standard was modified in 1957 to use 2% infected mouse brain homogenate with a total nitrogen content less than 0.4 mg/ml. Some purification procedures such as protamine sulfate, kaolin, and active carbon treatment could modify the standard to the total nitrogen content less than 0.2 mg/ml in 1962. The most remarkable improvement was achieved in 1965 by a purification procedure using either ultracentrifugation (Takaku et al., 1968) or alcohol–protamine precipitation (Nakamura, 1971). These technical achievements allowed for an improvement in the standard to a protein nitrogen content less than 0.02 mg/ml in 1965. Further technologic improvements improved the standard to reduce the protein nitrogen to less than 0.01 mg/ml in 1971; the final preparation became extremely pure virion (Fig. 1).

Vaccine Efficacy. Convincing evidence for the vaccine's efficacy was obtained by the field test performed in Taiwan; the result is summarized in Table 5 (Hsu et al., 1971). There was a significant difference between the morbidity from JE in the group that received two vaccine shots and placebo or the control group that received no vaccination. However, the difference between the group receiving a single shot and the control or placebo-treated group was not statistically significant. The result indicated that two shots of this type of inactivated JE vaccine was effective to

TABLE 4 Improvement of National Standard of JE Vaccine in Japan

Year	Preparation	Limit of Contaminant
1954	5% infected mouse brain homogenate supernatant	Total solid material less than 20 mg/ml
1957	2% infected mouse brain homogenate supernatant	Total nitrogen less than 0.4 mg/ml
1962	Treatment with protamine sulfate, kaolin, active carbon	Total nitrogen less than 0.2 mg/ml
1965	Purification by alcohol protamin precipitation or ultracentrifugation	Protein nitrogen less than 0.02 mg/ml
1971	Same as above	Protein nitrogen less than 0.01 mg/ml
1989	Vaccine strain changed from Nakayama to Beijing-1	Protein content/dose 40 microgram/0.5 ml inoculum volume

Source: Modified from Japanese Society of Biological Products.

TABLE 5 Efficacy Test of JE Vaccine in Taiwan, 1965

		No. of JE Cases		Morbidity Rate/100,000	
Group	No. of Population	Sero[a]	Sero + Clinic[b]	Sero	Sero + Clinic
Vaccinated					
Total	133,943	6	7	4.48 ± 3.58	5.23 ± 3.87
1 dose	22,194	2	2	9.01 ± 12.54	9.01 ± 12.54
2 doses	111,749	4	5	3.58 ± 3.51	4.47 ± 3.92
Placebo	131,865	24	31	18.20 ± 7.28	23.51 ± 3.92
Unvaccinated	140,514	35	52	24.91 ± 8.25	27.01 ± 10.05

[a]Serologic diagnosis.
[b]Clinical diagnosis.
Source: Modified from Hsu et al. (1971) by permission.

prevent human JE. The significant difference in JE morbidity between the placebo-treated group and the control group without any vaccination was considered to be the result of different educational standard in these two groups, which could be related to different living standards.

Another placebo-controlled double-blind test was performed in an epidemic area in Thailand (Kamphanphet province). The result clearly showed a significant difference between morbidity from JE in vaccinated and placebo-control groups (Hoke et al., 1988; Table 6). In this study, two vaccination groups were set up: one received a Nakayama monovalent vaccine and another with Nakayama + Beijing-1 bivalent vaccine. The theory behind this regimen was to cover different strains of JE virus that might be circulating in the study area. Even in the presence of antigenic differences among JE virus isolates, the efficacy of vaccine in preventing overt human JE was 91% in both vaccinated groups. The morbidity of dengue hemorrhagic fever, another serious mosquito-borne flavivirus disease, in the vaccinated group was slightly lower than that in the control group but the difference was not statistically significant. Follow-up studies on the protective efficacy of this vaccination showed that those vaccinated were protected until 1990 (Innis, personal communication).

Studies on the vaccination history of patients with JE in Japan showed that only 4.8% had been vaccinated, in contrast to 62.2% without vaccination, and the remaining 33% did not have a clear history of vaccination (Table 7; Kitano, 1990). An interesting figure deduced from these data is that the patient's outcome was not significantly different based on vaccination history. This observation may support the idea that JE vaccination

TABLE 6 Efficacy of Bivalent and Monovalent JE Vaccines in Preventing JE, Dengue Fever (DF), and Dengue Hemorrhagic Fever (DHF), in Kamphanphet Province, Thailand

		JE		DF		DHF	
Group	No. of Population	No. of Cases	MR[a]	No. of Cases	MR	No. of Cases	MR
Vaccinated							
Total	43,708	2	5	46	105	30	69
Bivalent	22,080	1	5	22	100	14	63
Monovalent	21,628	1	5	24	111	16	74
Placebo	21,516	11	51	29	135	23	107

[a]Morbidity rate/100,000.
Source: Modified from Hoke et al. (1988) by permission.

TABLE 7 Vaccination History and Outcome of JE in Japan, 1982–1988

Vaccination History of JE Vaccine	Outcome							
	Complete Recovery		Residual Sequelae		Dead		Total	
	N	%	N	%	N	%	N	%
Yes	3	30.0	5	50.0	2	20.0	10	4.8
No	46	35.4	67	51.5	17	13.1	130	62.2
Unknown	20	29.0	29	42.0	20	19.0	69	33.0
Total	60	33.0	101	48.3	39	18.7	209	100

Modified from Kitano (1990) by permission.

was effective in blocking the viremic phase by humoral antibodies, but would not be effective in modifying the disease outcome after neuroinvasion of the virus (Fig. 6). Other supportive evidence for the efficacy of JE vaccination in Japan is the change in age-specific JE morbidity before and after mass vaccination. The data in 1955, when vaccination was not performed extensively, showed the highest morbidity in 5–9-year-olds followed by 1–4-year-olds. In contrast, the figure in 1967 showed reduced morbidity in these young age groups, probably reflecting extensive vaccination, with increased morbidity in older age groups.

Duration of Immunity and Recommended Vaccination Schedule. Follow-up studies on the duration of neutralizing antibodies among JE vaccines in nonendemic Hokkaido were performed by Kanamitsu et al. (1970). Sufficient preventive level of neutralizing antibodies was produced by two successive vaccinations with a 1 week to 1 month interval. The titer gradually decreased to a marginally protective level above 1:10 after 1 year. The antibody titer was rapidly and significantly increased by booster immunization and was maintained above the protective level for at least 3 years. This augmentation of neutralizing antibody level could be repeated by booster immunization. Thus, the present recommendation for human JE vaccination in Japan is the primary vaccination with two shots with 1 week to 1 month interval followed by a booster in the following year. Then the immunity would be maintained by booster vaccination once every 3–4 years.

Safety of the Nakayama Strain JE Vaccine. The side effects of the Nakayama strain JE vaccine have been analyzed by Okinaka et al. (1967). Among a total of 12,016 vaccines, 0.75% (90 individuals) showed some side effects. The most frequent was headache (0.26%) followed by fever (0.16%), general malaise (0.12%), headache and general malaise (0.08%), and fever and general malaise (0.07%), with fewer than 0.03% experiencing abdominal pain, nausea, local erythema, palpitation, and dizziness. These complaints were relatively minor, however. The data on 60,629,250 vaccinees from 1977 to 1984 were issued by the Vaccination-Induced Health Damage Authorization Committee in Japan. This report described thirteen cases with nervous system involvement (three each of encephalitis and peripheral nerve paralysis; two each of meningitis and febrile convulsion; and each one of encephalopathy, convulsive disorders, and other CNS involvement), four cases of serious systemic reactions (three shock and one sudden death), seven local adverse reactions (three rash, two each of local reactions and abscess-phlegmon), and two other side effects that were not clearly documented. The total number of twenty-six cases with side effects (0.43 in 1 million vaccination), was less than the rate following immunization for measles (6.0), bacille Calmette-Guérin (1.55), diphtheria/pertussis/tetanus (0.99), and polio (0.62), similar to that of rubella (0.42), and more than that of influenza (0.35) vaccine.

Evaluation of the potency and safety of the Japanese-made purified JE vaccine was performed in the United States (Poland et al., 1990). The results showed that the neutralizing antibody conversion rate was 77% in the vaccinees who received two doses with a 1–2 week interval, and the rate increased to 99% by the third dose after 6–12 months. The following adverse reactions were reported: local pain (18%), headache (9%), erythema (6%), swelling (3%), and less than 5% incidence of dizziness, fatigue, somnolence, nausea, chills, fever, and lower back pain. The study recommended three doses of this vaccine to those at risk of JE virus infection, such as travelers to JE-endemic Asia (Denning and Kaneko, 1987).

Differences Among JE Virus Isolates and Vaccine Strains. It has been shown that some strain variation in pH dependency is present among various JE virus isolates (Okuno et al., 1965) and antigen adsorption in the HI (Okuno et al., 1968) or neutralization test (Oda, 1976). The antigenic variation was further analyzed by MCA and the HI test (Kobayashi et al., 1984, 1985). Genomic variation among JE virus isolates was shown by oligonucleotide fingerprint analysis (Hori et al., 1986; Hori, 1986), and recently by nt sequencing of the PreM gene region of the viral genome (Chen et al., 1990).

Of particular significance regarding the protective efficacy of JE vaccine against various JE virus isolates was the cross-neutralization test by immune mouse sera obtained by different strains of JE vaccine. The result showed that there appear to exist two antigenic subtypes in JE virus isolates: Nakayama and Beijing-1. Each subtype of vaccine could produce high titer neutralizing antibodies to the homologous subtype, but the cross-neutralization to the heterologous subtype was less, particularly by the Nakayama strain, which had been the only vaccine strain until recently in Japan (Oya, 1987). The first method devised to cover various JE virus isolates was to prepare bivalent vaccine by combining Nakayama and Beijing-1 vaccines. Since a single-strain vaccine was preferred to the bivalent vaccine in terms of production procedures and potency test, the National Institute of Health of Japan changed the vaccine strain from the classic Nakayama to Beijing-1 in 1989, with a consequent reduction of the immunizing dose to 0.5 ml (half of the previous volume), and protein content to less than 40 μg/dose (Table 4).

Production of Mouse Brain–Derived JE Vaccine in Asia. The Republic of Korea has been producing the Japanese-type mouse brain–derived JE vaccine. Their production scale appears to be more than sufficient to cover domestic demand and some of their product was said to be exported to other countries.

The technology of JE vaccine production has been transferred from Japan to India and Thailand, but their production scale is still far from sufficient to cover their demand.

Inactivated JE Vaccine Produced in China

China has been producing formalin-inactivated JE vaccine from hamster-infected kidney cell cultures since 1967 (Gu and Ding, 1987). This type of vaccine was originally described by Darwish and Hammon (1966), and its production was greatly increased since 1968 using P_3 strain JE virus. The production scale at the Beijing Institute of Biological Products in 1968 was 10,000,000 doses. The vaccine, supplemented with 0.1% human albumin, was stable for more than 2 years at 2–8°C. An epidemiologic survey showed 76–94% protective efficacy by this type of JE vaccination. The Expert Advisory Committee on JE of the World Health Organization (WHO) proposed an international standard to cover both the Japanese and Chinese type of inactivated vaccine in 1987. Accordingly, some concentration procedures were applied for Chinese-made JE vaccine and subsequent field tests showed 100% seroconversion rate in neutralizing antibody production.

Live-Attenuated JE Vaccine Developed in China

To cover the demand for JE vaccine, China has developed live-attenuated JE vaccine strains by repeated passage in hamster kidney cell cultures and plaque purification (Li, 1986; Ao et al., 1989). One of the candidate vaccines SA_{14}-14-2, was given to 1,026 children without untoward reactions and the seroconversion rate was 100% when vaccine was diluted 1:5 or less, while the seroconversion rate for 1:50 vaccine dilution was 83.3% (Yu et al., 1987, 1988). At present, there is no international standard for the live-attenuated JE vaccine and the SA_{14}-14-2 vaccine has been used exclusively in China.

Development of the Second-Generation JE Vaccine

To solve the problems of JE vaccination in developing Asian countries, particularly to provide inexpensive vaccine in unlimited amounts, WHO has proposed development of the second-generation JE vaccine using recombinant DNA technology. Since the E protein possesses neutralizing epitope, several attempts have been made to express the E protein gene in recombinant yeast (Fujita et al., 1986), *Escherichia coli* (Mason et al., 1987), baculovirus (Aira, 1987), and vaccinia virus (Haishi et al., 1988). These studies detected E gene products, which were generally of low immunogenicity and unsatisfactory as vaccine candidates. The result may be related to the fact that most of the E protein epitopes are conformational (Srivastava et al., 1987). Presence of disulfide bond in a minimum size of 95 amino acid peptide was essential for the E gene product to react with neutralizing and protective MCA (Mason et al., 1989). However this peptide expressed by recombinant *E. coli* was not immunogenic to induce neutralizing antibodies in mice.

Studies to express E gene product with authentic antigenicity were performed using recombinant baculovirus (Matsuura et al., 1989) or vaccinia virus (Yasuda et al., 1990). These investigators constructed several recombinants possessing varying sizes of inserted JE virus gene cDNA. The reactivity with a battery of MCA showed that the gene product made by the construct possessing not only E gene but also its upstream PreM and a part of C gene reacted with all MCA in almost the same way as the authentic E protein. This gene product was expressed on the surface of infected cells and immunization of such recombinant virus-infected cells induced neutralizing antibodies in experimental animals. However, the response was still less than that of the current vaccine, although its priming effect was observed (Matsuura et al., 1989). Immunization of rabbit with a recombinant vaccinia virus with this JE virus cDNA insert induced a high level of long-lasting neutralizing antibodies, and the same construct conferred protective immunity in mice (Yasuda et al., 1990). Similar recombinant vaccinia virus constructs that expressed not only E and NS1 but also PreM gene produced a particulate component associated with E and M proteins (Mason et al., 1991). This component was released into the medium and sedimented in almost the same way as SHA, and induced significant protective immunity in mice.

Another aspect of the study was to find a denaturation-resistant, and thus possibly linear neutralizing, E protein epitope. Examination of several peptide fragments cleaved from JE virus E protein by cyanogen bromide showed that an 8 kD fragment close to the C-terminal of E protein was immunogenic to induce neutralizing antibodies in mice (Srivastava et al., 1990a). Expression of E protein gene cDNA covering this 8 kd region by recombinant *E. coli* showed that the gene product was immunogenic and conferred protection against lethal challenge with JE virus in mice (Srivastava et al., 1990b).

Before any attempts are made to use recombinant virus gene product or recombinant infectious vaccinia virus in humans, extensive purification of the gene product and careful evaluation of the use of recombinant vaccinia virus should be performed, with the worldwide eradication of smallpox borne in mind.

IV. OVERWINTERING OF JE VIRUS: AN UNANSWERED QUESTION

Although epidemic cycles of JE virus transmission involving swine and *C. tritaeniorhynchus* have been studied extensively, this cycle does not appear to be essential for the maintenance of JE virus in nature. So far, all attempts to find out where and how JE virus exists in nature during the inter-epidemic season in a temperate climate have been unsuccessful. Identification of the basic cycle of JE virus transmission would not only be interesting from scientific standpoint but also important for the eradication of the virus from the environment. This problem was reviewed by Rosen (1986), who showed that JE virus could be transmitted transovarially to offspring mosquitoes under experimental conditions (Rosen et al., 1978). Attempts to isolate JE virus from overwintering *C. tritaeniorhynchus* were negative (Hayashi et al., 1978). No evidence has been obtained so far that JE virus-infected mosquitoes regularly introduced the virus from tropical areas to Japan.

In the case of vertebrate hosts, JE virus could persist as latent infection in T lymphocytes and be transmitted vertically to offsprings in mice (Chaturvedi et al.,1980; Mathur et al., 1982, 1986, 1987). Some species of bat can be infected experimentally with JE virus accompanied by sufficient viremia to infect vector mosquitoes and maintain the virus for 107 days under simulated hibernation (LaMotte, 1958). JE virus has also been transmitted transplacentally (Sulkin et al., 1964). Virus isolation and serologic survey showed that some species of bats were frequently infected with JE virus (Miura et al., 1970; Sulkin et al., 1970; Miura and Kitaoka, 1977). However, there is no definite evidence to connect bat infection with the *Culex*–swine epidemic cycle. Some kind of lizards were infected experimentally with JE virus and maintained it during the winter season until spring and were able to develop viremia after hibernation (Doi et al., 1983; Oya et al., 1983). However, examination of these lizards in nature could not isolate JE virus, although HI antibodies were found. Antibody surveillance of turtles indicated infection by JE virus but its implication for the survival of JE virus was not clarified (Shortridge et al., 1975).

Epidemiologic observation in the northern island of Japan, where JE is less endemic, showed that JE virus infection in several swine farms occurred focally, not continuously, indicating local virus persistence (Takashima et al., 1988). Future study would probably require modern technologies to demonstrate persistent viral genome not as infection virion, which would be a kind of special developmental stage of viral replication. Detection of latent viral gene and its activation under certain condition would provide further insight into the overwintering of JE virus and its natural ecology.

V. CONCLUSIONS

JE is among the most serious health problems in endemoepidemic areas in several Asian countries. Enlarged JE epidemics in these areas appear to be related to their economic and social development. Although human vaccination has been proven to be the most reliable method to control overt disease, international cooperation is essential for its better operation, including technology transfer and development of the basic virologic techniques. The basic maintenance and overwintering mechanism of JE virus in nature need to be clarified to eradicate JE virus and its disease from the environment.

ACKNOWLEDGMENTS

The author expresses his thanks to Professor Doctor Edouard Kurstak for his providing a chance to prepare this chapter. The kind assistance of Ms. S. Uchida, Ms. K. Jodai, and Mr. G. M. M. Shameem is also appreciated.

REFERENCES

Aihara, S., Chunming, R., Yu, Y-X., Lee, T., Watanabe, K., Kamiya, T., Sumiyoshi, H., Hashimoto, H., and Nomoto, A. (1991). *Virus Genes* 5: (in press).

Aira, Y. (1987). *Trop. Med. 29*:195–209.

Ao, J., Wu, P-F., Jia, R-Z., Yao, L-T., Yu, Y-X., and Li, H-N. (1989). *JE & HFRS Bull. 3*:7–13.

Buescher, E. L., Scherer, W. F., Rosenberg, M. Z., Gresser, I., Hardy, J. L., and Bullock, H. R. (1959). *Am. J. Trop. Med. Hyg. 8*:651–664.

Bundo, K., and Igarashi, A. (1985). *J. Virol. Methods 11*:15–22.

Burke, D. S., and Nisalak, A. (1982). *J. Clin. Microbiol. 15*:353–361.

Burke, D. S., Nisalak, A., and Ussery, M. A. (1982). *J. Clin. Microbiol. 16*:1034–1042.

Burke, D. S., Nisalak, A., Ussery, M. A., Laorakpongse, T., and Chantavibul, S. (1985a). *J. Infect. Dis. 151*:1093–1099.

Burke, D. S., Lorsomrudee, W., Leake, C. J., Hoke, C. H., Nisalak, A., Chongswasdi, V., and Laorakpongse, T. (1985b). *Am. J. Trop. Med. Hyg. 34*:1203–1210.

Burke, D. S., Chatiyanonda, K., Anandrik, S., Nakornsri, S., Nisalak, A., and Hoke, C. H. (1985c). *Bull. WHO. 63*:1037–1042.

Burke, D. S., Tingpalapong, M., Ward, G. S., and Leake, C. J. (1986). *JE & HFRS Bull. 1*:17–26.

Calisher, C. H., Karabatsos, N., Dalrymple, J. M., Shope, R. E., Porterfield, J. S., Westaway, E. G., and Brandt, W. E. (1989). *J. Gen. Virol. 70*:37–43.

Carey, D. E., Myers, R. M., and Reuben, R., and Webb, J. K. G. (1968). *J. Indian Med. Assoc.* 52:10–15.

Cecilia, D., and Gould, E. A. (1991). *Virology 181*:70–77.

Cecilia, D., Cadkari, D. A., Kedarnath, N., and Ghosh, S. N. (1988). *J. Gen. Virol. 69*:2741–2747.

Chaturvedi, U. C., Mathur, A., Chandra, A., Das, S. K., Tandon, H. O., and Singh, U. K. (1980). *J. Infect. Dis. 141*:712–715.

Chen, W.-R., Tesh, R. B., and Rico-Hesse, R. (1990). *J. Gen. Virol. 71*:2915–2922.

Cho, H. W. (1988). 22nd Joint Conference on Viral Diseases. Japan–U.S. Cooperative Medical Science Program, Tokyo.

Clarke, D. H., and Casals, J. (1958). *Am. J. Trop. Med. Hyg. 7*:561–573.

Clarke, D. H., and Casals, J. (1965). In: *Viral and Rickettsial Infections of Man*, F. L. Horsfall and I. Tamm (Eds.). J. B. Lippincott, Philadelphia and Montreal, pp. 606–658.

Darwish, M. A., and Hammon, W. McD. (1966). *J. Immunol. 97*:506–511.

DeMadrid, A. T., and Porterfield, J. S. (1974). *J. Gen. Virology* 23:91–96.

Denning, D. W., and Kaneko, Y. (1987). *Lancet* April 11, 853–854.

Dickerson, R. B., Newton, J. R., and Hansen, J. E. (1952). *Am. J. Med. 12*:277–290.

Doi, R., Oya, A., Shirasaka, A., Yabe, S., and Sasa, M. (1983). *Jpn. J. Exp. Med. 53*:125–134.

Edelman, R., and Pariyanonda, A. (1973). *Am. J. Epidemiol. 98*:29–38.

Fan, W., and Mason, P. W. (1990). *Virology 177*:470–476.

Fujita, H., Sumiyoshi, H., Mori, C., Manabe, S., Takagi, M., Yoshida, I., Morita, K., Fuke, I., Fukai, K., and Igarashi, A. (1986). *Bull. WHO 65*:303–308.

Gould, D. J., Edelman, R., Grossman, R. A., Nisalak, A., and Sullivan, M. F. (1974). *Am. J. Epidemiol. 100*:49–56.
Grossberg, S. E., and Scherer, W. F. (1966). Soc. Exp. Biol. Med. 123:118–124.
Grossman, R. A., Gould, D. J., Smith, T. J., and Johnsen, D. O., and Pantuwatana, S. (1973a). *Am. J. Epidemiol. 98*:111–120.
Grossman, R. A., Edelman, R., Chiewanich, P., Voodikul, P., and Siriwan, C. (1973b). *Am. J. Epidemiol. 98*:121–132.
Grossman, R. A., Edelman, R., Willhight, M., Puntawatana, S., and Udomsakdi, S. (1973c). *Am. J. Epidemiol. 98*:133–149.
Grossman, R. A., Edelman, R., and Gould, D. J. (1974). *Am. J. Epidemiol. 100*:69–76.
Gu, P. W., and Ding, Z.-F. (1987). *JE & HFRS Bull.* 2:15–26.
Haishi, S., Imai, H., Hirai, K., Igarashi, A., and Kato, S. (1988). *Acta Virol. 33*:497–503.
Halstead, S. B., and Grosz, C. R. (1962). *Am. J. Hyg. 75*:190–210.
Hammon, W. McD., Kitaoka, M., and Downs, W. G. (Eds.) (1971). *Immunization for Japanese Encephalitis*. Igaku Shoin, Tokyo.
Hase, T., Summers, P. L., and Cohen, W. H. (1989). *Arch. Virol. 108*:101–114.
Hashimoto, H., Nomoto, A., Watanabe, K., Mori, T., Takezawa, T., Aizawa, C., Takegami, T., and Hiramatsu, K. (1988). *Virus Genes 1*:305–317.
Hayashi, K., Mifune, K., and Schichijo, A. (1978). *Trop. Med. 20*:131–142.
Hoke, C. H., Nisalak, A., Sangkawhipa, N., Jatanasen, S., Laorakpongse, T., Innis, B. L., Kotchasenee, A., Gingrich, J. B., Latendresse, J., Fukai, K., and Burke, D. S. (1988). *N. Engl. J. Med. 319*:608–614.
Hori, H. (1986). *Trop. Med. 28*:179–190.
Hoshi, S., and Ito, T. (1951). *Report of the National Institute of Animal Health, Japan, 1*:1–42.
Hori, H., Morita, K., and Igarashi, A. (1986). *Acta Virol. 30*:353–359.
Hsu, T. C., Chow, L. P., Wei, H. Y., Chen, C. L., Hsu, S. T., Huang, C. T., Kitaoka, M., and Sunaga, H. (1971). In *Immunization for Japanese Encephalitis*, W. McD. Hammon, M. Kitaoka, and W. G. Downs (Eds.). Igaku Shoin, Tokyo, pp. 258–265.
Hsu, S. H., Huang, W. C., and Cross, J. H. (1978). *J. Med. Entomol. 14*:698–701.
Huang, C. H. (1957). *Acta Virol. 1*:36–45.
Huang, C. H. (1982). *Adv. Virus Res. 27*:71–101.
Huang, C. H., and Wong, C. (1963). *Acta Virol. 7*:322–330.
Igarashi, A. (1978). *J. Gen. Virol. 40*:531–544.
Igarashi, A. (1986). *Infect. Inflamm. Immunol. 16*:207–213.
Igarashi, A. (1988). *SE Asian J. Trop. Med. Public Health 19*:493–500.
Igarashi, A. (1991). *Prog. Med. Sci. 156*:782.
Igarashi, A., Kitano, H., and Fukai, K. (1963a). *Biken J. 6*:25–26.
Igarashi, A., Kitano, H., and Fukai, K. (1963b). *Biken J. 6*:21–23.
Igarashi, A., Fukunaga, T., and Fukai, K. (1964). *Biken J. 7*:111–119.
Igarashi, A., Buei, K., Ueba, N., Yoshida, M., Ito, S., Nakamura, H., Sasao, F., and Fukai, K. (1981a). *Am. J. Trop. Med. Hyg. 30*:449–460.
Igarashi, A., Sasao, F., Fukai, K., Buei, K., Ueba, N., and Yoshida, M. (1981b). *Ann. Virol. (Inst. Pasteur) 1 32E*:253–245.

Igarashi, A., Ogata, T., Fujita, N., Fukunaga, T., Mori, A., Uzuka, Y., Supawadee, J., Chiowanich, P., Peerakome, S., Leechanachai, P., Charoensook, O., and Chanyasanha, C. (1983). *SE Asian J. Trop. Med. Public Health 14*:470–480.
Johnsen, D. O., Edelman, R., Grossman, R. A., Muangman, D., Pomsdhit, J., and Gould, D. J. (1974). *Am. J. Epidemiol. 100*:57–67.
Joshi, D. D. (1986). *JE & HFRS Bull. 1*:5–15.
Joshi, D. D. (1987). *JE & HFRS Bull.* 2:1–10.
Kamimura, K., and Maruyama, Y. (1983). *Jpn. J. Sanit. Zool. 34*:33–37.
Kanamitsu, M., Hashimoto, N., Urasawa, S., Katsurada, M., and Kimura, H. (1970). *Biken J. 13*:313–328.
Ketel, W. B., and Ognibene, A. J. (1971). *Am. J. Med. Sci. 261*:271–279.
Kimoto, T., Yamada, T., Ueba, N., Kunita, N., Kawai, A., Yamagami, S., Nakajima, K., Akao, M., and Sugiyama, S. (1968). *Biken J. 11*:157–168.
Kimura-Kuroda, J., and Yasui, K. (1983). *J. Virol. 45*:124–132.
Kimura-Kuroda, J., and Yasui, K. (1986). *J. Gen. Virol. 67*:2663–2672.
Kimura-Kuroda, J., and Yasui, K. (1988). *J. Immunol. 141*:3606–3610.
Kitano, T. (1990). *Clin. Drug Ther. 9*:707–711.
Kitano, T., Suzuki, K., and Yamaguchi, T. (1974). *J. Virol. 14*:631–639.
Kitaoka, M., and Nishimura, C. (1965). *Jpn. J. Med. Sci. Biol. 18*:177–187.
Kobayashi, Y., Hasegawa, H., Oyama, T., Tamai, T., and Kusaba, T. (1984). *Infect. Immun. 44*:117–123.
Kobayashi, Y., Hasegawa, H., and Yamaguchi, T. (1985). *Microbiol. Immunol. 29*:1069–1082.
Konno, J., Endo, K., Agatsuma, H., and Ishida, N. (1966). *Am. J. Epidemiol. 84*:292–300.
Kos, K. A., Osborne, B. A., and Goldsby, R. A. (1975). *J. Virol. 15*:913–917.
LaMotte, L. C. (1958). *Am. J. Hyg. 67*:101–108.
Leake, C. J., Burke, D. S., Nisalak, A., and Hoke, C. H. (1986). *Am. J. Trop. Med. Hyg. 35*:1045–1050.
Lennette, E. H., and Koprowski, H. (1949). *J. Immunol. 49*:175–191.
Li, H-M. (1986). In *Virus Vaccines in Asian Countries*, K. Fukai (Ed.). University of Tokyo Press, Tokyo, pp. 159–165.
Mason, P. W. (1989). *Virology 169*:354–364.
Mason, P. W., McAda, P. C., Dalrymple, J. M., Fournier, M. J., and Mason, T. L. (1987). *Virology 158*:361–372.
Mason, P. W., Dalrymple, J. M., Gentry, M. K., McCown, J. M., Hoke, C. H., Burke, D. S., Fournier, M. J., and Mason, T. L. (1989). *J. Gen. Virol. 70*:2037–2049.
Mason, P. W., Pincus, S., Fournier, M. J., Mason, T. L., Shope, R. E., and Paoletti, E. (1991). *Virology 180*:294–305.
Mathur, A., Arora, K. L., and Chaturvedi, U. C. (1982). *J. Gen. Virol. 59*:213–217.
Mathur, A., Arora, K. L., Rawat, S., and Chaturvedi, U. C. (1986). *J. Gen. Virol. 67*:381–385.
Mathur, A., Kulshreshtha, R., and Chaturvedi, U. C. (1987). *J. Gen. Virol. 70*:461–465.
Matsuura, Y., Miyamoto, M., Sato, T., Morita, C., and Yasui, K. (1989). *Virology 173*:674–682.

McAda, P. C., Mason, P. W., Schmaljohn, C. S., Dalrymple, J. M., Mason, T. L., and Fournier, M. J. (1987). *Virology 158*:348–360.

Miles, J. A. R. (1960). *Bull. WHO* 22:339–371.

Ministry of Health and Welfare, Japan (1988). Statistics of communicable diseases, Japan.

Mitamura, A., Kitaoka, M., Mori, K., and Ohkubo, K. (1938). *Nihon Ijishinshi 62*: 820–824.

Mitchell, C. J., Chen, P.-S., and Okuno, T. (1974). *J. Formosan Med. Assoc. 73*:295–312.

Miura, T., and Kitaoka, M. (1977). *Arch. Virol. 53*:281–286.

Miura, T., Toyokawa, K., Allen, R., and Sulkin, E. (1970). *Am. J. Trop. Med. Hyg. 19*:88–93.

Miura, K., Onodera, T., Nishida, A., Goto, N., and Fujisaki, Y. (1990). *Arch. Virol. 112*:261–270.

Monath, T. P. (1986). In *The Togaviridae and Flaviviridae*, S. Schlesinger and M. J. Schlesinger (Eds.). Plenum Press, New York and London, pp. 375–440.

Monath, T. P. (1988). *N. Engl. J. Med. 319*:641–643.

Monath, T. P. (1990). In *Fields Virology*, B. N. Fields, D. M. Knipe, R. M. Chanock, M. S. Hirsch, J. L. Melnick, T. P. Monath, and B. Roizman (Eds.). Raven Press, New York, pp. 763–814.

Mori, H., and Nozima, T. (1965). *Acta Virol. 9*:392–396.

Nagasaki Prefectural Institute of Public Health and Environmental Sciences (1972). Annual Report.

Nakamura, M. (1961). *Nature 191*:624.

Nakamura, H. (1971). In *Immunization for Japanese Encephalitis*, W. McD. Hammon, M. Kitaoka, and W. G. Downs (Eds.). Igaku Shoin, Tokyo, pp. 147–148.

Nakamura, H., and Nakamura, J. (1963). *Jpn. J. Med. Sci. Biol. 16*:47–49.

National Institute of Virology, Pune, India (1989). Annual Report, 1988–1989.

Nishimura, C., and Tsukeda, H. (1971). *Jpn. J. Microbiol. 15*:309–316.

Nitayaphan, S., Grant, J. A., Chang, G.-J., and Trent, D. W. (1990). *Virology 177*: 541–552.

Nozima, T., Mori, H., Minobe, Y., and Yamamoto, S. (1968). *Acta Virol. 12*:296–300.

Oda, K. (1976). *Kobe J. Med. Sci.* 22:123–137.

Ogata, A., Nagashima, K., Hall, W. W., Ichikawa, M., Kimura-Kuroda, J., and Yasui, K. (1991). *J. Virol. 65*:880–886.

Okinaka, S., Toyokura, Y., Tsukagoshi, H., Kuroiwa, Y., Araki, S., Arima, M., Otani, S., Tsubaki, T., Shiraki, H., Takatsu, T., Narabayashi, H., and Yoshimura, S. (1967). *Adv. Neurol. Sci. 11*:410–424.

Okuno, T., Suzuki, M., Kondo, A., and Ito, T. (1965). *Jpn. J. Med. Sci. Biol. 18*:227–238.

Okuno, T., Okada, T., Kondo, A., Suzuki, M., Kobayashi, M., and Oya, A. (1968). *Bull. WHO 38*:547–563.

Ota, Z. (1965). *Virology* 25:372–378.

Oya, A. (1964). *Clin. Paediatr. 1*:32–40.

Oya, A. (1967). *Jpn. J. Med. Sci. Biol. 20*:26–30.

Oya, A. (1987). *JE & HFRS Bull.* 2:11–13.

Oya, A. (1988). *Acta Paediatr. Jpn. 30*:175–184.

Oya, A., Sakumoto, H., and Kobayashi, M. (1963). *Jpn. J. Med. Sci. Biol. 16*:50–52.
Oya, A., Doi, R., Shirasaka, A., Yabe, S., and Sasa, M. (1983). *Jpn. J. Exp. Med. 53*:117–123.
Oyanagi, S., Ikuta, F., and Ross, E. R. (1969). *Acta Neuropathol. 13*:169–181.
Poland, J. D., Cropp, C. B., Craven, R. B., and Monath, T. P. (1990). *J. Infect. Dis. 161*:878–882.
Rice, C. M., Lenches, E. M., Eddy, S. R., Shin, S. J., Sheets, R. L., and Strauss, J. H. (1985). *Science 229*:726–733.
Rosen, L. (1986). *Annu. Rev. Microbiol. 40*:395–414.
Rosen, L., Tesh, R. B., Lien, J. C., and Cross, J. H. (1978). *Science 199*:909–911.
Sabin, A. B. (1947). *JAMA 133*:281–293.
Sabin, A. B., Duffy, C. E., Warren, J., Ward, R., Peck, J. L., Jr., and Ruchman, I. (1943). *JAMA 122*:477–486.
Scherer, W. F., Buescher, E. L., and McClure, H. E. (1959a). *Am. J. Trop. Med. Hyg. 8*:689–697.
Scherer, W. F., Moyer, J. T., Izumi, T., Gresser, I., and McCown, J. (1959b). *Am. J. Trop. Med. Hyg. 8*:698–706.
Self, L. S., Ree, H. I., Lofgren, C. S., Shim, J. C., Chow, C. Y., Shin, H. K., and Kim, K. H. (1973a). *Bull. WHO 49*:353–357.
Self, L. S., Tonn, R. J., Bai, D. H., and Shin, H. K. (1973b). *Trop. Med. 15*:177–188.
Shameem, G. M. M., Morita, K., Bundo-Morita, K., and Igarashi, A. (1989). *Trop. Med. 31*:111–123.
Shapiro, D., Brandt, W. E., Cardiff, R. D., and Russel, P. K. (1971). *Virology 44*: 108–124.
Shapiro, D., Kos, K. A., and Russell, P. K. (1973). *Virology 56*:95–109.
Shegal, S. (1989). *JE & HFRS Bull. 3*:31–40.
Shope, R. E. (1980). In *The Togaviruses, Biology, Structure, Replication*, R. W. Schlesinger (Ed.). Academic Press, New York, pp. 47–82.
Shope, R. E. (1987). *JE & HFRS Bull. 2*:27–32.
Shope, R. E., and Sather, G. E. (1979). In *Diagnostic Procedures for Viral, Rickettsial and Chlamydial Infections*. E. H. Lennette and N. J. Schmidt (Eds.). ASM, Washington, DC, pp. 767–814.
Shortridge, K. F., Oya, A., Kobayashi, M., and Yip, D. Y. (1975). *SE Asian J. Trop. Med. Public Health 6*:161–169.
Southam, C. M. (1956). *J. Infect. Dis. 99*:163–169.
Srivastava, A. K., Aira, Y., Mori, C., Kobayashi, Y., and Igarashi, A. (1987). *Arch. Virol. 96*:97–107.
Srivastava, A. K., Morita, K., and Igarashi, A. (1990a). *Acta Virol. 34*:228–238.
Srivastava, A. K., Morita, K., Tanaka, M., Haishi, S., and Igarashi, A. (1990b). Abstracts VIII International Congress on Virology, Berlin, pp. 8–38.
Sugawara, S., Toshima, S., Ogata, M., Morimoto, T., Sugimori, T., and Fujisaki, Y. (1973). *Jpn. J. Vet. Med. 26*:558–560.
Sulkin, S. E., Sims, R., and Allen, R. (1964). *Am. J. Trop. Med. Hyg. 13*:475–481.
Sulkin, S. E., Allen, R., Miura, T., and Toyokawa, K. (1970). *Am. J. Trop. Med. Hyg. 19*:77–87.

Sumiyoshi, H., Morita, K., Mori, C., Fuke, I., Shiba, T., Sakaki, Y., and Igarashi, A. (1986). *Gene 48*:195–201.

Sumiyoshi, H., Mori, C., Fuke, I., Morita, K., Kuhara, S., Kondou, J., Kikuchi, Y., Nagamatsu, H., and Igarashi, A. (1987). *Virology 161*:497–510.

Takahashi, M. (1976). *J. Med. Entomol. 13*:275–284.

Takahashi, M., and Yasutomi, K. (1987). *J. Med. Entomol. 24*:595–603.

Takaku, K., Yamashita, T., Osanai, T., Yoshida, I., Kato, M., Goda, H., Takagi, M., Hirota, T., Amano, T., Fukai, K., Kunita, N., Inoue, K., Shoji, K., Igarashi, A., and Ito, T. (1968). *Biken J. 11*:25–39.

Takashima, I., Watanabe, T., Ouchi, N., and Hashimoto, N. (1988). *Am. J. Trop. Med. Hyg. 38*:420–427.

Takeda, H., Yamada, M., and Aoyama, Y. (1965). *Jpn. J. Med. Sci. Biol. 18*:111–120.

Takeda, H., Oya, A., Hashimoto, K., and Yamada, M. (1977). *Gen. Virol. 34*:201–205.

Takeda, H., Oya, A., Hashimoto, K., Yasuda, T., and Yamada, M. (1978). *J. Gen. Virol. 38*:281–291.

Takegami, T., and Hotta, S. (1989). *Virus Res. 13*:337–350.

Takegami, T., and Hotta, S. (1990). *Microbiol. Immunol. 34*:849–857.

Takegami, T., Miyamoto, H., Nakamura, H., and Yasui, K. (1982). *Acta Virol. 26*:312–320.

Takegami, T., Washizu, M., and Yasui, K. (1986). *Virology 152*:483–486.

Thongcharoeng, P. (1985). *J. Med. Assoc. Thailand 68*:534–545.

Thongcharoeng, P. (1989). Faculty of Tropical Medicine, Mahidol University, Bangkok.

Ueba, N., Maeda, A., Otsu, K., Mitsuda, B., Kimoto, T., Fujito, S., and Kunita, N. (1972). *Biken J. 15*:67–79.

Umenai, T., Krzysko, R., Bektimirov, A., and Assaad, F. A. (1985). *Bull. WHO 63*:625–631.

Vitarana, T., Jayasekera, N., Wdasinghe, N., Senaratne, A., Colombage, G., Kanapathipillai, M., Hettiaratchy, L., Ariyaratnam, N., Peiris, L., Aluthwatte, A., Gunasekera, H. D. N. (1988). In *Virus Diseases in Asia*, P. Thongcharoeng and E. Kurstak (Eds.). Mahidol University, Bangkok, pp. 193–196.

Watanabe, M. (1988). *Life Environ. 33*:33–38.

Westaway, E. G. (1969a). *Nature 219*:78–79.

Westaway, E. G. (1969b). *J. Immunol. 100*:569–580.

Westaway, E. G., Brinton, M. A., Gaidamovich, S. Y., Horzinek, M. C., Igarashi, A., Kaariainen, L., Lvov, D. K., Porterfield, J. S., Russell, P. K., and Trent, D. W. (1985). *Intervirology 24*:183–192.

Yamada, T., Rojanasuphot, S., Takagi, M., Wungkobkiat, S., Hirota, T., Yamashita, T., Ahandrik, S., Pisuthipornkul, S., Sawasdikosol, S., Tuchinda, P., Wacharothal, S., Jatanasen, S., Hiranniramon, S., Laosuthipongse, V., Chiowanich, P., Roberts, C. E., Jr., Oesawadi, P., Bukhavesa, S., Gaew-Im, M., Shimizum, A., and Kitaoka, M. (1971). *Biken J. 14*:267–296.

Yasuda, A., Kimura-Kuroda, J., Ogimoto, M., Miyamoto, M., Sata, T., Sato, T., Takamura, C., Kurata, T., Kojima, A., and Yasui, K. (1990). *J. Virol. 64*:2788–2795.

Yasui, K. (1987). *Jpn. J. Clin. Med.* 45:2390–2396.
Yasui, K., Nozima, T., Homma, R., and Ueda, S. (1971). *Acta Virol.* 15:7–18.
Yasutomi, K., and Takahashi, M. (1987). *J. Med. Entomol.* 604–608.
Yasuzumi, G., and Tsubo, I. (1965). *J. Ultrastructure Res.* 12:304–316.
Yoshida, I., Takagi, M., Inokuma, E., Goda, H., Ono, K., Takaku, K., Oku, J., Kunita, N., Amano, T., and Okuno, Y. (1981). *Biken J.* 24:47–67.
Yu, Y.-X., Zhang, G.-M., Guo, Y.-P., Ao, J., and Li, H.-M. (1987). *JE & HFRS Bull.* 2:33–38.
Yu, Y.-X., Zhang, G.-M., Guo, Y.-P., Ao, J., and Li, H.-M. (1988). *Am. J. Trop. Med. Hyg.* 39:214–217.

13

Dengue Virus Infections

Vaccines and Immunization Strategies

Kenneth H. Eckels *Walter Reed Army Institute of Research, Washington, D.C.*

I. INTRODUCTION

Four distinct serotypes (1–4) contribute to an estimated 100 million cases of dengue (DEN) fever annually (Halstead, 1988) with first infection in endemic regions usually acquired in childhood. Uncomplicated first episodes of dengue fever are rarely fatal, but in regions of high endemicity in which more than one DEN serotype may be circulating, the most serious and often fatal forms of infection, dengue hemorrhagic fever or shock syndrome, may occur (Halstead, 1988; Guzman et al., 1990). Success with vaccines for other flaviviruses including yellow fever, Japanese encephalitis, and tick-borne encephalitis has held out hope that DEN infections could be controlled with a protective vaccine. Problems particular to DEN have made this goal difficult for researchers. These problems include the lack of an animal model for DEN disease and relatively low yields of virus from cell cultures. Serotype-specific protection also demands that a vaccine be prepared for each serotype and combined as a tetravalent vaccine. It has been proposed by Halstead and others that previous infection with DEN predisposes individuals to more severe disease when they subsequently become infected with a second DEN serotype (Halstead, 1988). Therefore, a tetravalent DEN vaccine that would protect against all DEN infections is the most desirable formulation.

This chapter will summarize historical as well as more recent approaches to the preparation of DEN vaccines and DEN vaccination.

Gene cloning technology has rapidly expanded our knowledge of DEN genome organization and the molecular basis of immunogenicity. Although at this point no human trials have begun using genetically engineered subunit or vectored DEN vaccines, these approaches will also be discussed.

II. LIVE-ATTENUATED VACCINES

During World War II it was found that, similar to yellow fever (YF), serial mouse brain passage of DEN resulted in progressively greater neurovirulence in mice paralleled by dramatic attenuation in volunteers (reviewed in Schlesinger, 1977). Although never widely used, human vaccination with such live-attenuated mouse brain preparations of DEN (serotypes 1 and 2) consistently stimulated production of serotype-specific neutralizing antibody and provided considerable protection against experimental challenge with the unmodified virus. However, clinical reactions typical of mild dengue fever and evidence of neurovirulence in monkeys dampened enthusiasm for such vaccines.

Tissue culture-derived and cloned DEN variants that were all temperature-sensitive, of small-plaque phenotype, and caused diminished viremia in monkeys have been tested as candidate vaccines. However, despite these presumed markers of attenuation, typical viremic DEN fever developed in some vaccinees (Bancroft et al., 1984; Eckels et al., 1984; Innis et al., 1988; McKee et al., 1987).

Encouraging preliminary results have recently been reported after immunization of a small number of individuals with live, uncloned DEN-2 or DEN-4 vaccines attenuated by passage in primary dog kidney (PDK) cells at reduced temperature (Bhamarapravati et al., 1987; Hoke et al., 1990). PDK cell-propagated DEN-2 (53rd passage) stimulated neutralizing antibody production in each of 10 volunteers with only trivial side effects. Vaccination with DEN-4 passaged in diploid rhesus monkey lung cells after 20 PDK passages was equally well tolerated but resulted in seroconversion in only 5 of 8 vaccinees. Most recently, Bhamarapravati and Yoksan (1989) demonstrated that DEN-2 and DEN-4 PDK vaccines given simultaneously to human volunteers stimulated the production of serotype-specific antibodies.

III. EXPERIMENTAL SUBUNIT VACCINES

Protection experiments in mice involving passive transfer of monoclonal antibodies against flaviviral proteins or active immunization with native or recombinant flaviviral proteins has thus far conclusively demonstrated that antibody to the virion envelope proteins E and prM/M and, surprisingly, to the nonvirion glycosylated protein NS1, confers protection. Passive transfer experiments in mice employing monoclonal antibodies against the E protein of a number of flaviviruses (Heinz et al., 1983; Matthews and Roehrig, 1984; Brandriss et al., 1986; Gould et al., 1986; Kaufman et al., 1987) showed that those with high-titer neutralizing activity (as measured by in vitro plaque reduction) invariably protected against challenge with the homologous virus. Monoclonal antibodies for DEN-2 E protein were found to be consistently neutralizing, although of varying titer. However, some of these antibodies failed to protect mice in passive immunization experiments (Kaufman et al., 1987).

Immunization with purified, native E protein has been reported only with intact E protein from tickborne encephalitis virus (Heinz et al., 1981). Immunization with other flavivirus native E proteins, including DEN, would help to establish protection parameters using this protein as a subunit vaccine.

A vaccinia recombinant (VR) containing DEN-4 E was shown to be protective after immunization of mice with this recombinant (Bray et al., 1989). Although there was complete protection, no neutralizing antibodies were stimulated in these mice. Another DEN-4 VR construct that contained C-prM-E was also completely protective, while other DEN-4 constructs including C-prM-E-NS1-NS2a were incompletely protective (Falgout et al., 1990). For DEN-2, VR E alone was not protective while VR C-prM-E was completely protective (Lai et al., 1989). For another flavivirus, Japanese encephalitis, the inclusion of the prM protein in VR constructs was found to be essential to protect mice (Mason et al., 1990; Yasuda et al., 1990).

With the use of baculovirus recombinants (BR) for the production of DEN gene products in *Spodoptera frugiperda* (Spf) cells, a series of DEN-4 BR-infected Spf cell extracts was used to immunize mice who were then challenged with mouse-adapted DEN-4 virus (Zhang et al., 1988; Lai et al., 1989). DEN-4 BR C-prM-E-NS1-NS2a and RSVG-E preparations were completely protective for mice. (The latter construct contained truncated respiratory syncytial virus G protein to enhance secretion.) Rhesus monkeys receiving these same preparations were only partially protected (Lai et al., 1990). To date, it appears that DEN E alone or in combination with other structural or nonstructural proteins is protective in the mouse model. Whether the success in mice can be duplicated in primates is still undetermined.

Kaufman et al. (1989) demonstrated protection of mice with five monoclonal antibodies specific for prM/M protein of DEN-3 and DEN-4. Four of these protected against heterologous DEN challenge as well. Despite binding of each antibody to purified virions, only two exhibited plaque-reducing neutralizing activity (of low titer), even after addition of complement or antimouse immunoglobulin. Successful immunization with the prM/M protein has not been reported as yet.

The nonvirion glycoprotein NS1 is expressed on the surface of flavivirus-infected cells (Schlesinger et al., 1985). Antibodies against the NS1 protein do not react with virions and exhibit no neutralizing activity. It was therefore unexpected that passive transfer of some monoclonal antibodies directed to YF or DEN NS1 protected mice against lethal infection with the respective viruses (Schlesinger et al., 1985; Gould et al., 1986; Henchal et al., 1988). Active immunization of mice with YF or DEN-2 NS1 purified from infected cell cultures was protective (Schlesinger et al., 1985, 1987). YF NS1-immunized monkeys likewise exhibited marked reduction in the magnitude of YF viremia and were partially protected against fatal YF hepatitis (Schlesinger et al., 1986). A similar experiment in monkeys using DEN-2 NS1 did not result in protection against challenge (Eckels, unpublished data). Cloned DEN-4 NS1-NS2a in a vaccinia vector partially protected mice and stimulated the production of cytolytic antibodies (Falgout et al., 1990). A DEN-2 NS1-NS2a-NS2b VR was not able to protect mice against challenge (Falgout et al., 1990), while a similar yellow fever VR was partially protective for mice (Putnak and Schlesinger, 1990). These experiments demonstrate that NS1 in combination with NS2a plays a role in the protection of animals after infection. The cytolytic activity of NS1 antibodies is probably important for the recognition and destruction of viral-infected cells bearing NS1 (Schlesinger et al., 1985; Falgout et al., 1990).

As can be seen from this brief summary, protection against lethal flavivirus encephalitis in mice conferred by immunization with recombinant flavivirus proteins has varied widely and often unpredictably with the protein(s) of interest and with the particular flavivirus and expression vector. The mouse protection model has been invaluable for screening DEN immunogens, even though the intracerebral challenge, which this model uses, is an undesirable route of challenge. Several candidates need to be further evaluated in monkeys following purification and addition of adjuvants.

IV. FUTURE DIRECTIONS

Rapid advances in flavivirus molecular biology have provided an abundance of new information on genome organization, expression, and replication, and have facilitated the recognition and study of viral proteins important to the protective immune response. Although preliminary results suggest that production of efficacious subunit or more highly defined attenuated flavivirus vaccines is feasible, definitive answers to a number of questions will be needed to realize this goal fully. One of these questions for DEN is whether an E subunit vaccine would be desirable and effective. Neutralizing antibodies undoubtedly provide the initial and major barriers to the establishment of DEN virus infections. However, in situations where neutralizing antibodies are of insufficient concentration to prevent infection, a role for NS1 antibodies may be important through complement-mediated lysis of infected cells or possibly by antibody- dependent cell cytolysis. Other DEN virus proteins, including nonstructural proteins, may play similar roles in the elimination of viral-infected cells. The recent demonstration by Mason et al. (1990) that a noninfectious hemagglutinating particle for Japanese encephalitis virus from recombinant-infected cells is highly immunogenic and protective introduces a novel subunit vaccine for this flavivirus and possibly others. This kind of immunogen would circumvent the need for inactivation of live virus in an inactivated, whole virus vaccine. This particulate immunogen may also not require the addition of adjuvants that is probably essential for optimal immunization with other subunit flavivirus vaccines.

Recent construction of CDNA clones of 17D yellow fever capable of producing infectious RNA transcripts (Rice et al., 1989) offers researchers the opportunity to design live-attenuated vaccines specifically for various flaviviruses, including DEN. Site-directed deletions in the flaviviral genome may eventually result in stable, genetically defined vaccine candidates with acceptable attenuation characteristics. However, without a suitable animal model for DEN, these mutants would have to be tested in humans for acceptable attenuation. The opportunity also exists, through the same technology, to design chimeras that would represent all of the DEN serotypes combined into one genome. Such a vaccine would eliminate the need to mix monovalent vaccines into a tetravalent formulation.

Finally, success with the PDK-passaged DEN vaccines has increased the possibility that these empirically derived vaccines will soon be tested for efficacy in field trials. Well-designed trials to test the importance of prior flavivirus immunity are essential, especially in populations where the virus is endemic. A bivalent vaccine has already been tested in humans that stimulated the production of serotype-specific neutralizing antibodies in vaccinees. If this success can be repeated for tri- and tetravalent vaccines, the possibility of predisposing an individual to more severe illness by creating incomplete protection will be reduced.

ACKNOWLEDGMENT

The author thanks J. J. Schlesinger for reviewing the manuscript.

REFERENCES

Bancroft, W. H., Scott, R. McN., Eckels, K. H., Hoke, C. H., Simms, T. E., Jesrani, K. D. T., Summers, P. L., Dubois, D. R., Tsoulos, D., and Russell, P. K. (1984). *J. Infect. Dis. 149*:1005–1010.

Bhamarapravati, N., Yoksan, S., Chayaniyayothin, T., Angsubphakorn, S., and Bunyaratvej, A. (1987). *Bull. WHO 65*:189–195.

Bhamarapravati, N., and Yoksan, S. (1989). *Lancet 1*:1077.

Brandriss, M. W., Schlesinger, J. J., Walsh, E. E., and Briselli, M. (1986). *J. Gen. Virol. 67*:229–234.

Bray, M., Zhao, B., Markoff, L., Eckels, K. H., Chanock, R. M., and Lai, C.-J. (1989). *J. Virol. 63*:2853–2856.

Eckels, K. H., Scott, R. McN., Bancroft, W. H., Brown, J., Dubois, D. R., Summers, P. L., Russell, P. K., and Halstead, S. B. (1984). *Am. J. Trop. Med. Hyg. 33*: 684–689.

Falgout, B., Bray, M., Schlesinger, J. J., and Lai, C.-J. (1990). *J. Virol. 64*:4356–4363.

Gould, E. A., Buckley, A., Barrett, A. D. T., and Cammack, N. (1986). *J. Gen. Virol. 67*:591–595.

Guzman, M. G., Kouri, G. P., Bravo, J., Soler, M., Vasquez, S., and Morier, L. (1990). *Am. J. Trop. Med. Hyg. 42*:179–184.

Halstead, S. B. (1988). *Science 239*:476–481.

Heinz, F. X., Tuma, W., and Kunz, C. (1981). *Infect. Immun. 33*:250–257.

Heinz, F. X., Berger, R., Tuma, W., and Kunz, C. (1983). *Virology 126*:525–537.

Henchal, E. A., Henchal, L. S., and Schlesinger, J. J. (1988). *J. Gen. Virol. 69*:2101–2107.

Hoke, C. H., Jr., Malinoski, F. J., Eckels, K. H., Scott, R. McN., Dubois, D. R., Summers, P. L., Simms, T., Burrous, J., Hasty, S. E., and Bancroft, W. H. (1990). *Am. J. Trop. Med. Hyg. 43*:219–226.

Innis, B. L., Eckels, K. H., Kraiselburd, E., Dubois, D. R., Meadors, G. F., Gubler, D. J., Burke, D. S., and Bancroft, W. H. (1988). *J. Infect. Dis. 158*:876–880.

Kaufman, B. M., Summers, P. L., Dubois, D. R., and Eckels, K. H. (1987). *Am. J. Trop. Med. Hyg. 36*:427–434.

Kaufman, B. M., Summers, P. L., Dubois, D. R., Timchak, R. L., and Eckels, K. H. (1989). *Am. J. Trop. Med. Hyg. 41*:576–580.

Lai, C.-J., Zhang, Y.-M., Bray, M., Chanock, R. M., and Eckels, K. H. (1989). In *Vaccines, 1989*, R. A. Lerner, R. M. Chanock, and F. Brown (Eds.). Cold Spring Harbor Laboratory, Cold Spring Harbor, NY.

Lai, C.-J., Zhang, Y.-M., Bray, M., Chanock, R. M., Dubois, D. R., and Eckels, K. H. In *Vaccines, 1990*, F. Brown, R. M. Chanock, H. Ginsberg, and R. A. Lerner (Eds.). Cold Spring Harbor Laboratory, Cold Spring Harbor, NY.

Mason, P. W., Pincus, S., Fournier, M. J., Mason, T. L., Shope, R. E.,and Paoletti, E. (1990). *Virology 180*:294–305.

Matthews, J. H., and Roehrig, J. T. (1984). *J. Immunol. 132*:1533–1537.

McKee, K. T., Jr., Bancroft, W. H., Eckels, K. H., Redfield, R. R., Summers, P. L., and Russell, P. K. (1897). *Am. J. Trop. Med. Hyg. 36*:435–442.

Putnak, J. R., and Schlesinger, J. J. (1990). *J. Gen. Virol. 71*:1697–1702.

Rice, C. M., Struss, E. G., and Struss, J. H. (1986). In *The Togaviridae and Flaviviridae*, S. Schlesinger and M. J. Schlesinger (Eds.). Plenum Press, New York and London, pp. 279–326.

Schlesinger, R. W. S. (1977). In *The Dengue Viruses*, R. W. S. Schlesinger (Ed.). Springer-Verlag, Vienna and New York, pp. 104–113.

Schlesinger, J. J., Brandriss, M. W., and Walsh, E. E. (1985). *J. Immunol. 135*:2805–2809.

Schlesinger, J. J., Brandriss, M. W., Cropp, C. B., and Monath, T. M. (1986). *J. Virol. 60*:1153–1155.

Schlesinger, J. J., Brandriss, M. W., and Walsh, E. E. (1987). *J. Gen. Virol. 68*:853–857.

Yasuda, A., Kimura-Kuroda, J., Ogimoto, M., Miyamoto, M., Sata, T., Sato, T., Takamura, C., Kurata, T., Kojima, A., and Yasui, K. (1990). *J. Virol. 64*:2788–2795.

Zhang, Y., Hayes, E. P., McCarty, T. C., Dubois, D. R., Summers, P. L., Eckels, K. H., Chanock, R. M., and Lai, C.-J. (1988). *J. Virol. 62*:3027–3031.

Part VI

Respiratory and Diarrheal Virus Diseases

14

World Health Organization Program on the Control of Influenza

Yuri Ghendon *World Health Organization, Geneva, Switzerland*

I. INTRODUCTION

Influenza has long been recognized as a problem in both developed and developing countries. Recurring epidemics are known to have many consequences among different populations of the world; these include a high frequency of morbidity that disrupts work in schools, public services, and elsewhere, as well as other activities. During major epidemics it causes large numbers of persons to require medical treatment or hospitalization. In developed countries influenza is important as a cause of severe morbidity and mortality. Excess mortality often accompanies influenza epidemics, the vast majority affected being the elderly. The fastest growing sector of the populations of many countries is the elderly, whose numbers are projected to double by early in the next century. These changing trends in modern society, especially in developed nations, will lead to an increased awareness of the impact of influenza.

Influenza also occurs frequently in developing and tropical countries where the prevalence of individual virus variants is not substantially different from that in the industrialized countries. However, the relative impact of influenza as a cause of morbidity and mortality may be lower in the developing countries because of the high prevalence of other infectious diseases. Nevertheless, as general health standards improve and longevity increases, the numbers of elderly persons and consequently the number of high-risk individuals will increase in these countries, creating an increased need for effective vaccines against influenza and a well-considered prevention policy.

II. IMPACT OF INFLUENZA

As noted above, influenza infections are a predictable cause of excess mortality. For example, in the United States in 1957 the Asian strain of influenza virus caused an estimated 70,000 deaths; the Hong Kong virus that appeared in 1968 caused about 30,000 deaths in the United States alone. Even in years not associated with antigenic shift, many people die as a result of influenza infection. More than 10,000 excess deaths have been documented in the United States during each of 18 different epidemics from 1957 to 1985 (Prevention and control of influenza, 1989).

In the 1989–1990 epidemiologic season only, in the United Kingdom influenza has been responsible for about 8,000 deaths. The morbidity rate was also very high. At the peak of this outbreak in Scotland the highest general practitioners' consultation rate was 2,719:100,000. A large number of schools had to close and hospitals had difficulty coping with patients both due to their number and because staff were also ill (Curwen et al., 1990).

During the influenza outbreak, the morbidity is highest in children between 1 and 14 years (rate, 37:100 persons); in those aged 60 and over the rate is only 10:100 persons. Hospitalization rates are relatively uniform for ages 5–44 and are highest in age groups <5 and >65. At the same time, the death rate in children is low (2.7:100,000) and is highest in the over-65 age group (75.9:100,000) (New Vaccine Development, 1985; Couch et al., 1986). More than 80% of the excess deaths attributed to pneumonia and influenza during epidemics have occurred among persons 65 years of age or more. It should be stressed that excess mortality is a direct result not only of pneumonia but also of cardiopulmonary or other chronic diseases that are exacerbated during influenza infection.

Although mortality is the most important problem caused by influenza, the days lost by absenteeism from both school and work and the hospitalization required for complications all result in a very high cost of influenza to society. If the disease burden value and costs associated with disease treatment were normalized and influenza defined as 100%, all other diseases can be shown to have a burden value and cost associated with disease much lower than influenza (New Vaccine Development, 1985).

It was estimated that in the United States during an influenza outbreak about 70 million people catch influenza at a cost of about $4.5 billion. Most of these cases can be avoided by vaccination. After vaccination, approximately 80% of the population would be protected against influenza, at a saving of about $2.1 billion (New Vaccine Development, 1985).

Serious analysis of the economic cost of influenza was done recently in France (Levy et al., 1990). During the influenza outbreak in the 1988–1989 epidemiologic season, there were 4.5 million primary diagnoses of influenza and each diagnosis accounted for 3 drug prescriptions; 7,388 patients with influenza were hospitalized; more than 16.8 million work days were lost by the active population; and 7.5 million school days were lost by children due to influenza. Analysis of the economic impact of this influenza epidemic shows that consultation and visits to doctors cost about $81 million, the cost of drug prescriptions was about $105 million, the cost of hospitalization was about $19 million, the cost of absenteeism was about $73 million, and the total cost of this outbreak for society was about $27.5 billion.

In spite of influenza infection being a widespread problem in many countries, the existing influenza vaccines are among the least utilized vaccines available. The need for annual revaccination and misconceptions about the capabilities of the vaccines (many recipients expect them to prevent all respiratory infections) have led many physicians to conclude that vaccination against influenza is not worth the effort.

In fact, there are considerable data on the efficacy of influenza vaccines in the prevention of morbidity and mortality, especially in elderly people, and it was shown that influenza vaccines can protect not only individuals but, if used properly, 70–80% of vaccinees in the community as a whole.

III. CONTROL OF INFLUENZA WITH VACCINES

The problems of control of influenza were discussed at a World Health Organization (WHO) meeting on influenza vaccines (Progress in the development of influenza vaccines, 1987). The WHO experts stressed that the impact of influenza epidemics can be reduced, to some extent, by immunoprophylaxis with available influenza vaccines.

Two main objectives for influenza vaccination strategies have been identified. These are, first, to protect individuals who are at particular risk of diseases (e.g., elderly persons in nursing homes). The risk of death during an influenza epidemic is high in certain population groups such as the aged, the chronically sick (e.g., patients with rheumatic heart disease, cardiovascular disorders, bronchopulmonary disease, immunodeficiency, and diabetes mellitus) and persons residing in institutions under crowded conditions. It was noted by experts that in closed or semiclosed settings, maximum benefit from immunization is likely to be achieved when more than about three-quarters of the population are vaccinated so that the benefits of herd immunity can be exploited. The second strategy to reduce the impact of influenza includes mass vaccination of certain populations (e.g., schoolchildren, as in Japan, or working adults, as in the Soviet Union) to protect such persons and to reduce illness in the overall community. In this case, vaccination may have direct benefit for the individuals involved and for the community as a whole.

It is not realistic to expect to prevent the disease in the community as a whole as is feasible with vaccines against measles and poliomyelitis. However, the impact of influenza epidemics can be reduced by immunoprophylaxis with available vaccines made from the appropriate strains of influenza viruses and used at the right time.

For prophylaxis of influenza, two types of vaccines are available: inactivated vaccines and live attenuated vaccines. Inactivated vaccines are in routine use in many countries. Several different forms of inactivated influenza vaccine for parenteral injection are in use: whole virion vaccine, disrupted (split) virus vaccines, and surface antigen (subunit) vaccines (see Ghendon, 1990a).

In unprimed subjects of all ages the disrupted and surface antigenic vaccines are less immunogenic than whole virus inactivated vaccines (Bernstein et al., 1988). In primed subjects surface antigen vaccines are equal to whole virion vaccines in their capacity to evoke humoral antibody response (Clarke et al., 1983a,b). No differences in immunogenicity of disrupted or surface antigen vaccines were found for all age groups (Jennings et al., 1984).

Depending on the age group, the immune response to inactivated influenza vaccines is either a primary or a booster type (Couch and Kasel, 1983). Subjects who have not previously been exposed to influenza (mainly children) mount a primary antibody response and titers after their first dose of vaccine are low. After the second dose of vaccine, which provides a boost, antibody titers rise in these children. Most adults, unless they are being exposed to an entirely new antigen, will mount a booster antibody response even to strains in which antigens are marginally changed.

Antibodies to influenza vaccines are generally of the IgG class and they react against the hemagglutinin (HA) and neuraminidase (NA) of the vaccine strains. Antibody titers usually peak at 10–14 days after a vaccine boost, and then decline in ensuing months. Serum antibodies appear to be very important in protecting against infection with influenza viruses (see Ghendon, 1990b).

Many studies have revealed that normal children and adults have very good responses to inactivated influenza vaccines. Nearly all such persons have fourfold or greater antibody titer rises after immunization. Elderly individuals, whether debilitated or in good health, also show favorable responses, but the response is less than that found in normal younger individuals (Marine and Thomas, 1973). Underlying disease, for example, malignancy or chronic renal failure, does not by itself impair the antibody response. When active chemotherapy is being administered, or immunosuppressants such as drugs used for renal transplant recipients, responses are markedly diminished (Ruben, 1987).

Inactivated influenza vaccines vary in effectiveness but generally prevent about 70% of illness when the virus causing epidemics is closely related to the vaccine (Stuart-Harris and Schild, 1976).

Live attenuated influenza vaccines are administered to the upper respiratory tract, usually by the intranasal route. The viruses replicate in the respiratory tract, provoking an immune response. During the last decade, much progress has been achieved in the development of attenuated cold-adapted recombinant influenza vaccines, and it is now well established that suitable vaccine strains could be used to protect against influenza (see Ghendon, 1990a; Maassab et al., 1990).

It has been found that cold-adapted influenza viruses (i.e., viruses that grow well at 25°C but not at 37°C after serial passage at low temperatures) possess genes able to confer attenuation and ca and ts characteristics on their transfer to wild-type viruses (Ghendon, 1987; Wright and Karson, 1987). There is evidence that reassortants between cold-adapted master strains and wild influenza viruses that inherited five or six genes from the cold-adapted strain and HA and NA from wild virus are usually fully attenuated, immunogenic, do not spread, even between children, and are genetically stable (Ghendon, 1987).

In the Soviet Union ca donor strain A/Leningrad/134/17/57, which has ts mutation in three genes (P3, NP, and M), was used for obtaining reassortants for ca live influenza vaccine for adults and ca donor strain A/Leningrad/134/47/57, which has ts mutation in five genes (P1, P3, NP, M, NS) for children from 3 years of age (see Ghendon, 1987).

Reassortants obtained from the above donor should inherit at least five genes for nonglycosylated proteins from ca donor, including all genes containing ts mutation, and HA and NA from new antigen variants of influenza viruses.

The use of cold-adapted reassortants of influenza A viruses could allow the use of two components with different HA and NA antigenic specificity (e.g., H1N1 and H3N2) and even three components (H1N1, H3N2, B).

Considerable progress on the development and clinical evaluation of ca donors and reassortants of influenza A virus as an attenuated live influenza vaccine has also been achieved in the United States (see Maassab et al., 1990).

A very important question is protection afforded by inactivated and live influenza virus. One of the first comparative studies of protective effects of live and inactivated influenza vaccine (H1N1) was done by Clarke et al. (1983a,b). In a study of short-term immunity, young adults were vaccinated with ca live vaccine or inactivated vaccine. One month after vaccination, protection against challenge with homologous ca live vaccine was equivalent in the two groups as assessed by rises in titers of HAI antibody. The same data were obtained in a study of long-term immunity when groups of young adults were challenged 3 months after vaccination. It should be noted that this study did not include investigation of local antibody and viral shedding data.

Clements et al. (1984), in comparative studies on seronegative adult volunteers who were vaccinated with ca live vaccine or inactivated vaccine, showed that after challenge with the homologous wild-type virus 5–8 weeks after vaccination, recipients of live vaccine were completely protected against illness compared with a 72% efficacy rate in the inactivated vaccine recipients. Wild-type virus was recovered from only 13% of live vaccine vaccinees compared with 63% of inactivated vaccine vaccinees. The few infected vaccinees immunized with ca live vaccine shed 1,000 times less wild-type virus than did infected inactivated vaccine vaccinees or unvaccinated controls. This striking reduction in virus shedding suggests that influenza transmission may be more efficiently interrupted with live than with inactivated vaccine.

In subsequent studies by Clements et al. (1986) of resistance of vaccinees to challenge with influenza wild-type virus 7 months after vaccination, it was found that vaccine efficacy, measured by reduction in febrile or systemic illness in vaccinees, compared with that in controls, was 100% for ca live H3N2 vaccine, 87% for inactivated H3N2 vaccine, 79% for ca live H1N1 vaccine, and 67% for inactivated H1N1 vaccine. The authors concluded that ca live influenza vaccine induced significantly greater resistance to wild-type influenza virus 1–2 months after vaccination, but at 7 months postvaccination the resistance induced by live vaccines is only slightly greater than that induced by inactivated vaccine. It should be noted that in the studies of Johnson et al. (1986) and Wright et al. (1986), vaccinees immunized with ca live (H3N2) or inactivated vaccine and challenged with homologous live ca vaccine or natural challenge with wild-type influenza virus 12 months after vaccination, live ca vaccine significantly reduced ca virus shedding after challenge compared with inactivated vaccine.

As to the efficacy of inactivated or live influenza vaccines, it should be noted that at the moment there are no published comparative studies on the efficacy of the two types of vaccines during the same field trials. However, as many studies have shown, adults who have experienced one or more infections by influenza virus and have been immunized with inactivated vaccines may have protection against antigenically homologous influenza virus for at least 1–2 years. In unprimed individuals, usually young children, this immunization is less protective, probably because of the poor ability of parenterally administered inactivated virus to prime for a local humoral or T cell call response (Ada and Jones, 1986).

The efficacy of live influenza vaccines in primed adults is more or less similar to the efficacy of inactivated vaccines. Efficacy studies of ca live vaccines on unprimed children have shown (Wright et al., 1982; Belshe et al., 1984) that children receiving a H3N2 ca live vaccine appeared to be protected against subsequent natural infection with related strains of influenza virus. Ca live influenza A vaccine was studied in a controlled field trial among more than 16,000 children between 3 and 15 years of age vaccinated with bivalent vaccine (H1N1 + H3N2) (Alexandrova et al., 1986). Protective efficacy of both components of the vaccine was evident in the twofold decrease in morbidity of vaccinees during outbreaks of influenza A/H1N1 and A/H3N2.

Another important problem related to the efficacy of influenza vaccines is the protective effect of vaccine against drift variants of influenza virus. Hoskins et al. (1979) showed that the protective effect of inactivated influenza vaccine was limited to nonimmune schoolchildren who were vaccinated for the first time with the inactivated vaccine made from the prevailing strain of influenza virus. Revaccination with inactivated vaccine produced from the later prevailing strain did not provide protection against a new drift variant. On the other hand, natural infection with live influenza virus afforded almost complete protection during successive outbreaks involving drift variants for more than 4 years. Since the specificity of the antibody response after vaccination with inactivated vaccine and after infection with live virus is similar, differences in the extent of cross-reactive T-lymphocyte responses to vaccination and infection may account for the lesser degree of heterotypic protection seen after vaccination with inactivated vaccine. Taking the above into account it is possible to suggest that live influenza vaccine may have an advantage over inactivated vaccines in protecting against new drift variants of influenza viruses.

In conclusion, the inference that live intranasal vaccination may provide better and more durable protection than inactivated intramuscular vaccination remains unproven, and the factors responsible for protection should be defined more clearly. Nevertheless, with our present knowledge it is possible to suggest that local administration of live attenuated influenza vaccines can mimic natural influenza infection and may provide more natural and cross-reactive immunity to this disease than vaccination with inactivated vaccine, especially in the protection of seronegative children.

IV. WHO SHOULD BE VACCINATED?

In most countries influenza vaccines are recommended for persons with chronic disease and for other risk groups and in some countries for mass vaccination of healthy adults or children. In fact, only a small percentage of the high-risk groups of people are vaccinated against influenza. For example, in the United States 43 million Americans are at risk of death from influenza by virtue of their underlying medical illnesses and should be immunized. In reality, almost 8 million members of this group do receive vaccine (Mostow, 1986). In Great Britain, the high-risk groups include 10 million people, but only a small proportion of these are vaccinated (Volunteers in test of flu vaccine, 1987).

In the majority of countries, vaccination of high-risk persons each year before the influenza season is the most important measure for reducing the impact of influenza. Vaccination can be highly cost-effective when it is aimed at individuals who experience the most severe consequences and who have a higher than average risk of infection. Also, when administered to high-risk individuals during routine health care visits before the influenza season, vaccination can obviate the need for special visits to general practitioners.

Groups at greater risk of influenza-related complications include (Prevention and control of influenza, 1989): adults and children with chronic disorders of the pulmonary or cardiovascular systems requiring regular medical follow-up or hospitalization during the preceding year, including children with asthma; and residents of nursing homes and other chronic-care facilities housing patients of any age with chronic medical conditions.

Groups at moderate risk of influenza-related complications are otherwise healthy persons >65 years; adults and children who have required regular medical follow-up or hospitalizations during the preceding year because of chronic metabolic diseases (including diabetes mellitus), renal dysfunction, hemoglobinopathies, or immunosuppression; and children and teenagers (6 months–18 years) who are receiving long-term aspirin therapy and, therefore, may be at risk of contracting Reye's syndrome after an influenza infection.

Groups potentially capable of nosocomial transmission of influenza to high-risk persons should also be immunized. Individuals attending high-risk persons can transmit influenza infections to them while they are themselves incubating infection, undergoing subclinical infection, or working despite the existence of symptoms. Some high-risk persons (e.g., the elderly, transplant recipients, or persons with acquired immunodeficiency syndrome) can have relatively low antibody responses to influenza vaccine. Efforts to protect them against influenza may be improved by reducing the chances that their care providers may expose them to influenza. Therefore, the following groups should be vaccinated:

1. Physicians, nurses, and other personnel who have extensive contact with high-risk patients (e.g., primary care and certain specialty clinicians and staff of chronic-care facilities and intensive care units, particularly neonatal intensive care units).
2. Providers of home care to high-risk persons (e.g., visiting nurses, volunteer workers) as well as all household members of high-risk persons, including children, whether or not they provide care. Other groups who should be considered for vaccination are discussed below.

Physicians should administer influenza vaccine to any person who wishes to reduce his or her chances of acquiring influenza infection. Persons who provide essential community services may be considered for vaccination to minimize the disruption of essential activities during severe epidemics.

Pregnancy has not been shown to be a risk factor for severe influenza infection, except in the largest pandemics of 1918–1919 and 1957–1958. However, pregnant women who have medical conditions that increase their risks of complications from influenza should be vaccinated, since the inactivated vaccine is considered safe for pregnant women. Administering the vaccine after the first trimester is a reasonable precaution to minimize any concern over the theoretical possibility of teratogenicity. However, it is undesirable to delay vaccination of pregnant women with high-risk conditions who will still be in the first trimester of pregnancy when the influenza season begins.

Increases in infections and complications caused by various respiratory pathogens have been observed in persons infected with human immunodeficiency virus (HIV). However, similar increases due to influenza have not been reported during recent epidemics. Nevertheless, because influenza may result in serious illness and complications in some HIV-infected persons, vaccination is a prudent precaution.

Immunization with influenza vaccines is contraindicated for persons who have an anaphylactic hypersensitivity to eggs and persons with acute febrile illnesses until their temporary symptoms have abated.

Special attention should be paid to elderly people, who are most likely die of influenza. Of the about 500,000 influenza-related deaths in the past 20 years, most have occurred in older people. The elderly are also more likely than younger people to experience serious complications following influenza infection. Reasons for the more serious morbidity and higher mortality in the elderly include impaired host defenses, decreased immune response, and the chronic underlying medical conditions that often accompany aging.

In the elderly population living in the community, hospitalization rates during influenza epidemics have been shown to be almost three times higher than rates for younger individuals (McGlone and Arden, 1987). With respect to the nursing home population, it should be noted that in the United States 60% of residents may be affected during an outbreak, and up to 25% of patients die or develop life-threatening complications (Arden et al., 1986). Inactivated vaccines may be less immunogenic in the older people, but data exist to show that even in these cases protection against influenza and its complications is produced.

There are several examples of the efficacy of influenza vaccines in the prevention or morbidity and especially of mortality in older people. Studies in the United States in a large metropolitan population of noninstitutionalized ambulatory elderly persons during several recent influenza epidemics have consistently shown a reduction in morbidity of approximately 70% among vaccinees when the virus inducing the outbreak and the virus used for the production of influenza vaccine are immunologically closely related (Barker and Mullooly, 1986). This effect was shown for subgroups both with and without high-risk chronic conditions and appears broadly generalizable to the 90–95% of the elderly who live in the community at large.

As noted above, in the elderly vaccine efficacy is often substantially lower than that estimated for young adults. One of the reasons is that most young adults develop HAI titers of 40 or greater following vaccination (a level associated with protection against influenza infection) but only about one-half of nursing home residents develop such titers (Arden et al., 1986).

Nevertheless, mathematical models of herd immunity suggest that it is still theoretically possible, even in the face of poor antibody responses, to reduce the incidence of illness, provided that a large enough proportion of residents in a given nursing home are vaccinated (Fox et al., 1971). In fact, some studies of influenza outbreaks in nursing home populations showed evidence of influenza vaccine efficacy (Arden et al., 1986). In some of these studies it was found that an important phenomenon worthy of consideration is the potential for "herd immunity" to play a role in determining the spread of influenza virus in the institutional setting. Patriarca et al. (1986) compared a series of nursing homes that experienced sustained spread of influenza with a series of homes in which only sporadic cases occurred, and found that the former had significantly lower levels of vaccination (median of 51% vs. 81% of residents vaccinated). This suggests that herd immunity may be achieved with institutional vaccination rates of 70–80%.

It should be noted that the number of vaccinated persons in nursing homes usually is less than 80%. For example, in the United States, the vaccination rate varies from about 90%, with an average of about 60% (Barker and Mullooly, 1986).

Although the efficacy of influenza vaccines in preventing illness in nursing homes with low vaccination rates is low, larger studies have consistently shown that the efficacy in reducing the severity of illness and in preventing hospitalization, pneumonia, and death is significantly higher, ranging from 47% to 95% (Arden et al., 1986). That study reported a 50% reduction in the duration of illness, a 90% reduction in the incidence of complications, and 95% reduction in mortality in the vaccinated group compared with the unvaccinated group (Serie et al., 1977). Another study (Saah et al., 1986) found that the attack rate of pneumonia did not differ significantly between vaccinated and unvaccinated elderly people, but the risk of death from pneumonia in the unvaccinated group was threefold higher than in the vaccinated group. In studies by Gross et al. (1988) 7.9% of elderly vaccinees died during the influenza epidemic compared with 17.7% in an unvaccinated control group.

Data have also illustrated the benefits of influenza vaccination and support the use of amantadine hydrochloride 100 mg daily for outbreak control among elderly persons (Arden et al., 1988).

The best strategy for controlling influenza in elderly people is to induce herd immunity, which may be achieved with institutional vaccination rates in the vicinity of 80%, as recommended by the Immunization Practices Advisory Committee (Prevention and control of influenza, 1987). The cost and benefits of annual immunization of persons of 65 years of age and older against influenza in Ontario, Canada, were studied. The cost of the program was $1,337,000. The benefits of the program considered were hospitalization, physician, and prescription costs averted by preventing influenza; the figure reached was $2,021,267 (Helliwell and Drummond, 1988).

In the prevention of influenza with currently available inactivated vaccines, satisfactory anti-HA antibody titers 40 (Potter and Oxford, 1979) may be achieved in antigenically primed recipients given one dose of any type of inactivated vaccine containing approximately 15 μg HA.

The Immunization Practices Advisory Committee of the United States has recommended use of all types of inactivated influenza vaccines for children aged 3–12 years and for adults in doses of 15 μg of each component (HA) of vaccines that usually are administered trivalently. For children aged 6–35 months of age, 7.5 μg of each component is recommended (Prevention and control of influenza, 1989). In several other countries, 7 μg of inactivated influenza vaccine is used for the vaccination of children and adults.

In the opinion of WHO experts (Requirement for influenza vaccines, 1979), the formulation of a permanent and inflexible recommendation for the quantity of specific antigen of the A and B components of inactivated influenza vaccines is inappropriate. This is because of the antigenic variability of the viruses and the fact that, for new variants, different amounts of antigen will be required to induce antibody levels consistent with immunity. The antibody response depends on the age of the vaccinated person, the presence or absence of previous immunologic experience with viruses possessing HA (and NA) antigens related to that of the vaccine strain, and the number of doses and type of vaccine given (whole virion, disrupted virus, or surface antigen vaccines). Vaccine potency should be based on the results of clinical trials, particularly on the emergence of new variant strains. The trials should include studies of antibody response to vaccination, clinical reactions, and, where possible, the protective efficacy of the vaccine against infection by natural or artificial challenge.

As to the number of influenza vaccine injections, the WHO experts recommended only one injection of inactivated influenza vaccines for children and adults (primed) and two doses for children less than 12 years of age who are receiving influenza vaccine for the first time (Recommended composition of influenza virus vaccines, 1991).

With reference to the cold-adapted live influenza vaccines, it was found that the percentage of vaccines inducing a fourfold antibody rise after one or two doses of vaccine is the same, but geometric mean antibody titers were two times lower after the single-dose vaccine than after two doses (Alexandrova et al., 1984); therefore, two doses of live vaccinia may be desirable.

V. SURVEILLANCE OF INFLUENZA AND STRAINS FOR VACCINE PRODUCTION

The main objectives of influenza surveillance are:

To collect and analyze epidemiologic information on influenza morbidity and mortality in order to estimate the impact of disease

The early detection of influenza epidemics, enabling immunization of persons not previously vaccinated and notification of health providers to prepare for the possible impact on clinical workloads and hospital admissions

To identify high-risk areas and population groups for whom additional immunization input may be needed

To identify epidemiologic factors involved in influenza outbreaks (e.g., age groups, behavioral patterns, presence of domestic animals, etc.)

To collect influenza isolates and analyze antigenic characteristics of influenza viruses, including outbreaks or sporadic cases of influenza, to determine which antigenic variant should be used for the production of influenza vaccines during the next epidemiologic season

It is well known that influenza viruses are variable and can change antigenic specificity of their envelope proteins: hemagglutinin and neuraminidase. Such variants escape the protective antibodies that were developed through previous infection or vaccination. This last objective of influenza surveillance is very important for the control of influenza with vaccines.

The WHO Program on Influenza Surveillance was established in 1947. Essentially, this program consists of the rapid isolation and characterization of new strains of influenza viruses to make available for research and production laboratories those showing substantial variation from the current strains.

Recommendations on the composition of the influenza virus strains that should be used for the production of influenza vaccines for the forthcoming epidemiologic season have been drawn up by WHO.

The resulting WHO recommendation is based on various information sources, including epidemiologic data, serum surveys, data from vaccine trials, and results of the analysis of antigenic characteristics of thousands of strains of influenza viruses isolated in different countries during influenza outbreaks or from sporadic cases. The last studies involved 118 WHO-recognized National Institutions for Influenza designated by governments in 81 countries and 3 WHO Collaborating Centers for Reference and Research on Influenza at the Centers for Disease Control

(Atlanta, GA), the National Institute for Medical Research (London, UK), and the Commonwealth Serum Laboratories (Parkville, Australia).

Each year at the end of February, WHO holds a consultation on recommendations for influenza vaccines composition for the forthcoming epidemiologic season. These recommendations are published in the WHO *Weekly Epidemiological Record* at the end of February. At the end of September a review of the prevalence of influenza viruses in the world is published in the *Weekly Epidemiological Record* for consideration in parallel with the recommendations for the composition of influenza vaccines for use in the Southern Hemisphere.

For production of the inactivated influenza vaccines, the high-yield recombinants (reassortants) of new variants are used. It was shown about 25 years ago that reassortment of a high-yielding laboratory strain A/PR8/34 (H1N1) with low-yielding H2N2 strains freshly isolated from human subjects produced high-yielding virus-bearing surface antigens of the H2N2 subtype. After the 1968 pandemic, routine use of such reassortants in vaccines was advocated (Kilbourne, 1969). The method has been generally successful, and virtually all production of contemporary inactivated influenza vaccines is based on such reassortant high-yield viruses.

Two high-yield parental strains have been most commonly used to induce high-yield reassortants: A/PR8/34 (H1N1) and X-31, itself a high-yield reassortant between A/PR8/34 and A/Aichi/68 (H3N2), having all genes except those coding for HA and NA derived from A/PR8/34 virus (Kilbourne, 1987).

The selection of high-yielding reassortant usually involves cloning of the virus. Consequently, reassortant viruses may show slight antigenic differences from wild-type influenza virus detectable with monoclonal antibodies (Downie, 1984). Differences in virus passage history may lead to similar minor antigenic variations of reassortant from wild-type virus (Pemberton et al., 1985). In the opinion of specialists, however, the extent of these differences is probably of no practical significance (Kilbourne, 1987).

As to the live attenuated influenza vaccines, reassortment between an attenuated cold-adapted donor strain and a new antigenic variant of influenza virus has been considered recently as the most appropriate method for obtaining cold-adapted live attenuated vaccine strains.

The reassortants obtained by reassortment of cold-adapted donor strains with new antigenic variants of influenza viruses should inherit from the cold-adapted parent at least five genes encoding for nonglycosylated proteins, including all genes containing ts mutations.

VI. CONTROL OF INFLUENZA WITH ANTIVIRAL DRUGS

Besides vaccines, several good antiviral agents against influenza are available.

The WHO meeting of a Scientific Group on Progress in Development and Use of Antiviral Drugs and Interferon (Progress in the development and use of antiviral drugs and interferon, 1987) noted that amantidine and rimantadine have been shown in m any controlled trials to be effective against influenza A infections. In prophylactic trials a 70–90% reduction has often been achieved in laboratory-confirmed influenza A compared with the placebo-treated group (see also Douglas, 1990; Mostow, 1987). It should be noted, however, that while amantadine can induce side effects (e.g., dizziness, nervousness, failure to concentrate), rimantadine seems not to produce any side effects.

The WHO experts from this Scientific Group stressed that considering the effectiveness of these drugs, it was unfortunate that they were so little used in the treatment of influenza A infections.

Ribavirin has also been shown to be active against influenza A and B. Since it has to be administered by aerosol, its usefulness will probably be restricted to hospitalized patients with influenza B infection (Bernstein et al., 1988).

The development of influenza virus variants resistant to amantadine/ rimantadine can be an important problem for wide use of these antivirals (Belshe et al., 1989). The emergence of drug-resistant influenza virus mutants should be closely surveyed and monitored.

VII. CONCLUSION

Influenza continues to be an important disease known to cause high levels of morbidity in developed countries at unpredictable intervals, usually every few years. Complications are most common in certain high-risk persons. The extent of influenza in developing countries is less clear, but in pandemics all countries are involved. While prevention of epidemics is not feasible, largely due to the emergence of antigenic variants, the impact of epidemics can be reduced to some extent by immunoprophylaxis with available vaccines.

Different goals may be considered for the control of influenza. Prevention of all influenza infections would have obvious advantages, but this seems an unreasonable goal at this time. A more limited goal would be the prevention of influenza epidemics, so that the excessive morbidity and mortality that accompany these epidemics are minimized. The population to be vaccinated would be limited in this case, but it would still be large.

The policy of many countries at present calls for use of influenza vaccines to prevent serious disease and death. This goal, however, has never been effectively implemented. A more effective application of this policy represents the least that medicine should do toward the control of influenza at present.

It is clear that the priorities of individual countries in developing a program of immunization against influenza will depend on the impact of influenza relative to the incidence of other diseases. National policies on the use of influenza vaccines vary widely from country to country. It is important to stress that immunity to influenza can be both solid and long-lasting, as shown by the resistance of the population to H1N1 infection after the reappearance of viruses of this subtype in 1977–1978. As a consequence of antigenic drift, however, reinfection by antigenically different viruses occurs frequently and may result in epidemics. The currently available vaccines are of variable efficacy because of the unpredictable antigenic variability of influenza viruses and their epidemiologic behavior.

As noted above, two types of influenza vaccines are available now for the control of influenza: inactivated and live attenuated. Although data are not available at present to indicate a clearly superiority of live vaccines over inactivated vaccines for this purpose, a live vaccine will be more desirable if it is effective for 3–5 years. In the opinion of some specialists (Fedson, 1987), live attenuated vaccine should be given to children in school or day care; to close and semiclose groups of healthy persons who experience very high attack rates, such as those in boarding schools, prisons, and the military; to healthy persons in industry who work indoors in groups; and to medical personnel in contact with persons at high risk. It seems appropriate to continue use of inactivated vaccine for high-risk persons.

Expanded educational programs have been advocated as one method of encouraging better performance in the delivery of the influenza vaccine. It is clear also that administrative and organizational changes can greatly improve immunization rates for high-risk patients and secure vaccination of more than 75% of people in a community, especially in closed and semiclosed communities, so that the benefits of herd immunity can be exploited.

Other strategies to reduce the impact of influenza include mass immunizations of certain populations (e.g., schoolchildren or working adults), not only to protect such persons but also to reduce illnesses in the overall community. Adequate studies have not yet been undertaken to conclude whether the desired reduction in community-wide illnesses results from such targeted mass immunization programs.

Influenza is not a trivial disease. It kills thousands of patients every year, and its cost to a country's economy is enormous. But influenza is preventable. With the aid of vaccines and antivirals it is possible to protect both high-risk individuals and defined subsets of the population. Of course, many questions related to the efficacy of vaccines, optimal strategies for their application, problems of drug-resistant virus mutants, and others, need further investigation. If the vaccines are prepared and used correctly, vaccination may protect many millions of people, and will save the lives of thousands of people, especially elderly persons.

REFERENCES

Ada, G., and Jones, P. (1986). *Curr. Topics Microbiol. Immunol. 128*:1–55.

Alexandrova, G., Polezhaev, F., Budiliovsky, G., Gromashova, L., Topuria, N., Egorov, A., Romeiko-Gurco, Y., Koval, T., Kisovskaya, K., Klimov, A., and Ghendon, Y. (1984). *Infect. Immun. 44*:734–739.

Alexandrova, G., Budilovsky, G., Koval, T., Polezhaev, F., Garmashova, L., Ghendon, Y., Romanova, Y., and Smorodintsev, A. (1986). *Vaccine* 4:114–118.

Arden, N., Patriarca, P., and Kendal, A. (1986). In *Option for the Control of Influenza,* A. Kendal and P. Patriarca (Eds.). Alan R. Liss, New York, pp. 155–198.

Arden, N., Patriarca, P., Fasano, M., Liu, K., Harmon, M., Kendal, A., and Rimland, D. (1988). *Arch. Intern. Med. 148*:865–868.

Barker, W., and Mullooly, J. (1986). In *Option for the Control of Influenza,* A. Kendal and P. Patriarca (Eds.). Alan R. Liss, New York, pp. 169–171.

Belish, R., Van Voris, L., Bartram, J., and Crookshanks, F. (1984). *J. Infect. Dis. 150*:834–840.

Belshe, R., Burk, B., Newman, F., Cerruti, R., and Sim, I. (1989). *J. Infect. Dis. 159*:430–435.

Bernstein, D., Zahradnik, J., DeAngelis, C., and Cherry, J. (1982). *Am. J. Dis. Child. 36*:513–517.

Bernstein, D., Reuman, P., Sherwood, J., Young, E., and Schiff, G. (1988). *Antimicrob. Agents. Chemother.* 32:761–764.

Clarkc, K., Potter, C., Jennings, R., Nicholl, J., Langrick, K., Schild, G., Wood, D., and Tyrrell, D. (1983a). *J. Hyg. (London) 90*:351–359.

Clarke, A., Potter, C., Jennings, R., and Nicholl, J. (1983b). *J. Hyg. (London) 90*: 361–370.

Clements, M., Betts, R., and Murphy, B. (1984). *Lancet 1*:705–708.

Clements, M., Betts, R., Tierney, E., and Murphy, B. (1986). *J. Clin. Microbiol. 23*:73–76.

Couch, R., and Kasel, J. (1983). *Annu. Rev. Microbiol. 37*:529–531.

Couch, R., Kasel, J., Glezen, W., Cate, T., Six, H., Taber, L., Frank, A., Greenberg, S., Zahradnik, J., and Keitel, W. (1986). *J. Infect. Dis. 153*:431–440.
Curwen, M., Dunnell, K., and Ashley, J. (1990). *Br. Med. J. 300*:896.
Douglas, G. (1990). *N. Engl. J. Med.* 322:443–450.
Downie, J. (1984). *J. Biol. Stand.* 12:101–104.
Fedson, D. (1987). *Am. J. Med. 82*(Suppl. 6A):42–47.
Fox, J., Elveback, L., Scott, W., Gatewood, L., and Ackerman, E. (1971). *Am. J. Epidemiol. 94*:175–189.
Ghendon, Y. (1987). *Sov. Med. Rev. Virol. 1*:269–314.
Ghendon, Y. (1990a). *Adv. Biotechnol. Proc. 14*:159–201.
Ghendon, Y. (1990b). *Acta Virol. 34*:295–304.
Gross, P., Rodstein, M., LaMontagne, J., Kaslow, M., Saah, A., Wallenstein, S., Neufeld, R., Denning, C., Gaerlan, P., and Quinnon, J. (1988). *Arch. Intern. Med. 148*:559–561.
Helliwell, B., and Drummond, M. (1988). *Can. J. Public Health 79*:175–177.
Hoskins, T., Davis, J., Smith, A., Miller, C., and Allchin, A. (1979). *Lancet 1*:33–35.
Jennings, R., Smith, T., Spencer, R., Mellersh, A., Edey, D., Fenton, P., and Potter, C. (1984). *Vaccine* 2:75–80.
Johnson, P., Feldman, S., Thompson, J., Mahoney, J., and Wright, P. (1986). *J. Infect. Dis. 154*:121–157.
Kilbourn, E. (1969). *Bull. WHO 41*:643–648.
Kilbourn, E. (1987). In *Influenza.* Plenum, New York/London, p. 291.
Levy, E., Levy, P., and Lafarge, H. (1990). Abstracts, 4th European Meeting on Influenza and its Prevention, Paris, 20–21, Step.
Maassab, H., Heilman, C., and Herlocher, M. (1990). *Adv. Biotechnol. Proc. 14*: 203–242.
Marine, W., and Thomas, J. (1973). *Postgrad. Med. J. 49*:164–167.
McGlone, F., and Arden, N. (1987). *Am. J. Med. 82*(Suppl. 6A):55–57.
Mostow, S. (1986). *Am. Rev. Respir. Dis. 134*:1.
Mostow, S. (1987). *Am. J. Med. 82*(Suppl. 6A):35–41.
New Vaccine Development, Establishing Priorities. I. Disease of importance in the United States. (1985). National Academy Press, Washington, DC:55.
Patriarca, P., Weber, J., Parker, P., Orenstein, W., Hall, W., Kendal, A., and Schonberger, L. (1986). *Am. J. Epidemiol. 124*:114–119.
Pemberton, R., Jennings, R., and Smith, T. (1985). *J. Hyg. (London) 94*:229–232.
Potter, C., and Oxford, J. (1979). *Br. Med. Bull. 35*:69–75.
Prevention and control of influenza (1987). *MMWR 36*:273.
Prevention and control of influenza (1989). *MMWR 38*:317–325.
Progress in the development of influenza vaccines: memorandum from a WHO meeting. (1987). *Bull. WHO 65*:289–293.
Progress in the development and use of antiviral drugs and interferon. (1987). *WHO Techn. Rep. Ser.* 754.
Recommended composition of influenza virus vaccines for use in the 1991–1992 season. (1991). *WHO Wkly. Epidemiol. Rec. 9*:57–64.
Requirements for influenza vaccines. (1979). *WHO Techn. Rep. Ser. 638*:149.

Ruben, F. (1987). *Am. Med. J. 82*(Suppl. 6A):31–34.
Saah, A., Neufeld, R., Rodstein, M., LaMontagne, J., Blackwelder, W., Gross, P., Quinnan, J., and Kaslow, R. (1986). *Arch. Intern. Med. 146*:2353–2355.
Serie, C., Barme, M., and Hannoun, C. (1977). *Dev. Biol. Stand. 39*:317–321.
Stuart-Harris, C., and Schild, J. (1976). In *Influenza, the Virus and the Diseases*. Edward Arnold, London, pp. 164–173.
Volunteers in the test of flue vaccine. (1987). *The Times*, 16 July.
Wright, P., and Karson, D. (1987). *Progr. Med. Virol. 34*:70–88.
Wright, P., Okabe, N., McKee, K., Maassab, H., and Karson, D. (1982). *J. Infect. Dis. 146*:71–79.
Wright, P., Johnson, P., and Karson, D. (1986). In *Option for the Control of Influenza*. A. Kendal and P. Patriarca (Eds.). Alan R. Liss, New York, pp. 243–253.

15

World Health Organization Acute Respiratory Viruses Vaccine Development Program

Yuri Pervikov *World Health Organization, Geneva, Switzerland*

I. INTRODUCTION

In 1987 the World Health Organization established the Programme for Vaccine Development (PVD) with the objective of providing the means to reduce the high morbidity and mortality due to viral and bacterial diseases of childhood in developing countries, through the improvement of existing vaccines and development of new ones. The development of vaccines against diseases caused by respiratory syncytial virus (RSV) and parainfluenza virus type 3 (PIV3) was given high priority. It is estimated that RSV is the cause of 20–25% of cases of pneumonia and 40–50% of cases of bronchiolitis in hospitalized children (Heilman, 1990). This virus is also an important cause of respiratory disease in elderly and immunocomprised individuals. About 90,000 patients with RSV cases are hospitalized annually in the United States and the cost of these cases is estimated at $300 million (Heilman, 1990). All four serotypes of parainfluenza virus can induce acute respiratory tract infection. However, PIV3 is the most virulent type and is an important cause of bronchiolitis and pneumonia in infants. RSV and PIV3 are prevalent worldwide; for example, in several developing countries RSV had been isolated from 11–37% of children with signs of acute lower respiratory infection (Selwyn, 1990). Therefore, safe and effective vaccines for prevention of diseases caused by these viruses would be used in many countries.

All attempts to prepare killed and live vaccines have so far been unsuccessful. Several inactivated mono- and trivalent parainfluenza virus candidate vaccines induced antibodies in children but had a low protective effect. An inactivated RSV vaccine, prepared by formalin treatment of the virus, stimulated formation of antibodies and cell-mediated immunity in seronegative infants. However, it did not induce protection against natural RSV infection, but increased the frequency and severity of lower respiratory diseases during subsequent RSV infection in children 6–23 months of age. A live RSV vaccine was prepared by cultivation of the virus at low temperature and through chemical mutagenesis. Several vaccines prepared in this way were tested in children, but none could be recommended for use in medical practice because of either high residual virulence or overattenuation. The development of safe and effective RSV and PIV3 vaccines, therefore, remains a priority area for medical research.

II. MANAGEMENT OF THE PROGRAM

The development of RSV and PIV3 vaccines under the auspices of the WHO/UNDP Program for Vaccine Development is managed by a Steering Committee (SC) on Acute Respiratory Viruses and Measles, which is composed of leading international scientists in the area. The Steering Committee decides on research priorities, recommends research projects for financial support, and promotes collaborative research. The recommendations of the SC are subject to discussion and approval by the Scientific Advisory Group of Experts (SAGE), which decides on the general orientation of the Program and reviews its implementation. The WHO Secretariat (Microbiology and Immunology Support Services [MIM]), within the Division of Communicable Diseases, is responsible for the operational management and administration of the Program.

The SC attempts to attract to the Program the best researchers from the relatively large group of scientists studying RSV and PIV3. Thirty-nine research projects from seven countries have been granted during 1985–1990. Review of the status of RSV and PIV3 vaccine development below includes information from other sources, as well as the PVD. An important role of the SC is to coordinate activities of different laboratories through workshops and technical meetings, which offer insights into current research and a foundation for PVD decisions and strategies. To help research groups dealing with RSV and PIV3, one project has established a bank of reagents, including a selection of monoclonal antibodies for antigenic sites of RSV and PIV3 proteins, and a panel of vaccinia virus recombinants for each of the gene products of RSV and PIV3. These reagents are provided, upon request, to institutes and laboratories for research purposes.

III. RSV VACCINE DEVELOPMENT

The genome of RSV has now been completely sequenced. The viral F and G surface glycoproteins have been identified as the main protective antigens, and therefore, should be components of future vaccines against diseases caused by RSV.

Many studies have been performed to evaluate the protective role of humoral and cell-mediated immunity in RSV infection. It has been shown that passive transfer of anti-RSV sera or monoclonal antibodies for F and G RSV surface glycoproteins reduced virus replication in lungs of infected mice and cotton rats (Taylor et al., 1984; Prince et al., 1985). However, the injected monoclonal antibodies against the N protein did not show protective activity. The antibody-mediated clearance of RSV observed in cotton rat lungs could have occurred without involvement of complement and cell-mediated mechanisms (Prince et al., 1990). Conflicting results have been obtained from studies on the protective role of antibodies in children. Early work suggested that maternally transmitted antibody was not protective (Chanock et al., 1988). However, subsequent observations have shown that the amount of serum antibody to RSV correlates with resistance against severe RSV disease. There is also a correlation between the age of first infection and the level of antibody at birth (Glezen et al., 1981; Ward et al., 1983). In addition, immune therapy with anti-RSV IgG immunoglobulin enhanced clearance of virus from respiratory tract and improved clinical response (Hemming et al., 1987).

RSV infection induces synthesis of IgG, IgM, and IgA antibodies in the respiratory tract of infants. Appearance of anti-RSV IgA antibodies in the mucosa of the respiratory tract during primary infection correlates closely with the disappearance of virus from the lung of infected mice. In adult volunteers, resistance to infection correlates with the level of antibodies in the respiratory tract, but not with the level of neutralizing antibodies in blood (Mills et al., 1971). These results confirm the importance of local humoral immunity and imply that an effective vaccine should induce formation of antibodies in the respiratory tract. A vaccine for intranasal application seems more promising than a parenteral vaccine since intramuscular administration of live vaccine failed to induce a mucosal antibody response in calves (Kimmen and Westernbrink, 1990).

RSV infection induces anti-RSV cytotoxic T-cell (Tc) responses in mice (Nicholas et al., 1990) and humans (Isaacs et al., 1987). It also induces rapid production of interferon in lungs of BALB/c mice, accompanied by a rise in pulmonary natural killer cell cytotoxic activity (Anderson et al., 1990). The cytotoxic T-lymphocyte response observed after intranasal RSV infection in mice correlates with viral clearance and recovery (Taylor et al., 1985). Infants in their first months of life rarely exhibit cell-mediated RSV immunity and are at greatest risk of severe RSV infection (Isaacs et al., 1987; Chiba et al., 1989). Passive transfer of memory T cells was effective in clearing persistent RSV infection in immunodeficient mice (Cannon et al., 1987). Infants and mice with a defective cell-mediated response are unable to eliminate RSV infection (Fishaut, 1980). However, T8 cytotoxic lymphocytes are involved not only in clearance of infection but also in enhancing the pathologic changes in lungs of RSV-infected mice (Cannon et al., 1988).

The interest of researchers in the immunopathology of RSV infection was triggered by the enhancement of RSV disease observed in children vaccinated with the formalin-inactivated vaccine used in the 1960s. Analysis of this phenomenon showed that children who received a formalin-inactivated vaccine had high titers of "nonfunctional" antibodies that lacked neutralizing and syncytial-inhibiting activities (Murphy et al., 1986). These "nonfunctional" antibodies were ineffective at preventing infection. It remains unknown whether the nonfunctional antibody directly enhanced pulmonary disease through a mechanism such as the Arthus phenomenon. An additional potential factor in the enhance effect was identified by Dr. H. Gimenez and colleagues (1989), who demonstrated that human RSV specific antibodies considerably enhance RSV infection in a macrophage cell line. The titer of enhancing antibodies in selected sera correlated with the titer of RSV-neutralizing antibodies and it is now difficult to conclude whether neutralization and enhancement are caused by different subpopulations of antibodies or whether the same antibodies may be responsible for both effects. A more detailed analysis of the immune response would allow a better definition of protective and potentially injurious responses.

All types of modern technologic approaches have been used for the development of RSV vaccines. A subunit vaccine made from surface proteins absorbed to the adjuvant Quil A induced neutralizing antibodies in guinea pigs (Trudel et al., 1989). A protective effect was also provided by immunization with F and G glycoproteins, but not with 22K and P proteins (Routledge et al., 1988). F and G glycoproteins purified by affinity chromatography alone or in combination also protected cotton rats against lung RSV infection (Heilman, 1990). Testing in healthy adult volunteers has shown that these proteins are safe and immunogenic.

The first unsuccessful attempts with attenuated strains as vaccine did not discourage researchers. One study tested four temperature-sensitive (ts) mutants with well-characterized changes in their genomes in adult volunteers (Watt et al., 1990). All mutants showed a reduction in virulence. Mutant Ts1B with double changes in the genome caused few disease symptoms or asymptomatic infection, and induced an immune response comparable to wild-type RSV. It was suggested that Ts1B might be developed further to produce a live-virus vaccine.

Attempts to prepare synthetic peptides mimicking epitopes of RSV proteins have been undertaken by two research groups. One prepared a set of overlapping synthetic peptides representing the extramembranous part of the F and G glycoproteins (Norrby et al., 1987). The capacity of the G peptides to react with hyperimmune sera and anti-G monoclonal antibodies varied considerably from one protein to another. Analysis of several peptides representing parts of the F1 protein allowed identification of the decopeptide that mimicked either the whole or a major part of the neutralizing epitope (Trudel et al., 1987).

F and chimeric (FG) glycoproteins have been produced in insect cells infected with baculovirus expression vector (Wathen et al., 1989; Brideau et al., 1989). F glycoprotein was expressed as intact protein and as a truncated (Ft) glycoprotein in which the COOH-terminal anchor region was deleted. Ft protein induced neutralizing antibodies in cotton rats and protected vaccinated animals from challenge with RSV. Chimeric FG glycoprotein contained the signal and extracellular regions of the F glycoprotein linked to the extracellular region of the G glycoprotein. Vaccination of the cotton rats provided protection against challenge with either serogroup A or B strains of RSV. Testing of FG as vaccine in volunteers has shown its safety and immunologic efficacy.

Two groups of researchers developed a panel of vaccinia–RSV recombinants by inserting the genes for RSV structural proteins into the thymidine kinase (TK) gene of vaccinia virus (Ball et al., 1986; Olmsted et al., 1986; Stott et al., 1987; Wertz et al., 1987). Immunization of rodents with different recombinants demonstrated that F and G proteins induce neutralizing antibodies and protection against challenge with RSV (Elango et al., 1986; King et al., 1987; Stott et al., 1986; Walsh et al., 1987). Mice and cotton rats immunized with vaccinia virus recombinants that expressed the G protein of RSV strain from subgroup A were protected against subsequent inoculation with strains of the same subgroup. Those immunized with vaccinia virus recombinants that expressed F protein were protected against challenge with strains of both subgroups (Stott et al., 1987). Mice immunized with vaccinia virus recombinants which expressed either M2 or N proteins of RSV virus, exhibited significant but not total resistance, which appeared to wane rapidly with time (Connors et al., 1991). The recombinants that expressed other RSV proteins did not induce detectable resistance to RSV challenge. These results indicate that the F and G glycoproteins are the most important protective antigens. The vaccinia–RSV recombinants were satisfactorily immunogenic and protective in four species of lower primates (Chanock et al., 1988) but induced a negligible level of RSV-neutralizing serum antibody and little effect on the restriction of virus replication in chimpanzees (Collins et al., 1990). Further attempts to use vaccinia virus as a vector for a safe live vaccine could be directed to the development of recombinants with a considerably higher level of expression of RSV F and G glycoproteins during infection, and selection of vaccinia virus strains that are most acceptable in inoculating human beings.

A study was performed to develop anti-idiotypic (anti-Id) antibodies against anti-RSV monoclonal antibodies and to use them to stimulate anti-RSV immune response. Anti-Id were produced by immunizing rabbits with different monoclonal antibodies for RSV G and F glycoproteins (Palomo et al., 1990). Some sera of the immunized animals inhibited the binding of RSV with immunizing monoclonal antibodies and neutralized viral infectivity. The rabbits were then inoculated with affinity-purified anti-Id antibodies. Antibodies reacting with G glycoprotein and able to neutralize RSV strains of both A and B subtypes, were obtained from one of the rabbits.

IV. PIV3 VACCINE DEVELOPMENT

Progress in elucidating the molecular biology, immunology, and epidemiology of PIV3 provides the basis for the development of new vaccines against diseases caused by this virus. The surface glycoproteins, hemagglutinin–neuraminidase (HN) and fusion (F) proteins, which mediate the attachment and penetration of the virus into the host cell, have been identified as the main protective antigens. Antibodies to these glycoproteins neutralize virus infectivity, and antibodies to the F glycoprotein can also prevent cell to cell viral spread. In hamsters immunized with individual PIV3 proteins, a significant degree of protection was achieved only through immunity to both the HN and F glycoproteins (Ray et al., 1988). High titers of antibody to PIV3 induced by natural infection seemed to prevent infection and reinfection in children. However, the protection was not absolute and one-third of infants were susceptible to reinfection (Chanock and McIntosh, 1990).

The protective role of local immunity in the respiratory tract has been shown in several studies. Individuals without antibodies in the respiratory tract are not protected against PIV3 infection. The presence of anti-PIV1 or anti-PIV2 IgA neutralizing antibodies in nose secretions appears to be a more reliable indication of resistance to these viruses than the presence of neutralizing antibodies in serum (see Chanock and McIntosh, 1990). Adults infected with PIV1 respond by producing local nasal secretory neutralizing IgA antibodies. In contrast, the synthesis of local neutralizing antibodies is poor in infants during primary infection, which may explain why they can be reinfected later. Little is known about the protective role of T-cell-mediated immunity. Infection of the lungs of immunodeficient mice with paramyxovirus simian virus (SV5), which is closely related to PIV2, was prolonged compared with the infection in immunocompetent mice (Young et al., 1990). Adoptive transfer of immune lymphocytes increased the spread of clearance of SV5 from immunodeficient mice. Depletion of CD8+ cells, but not B cells, from the population of immune lymphocytes reduced their ability to clear the virus infection. Children with deficiencies of T-cell function excrete PIV3 for months and many die from disseminated PIV infection (Fishaut et al., 1980; Frank et al., 1983). It has been proposed that immunization with viral proteins or their fragments, which are immunogenic for T cells, could increase resistance to PIV3. The identification of PIV3 proteins that could stimulate T-cell response without an immunopathologic effect is, therefore, an important research component of PIV3 vaccine development.

Three experimental subunit vaccines that contain a mixture of HN and F glycoproteins of PIV3 have been prepared (Morein et al., 1983, 1984). The glycoproteins were in different forms with sedimentation coefficient 4S, 18S, and 30S. Both multimeric complexes were highly immunogenic in mice. The 30S protein micelles in oil adjuvant induced antibody response and protection against PIV3 in lambs. A mixture of HN and F glycoproteins administered in complex with Quil A induced at least a 10 times higher antibody response in animals than micelles formed by aggregation of the same glycoproteins alone (Morein et al., 1984). No adverse effects of the vaccine have been observed. In other work, purification of the HN and F glycoproteins was performed by affinity chromatography with specific monoclonal antibodies coupled to a Sepharose 4B matrix (Ray and Compans, 1987). Immunization of hamsters with the purified HN or F alone induced an antibody response to the respective glycoproteins but did not provide a significant level of protection. However, a mixture of HN and F induced a higher level of virus-neutralizing activity in bronchial lavages and complete protection at the subsequent challenge (Ray et al., 1988).

To develop attenuated live vaccine, the wild strain of PIV3 was adapted for propagation in simian cell culture at 20°C (Belshe and Hissom, 1982; Crookshanks-Newman and Belshe, 1986). Several clones, selected after 7, 12, 18, and 45 passages at 20°C, have been evaluated for stability, attenuation for rodents, and protective activity. The degree of protection induced by vaccination of hamsters with cold-adapted mutants is inversely related to the number of passages of the original strain in the cold. Mutants selected after 12 and 18 passages of the wild strain were declared suitable for future testing in children and have been passaged and cloned in cell lines approved for the preparation of vaccines to be administered to volunteers. Studies in adults and children with cp12 and cp18 have been initiated.

Another approach to the development of PIV3-related vaccine is through the bovine PIV3, which is antigenically related to the human virus and is not pathogenic for human beings. The human and bovine PIV3 strains are 25% related antigenically by reciprocal neutralization assay test (Coelingh et al., 1988). The human and bovine PIV3 hemagglutinins share three epitopes in the antigenic site A and two epitopes in the antigenic sites D and F (Coelingh et al., 1986, 1987). However, nine epitopes of the human PIV3 hemagglutinin are not identified in the structure of the bovine PIV3 HN. The homology of the amino acid sequence of NP, P, C, and N proteins of both viruses varies from 62 to 86% and homology of F and HN glycoproteins is 80% and 77%, respectively (Sakai et al., 1987; Suzu et al., 1987). Immunization of rodents with bovine PIV3 induces resistance to challenge with human PIV3. Intratracheal inoculation of bovine PIV3 to squirrel monkeys causes production of antibodies to both viruses and partial protection of the respiratory tract against further challenge with the human PIV3 (Murphy, 1988). The restricted replication of bovine PIV3 in rhesus monkeys and chimpanzees was considered as evidence of attenuation. However, despite this restricted replication, bovine PIV3 induces a high titer of antihuman PIV3 antibodies in rhesus monkeys and chimpanzees (Coelingh et al., 1988).

Baculoviruses have been used as vector for the HN glycoprotein of PIV3. The HN gene of PIV3 was inserted in *Autographa californica* nuclear polyhedrosis virus under the control of the polyhedrin promoter (Coelingh et al., 1988). Hemagglutinin produced in insect cells infected by the recombinant was glycosylated and had biological activities characteristic for viral cells in the HN glycoprotein. It was shown with the panel of monoclonal antibodies that all epitopes of the viral HN involved in the expression of neuraminidase and hemagglutination activities were conformationally unaltered in the recombinant protein. Immunization of cotton rats with the recombinant HN induced protection against further challenge with PIV3. The next step is to purify the HN glycoprotein and assess its suitability as an immunogen (Murphy, 1988).

An attempt was undertaken to use vaccinia virus as a vector for expression of PIV3 glycoproteins (Spriggs et al., 1987). F or HN genes were inserted into the thymidine kinase gene of vaccinia virus under control of the P7,5 early–late vaccinia virus promoter. The HN and F proteins expressed in cells infected with recombinants appeared to have the same biochemical and immunologic characteristics as the virus proteins. Inoculation of each of the recombinants to cotton rats induced neutralizing antibodies and protection against challenge with PIV3. However, the restriction of virus reproduction in the respiratory tract of the immunized animals indicated that vaccinia-PIV3 HN induced a better protective effect than the vaccinia-PIV3 F recombinant.

Human adenovirus type 5 (Ad5) has also been used as vector to express F glycoprotein of human PIV3. Following two different procedures (Prevec, L., and Graham, F. L., personal communication), one approach has been to insert the DNA corresponding to the F protein structural gene into a cassette between the SV40 promoter and the SV40 polyA addition sequences and then to insert the whole cassette into the E3 region of Ad5 to allow transcription of the gene from the E3 promoter or major late promoter. The second approach was to insert the F gene directly into adenovirus sequences to replace a fragment of the E3 region. In HeLa cells the recombinants expressed proteins that corresponded in size to those of the F0 and F1 glycoproteins of PIV3. Inoculation of the recombinants in BALB/c mice induced anti-PIV3 antibodies that have the capacity to interact with viral F0 and F1 glycoproteins and to neutralize infectivity of PIV3 as measured by plaque reduction assay. The next step is to study the protective effect of the recombinants using cotton rats as model animals.

V. FUTURE PROSPECTS

Remarkable developments in molecular biology and immunology during the past decade have generated much new information about RSV and PIV3. The genomes of both viruses have been sequenced, their gene products and protective antigens have been identified, and the antigenic structure of some fragments of proteins has been determined in detail. Some of the objectives of the strategic plan proposed at the beginning of the WHO/UNDP Program for Vaccine Development, have been reached. The Steering Committee on Acute Respiratory Viruses, therefore, revised the Strategic Plan for RSV and PIV3 vaccines in 1990. The goals of the revised plan for the next several years are to develop live attenuated and subunit vaccines; to explore the utility of vectors of viral antigens to protect against diseases caused by RSV and PIV3; to identify the protective immune response. As mentioned above, in recent years major progress has been achieved in the development of RSV candidate vaccines, and some RSV vaccines have been submitted for testing in clinical trials. In view of this, the PVD has taken essential steps to accelerate the final stages of RSV vaccine development. For this purpose a project has been established to improve further and define better the experimental models for assessment of safety and protective activity of candidate vaccines; study the mechanism of the enhancing effect, and establish appropriate guidelines to complete the final stages of RSV vaccine development. As part of this project, a task force has been established composed of immunopathologists and members of regulatory agencies.

A proposal from the WHO Expanded Programme on Immunization (EPI) to include measles vaccine in the activity of the Steering Committee on Acute Respiratory Viruses was supported by SAGE in 1990. The recommendation was based on the fact that current measles vaccines cannot be used for immunization of infants in their first months of life, when about 20% of measles cases occur in many developing countries. The current vaccines would, therefore, not permit a move towards global control of measles. Financial support has been granted by PVD for research projects in the following areas of new measles vaccines for early infancy: genetic basis of attenuation; appropriate animal models for assessment of vaccines; circumvention of the negative effects of passively transferred antibodies; subunit and live vector-based vaccines; influence of host cell on subsequent vaccine infectivity.

REFERENCES

Anderson, J. J., Norden, J., Saunders, D., Toms, G. L., and Scott, R. (1990). *J. Gen. Virol. 71*:1561–1570.

Ball, L. A., Young, K., Anderson, K., Collins, P., and Wertz, G. W. (1986). *Proc. Natl. Acad. Sci. 83*:246.

Belshe, R. B., and Hissom, F. K. (1982). *J. Med. Virol. 10*:235–242.

Belshe, R. B., Bernstein, J. M., and Dansby, K. N. (1984). In *Textbook of Human Virology*. PSG Publishing, Littleton, MA, pp. 361–383.

Brideau, R. J., Walters, R. R., Stier, M. A., and Wathen, M. W. (1989). *J. Gen. Virol. 70*:2637–2644.

Cannon, M. J., Stott, E. J., Taylor, G., and Askonas, B. A. (1987). *Immunology 62*:133–138.

Cannon, M. J., Openshaw, P. J. M., and Askonas, B. A. (1988). *J. Exp. Med. 168*:1163–1168.

Chanock, R. M., Murphy, B. R., Collins, P. L., Coelingh, K. V. W., Olmsted, R. A., Snyder, M. H., Spriggs, M. K., Prince, G. A., Moss, B., Flores, J., Gorziglia, M., and Kapikian, A. Z. (1988). *Vaccine 6*:129–133.

Chanock, R. M., and McIntosh, K. (1990). In *Virology*, 2nd ed., B. N. Fields, D. Knipe, et al. (Eds.). Raven Press, New York, pp. 963–988.

Chiba, Y., Higashidate, Y., Suga, K., Honjo, K., Tsutsumi, H., and Ogra, P. L. (1989). *J. Med. Virol. 28*:133–139.

Coelingh, K. J., Winter, C. C., Murphy, B. R., Rice, J. M., Kimball, P. C., Olmsted, R. A., and Collins, P. L. (1986). *J. Virol. 60*:90–96.

Coelingh, K. V. W., Winter, C. C., and Murphy, B. R. (1897). In *Vaccines 87*: *Modern Approaches to New Vaccines Including Prevention of AIDS*. R. Chanock and R. Lerner (Eds.). Cold Spring Harbor Laboratory, Cold Spring Harbor, NY, pp. 296–301.

Coelingh, K., Collins, P. L., Murphy, B., Battey, J., and Leback-Verheyden, A. (1988a). In *Vaccine 88*, H. Ginsberg, F. Brown, et al. (Eds.). Cold Spring Harbor Laboratory, Cold Spring Harbor, NY, pp. 171–177.

Coelingh, K. V. W., Winter, C., Tierney, E., London, W. L., and Murphy, B. (1988b). *J. Infect. Dis. 157*:655–662.

Collins, C., Connors, P., Prince, G. M., Hung, G., Chanock, R., and Murphy, B. (1990). In *Abstracts of VIIIth International Congress of Virology*, Berlin, W38-5, 72.

Connors, M., Collins, P. L., Firestone, C. Y., and Murphy, B. R. (1991). *J. Virol. 65*:1634–1637.

Crookshanks-Newman, F. K., and Belshe, R. B. (1986). *J. Med. Virol. 18*:131–137.

Elango, N., Prince, G. A., Murphy, B. R., Venkatesan, S., Chanock, R. M., and Moss, B. A. (1986). *Proc. Natl. Acad. Sci. USA 83*:1906–1910.

Fishaut, M., Tubergen, D., and McIntosh, K. (1980). *J. Pediatr. 96*:179–186.

Frank, J. A., Warren, R. W., Tucker, J. A., Zeller, J., and Wilfert, C. M. (1983). *Am. J. Dis. Child. 137*:1172.

Gimenez, H. B., Keir, H. M., and Cash, P. (1989). *J. Gen. Virol. 70*:89–96.

Heilman, C. (1990). *J. Infect. Dis. 161*:402–406.

Hemming, V. G., Rodriguez, W., Kim, H. W., Brandt, C. D., Parrott, R. H., Burch, B., Prince, G. A., Baron, P. A., Rink, R. J., and Risaman, G. (1987). *Antimicrob. Agents Chemother. 31*:1882–1886.

Isaacs, D., McMichael, A. J., and Bangham, C. R. M. (1987). Cell-mediated cytotoxic response to respiratory syncytial virus in infants with bronchiolitis. *Lancet* 2:769–771.

Kimman, T. G., and Westernbrink, F. (1990). *Arch. Virol. 112*:1–25.

King, A. M. Q., Stott, E. J., Langer, S. J., Young, K. K-Y., Ball, L. A., and Wertz, G. W. (1987). *J. Virol. 61*:2885–2890.

Mills, J., van Kirk, J. E., Wright, P. F., and Chanock, R. M. (1971). *J. Immunol. 107*:123–130.

Morein, B., Sharp, M., Sundquist, B., and Simons, K. (1983). *J. Gen. Virol. 64*:1557–1569.

Morein, B., Sundquist, B., Hoglund, S., Dalsgaard, K., and Osterhaus, A. (1984). *Nature 308*:457–460.

Murphy, B. R. (1988). *Bull. WHO 66*:391–397.

Murphy, B. R., Prince, G. A., Walsh, E. E., Kim, H. W., Parrott, R. H., Hemming, V. G., Rodriguez, W. J., and Chanock, R. M. (1986). *J. Clin. Microbiol. 24*:197–202.

Nicholas, J., Rubino, K., Levely, M., Adams, E., and Collins, P. (1990). *J. Virol. 64*:4232–4241.

Norrby, E., Mufson, M., Alexander, H., Houghten, R., and Lerner, R. (1987). *Proc. Natl. Acad. Sci. USA 84*:6572–6576.

Olmsted, R. A., Elango, N., Prince, G. A., Murphy, B. R., Johnson, P. R., Moss, B., Chanock, R. M., and Collins, P. L. (1986). *Proc. Natl. Acad. Sci. USA 83*:7462–7466.

Palomo, C., Albar, J., Garcia-Barreno, B., and Melero, J. (1990). *J. Virol. 64*:4199–4206.

Prince, G. A., Horswood, R. L., and Chanock, R. M. (1985). *J. Virol. 55*:517–520.

Prince, G., Hemming, V., Horswood, R., Baron, P., Murphy, B., and Chanock, R. (1990). *J. Virol. 64*:3091–3982.

Ray, B., and Compans, R. (1987). *J. Gen. Virol. 68*:409–418.

Ray, R., Glaze, B. J., and Compans, R. W. (1988). Role of individual glycoproteins of human parainfluenza virus type 3 in the induction of a protective immune response. *J. Virol. 62*:783–878.

Routledge, E. G., Willcocks, M. M., Samson, A. C. R., Morgan, L., Scott, R., Anderson, J. J., and Toms, G. L. (1988). *J. Gen. Virol. 69*:293–303.

Sakai, Y., Suzu, S., Shioda, T., and Shibuta, H. (1987). *Nucleic Acids Res. 15*:2927–2944.

Selwyn, B. J. (1990). *Re. Infect. Dis. 12*(Suppl. 8):5870–5888.

Spriggs, M., Murphy, B., Prince, G., Olmsted, R., and Collins, P. (1987). *J. Virol. 61*:3416–3423.

Stott, E. J., Ball, L. A., Young, K. K.-Y., Furze, J., and Wertz, G. W. (1986). *J. Virol. 60*:607–613.

Stott, E. J., Taylor, G., Ball, L. A., Anderson, K., Young, K. K.-Y., King, A. M. Q., and Wertz, G. W. (1987). *J. Virol. 61*:3855–3861.

Suzu, S., Sakai, Y., Shioda, T., and Shibuta, H. (1987). *Nucleic Acids Res. 15*:2945–2958.

Taylor, G., Stott, E. J., Bew, M., Ferni, B. F., Cote, P. J., Collins, A. P., Hughes, M., and Jebbett, J. (1984). *Immunology 52*:137–142.

Taylor, G., Stott, E. J., and Hayle, A. J. (1985). *J. Gen. Virol. 66*:2533–2538.

Trudel, M., Nadon, F., Seguin, C., Dionne, G., and Lacroix, M. (1987). *J. Gen. Virol. 68*:2273–2280.

Trudel, M., Nadon, F., Seguin, C., Simard, C., and Lussier, G. (1989). *Vaccine 7*:12–15.

Walsh, E. E., Hall, C. B., Briselli, M., Brandriss, M. W., and Schlesinger, J. J. (1987). *J. Infect. Dis. 155*:1198–1204.

Ward, K. A., Lambden, P. R., Ogilvie, M. M., and Watt, P. J. (1983). *J. Gen. Virol. 64*:1867–1876.

Wathen, M. W., Brideau, R. J., and Thomsen, D. R. (1989). *J. Infect. Dis. 159*:255–264.

Watt, P. J., Robinson, B. S., Pringle, C. R., and Tyrrell, D. A. J. (1990). *Vaccine 8*:231–235.

Wertz, G., Stott, E., Young, K., King, A., Bangham, C., and Ball, L. (1987). In *Vaccine 87*, R. Chanock, R. Lerner, and H. Ginsberg (Eds.). Cold Spring Harbor Laboratory, Cold Spring Harbor, NY, pp. 350–355.

Young, D. F., Randall, R. E., Hoyle, J. A., and Souberbielle, B. E. (1990). *J. Virol.* *64*:5403–5411.

16

ROTAVIRUS VACCINOLOGY

Current Approaches in Rotavirus Vaccine Development

Mark J. Redmond *Veterinary Infectious Disease Organization, Saskatoon, Saskatchewan, Canada*

Marta I. Sabara* *Praxis Biologics Inc., Rochester, New York*

Lorne A. Babiuk *Veterinary Infectious Disease Organization, Saskatoon, Saskatchewan, Canada*

I. INTRODUCTION

Acute diarrheal diseases continue to constitute a human and animal health problem throughout much of the world today. Epidemiologic studies have demonstrated that rotaviruses are the single most important group of pathogens causing diarrhea in both developed and developing countries. The disease is particularly prevalent in children under 2 years of age. Many factors, most significantly the nutritional and immunologic status of the individual, can influence the outcome of an infection and also the "take" of a vaccine. In developed countries, rotaviruses are frequently responsible for 40–60% of the cases of diarrhea requiring hospitalization (Ho et al., 1988; Institute of Medicine, 1985). In developing countries rotavirus infections are equally common, but the proportion of all diarrheal episodes caused by rotavirus is smaller, owing to the higher incidence of bacterial and parasitic diarrheas. Under these circumstances rotavirus diarrhea is more serious, accounting for 20–40% of cases of severe diarrhea (Black et al., 1981; Institute of Medicine, 1986; Sack et al., 1991). These findings emphasize the need for a vaccine to prevent rotaviral

**Present affiliation*: SmithKline Beecham Animal Health, Lincoln, Nebraska.

gastroenteritis during the first 2 years of life when the consequences of such illness can be fatal. It is estimated that an effective rotavirus could reduce all diarrheal deaths by 30%, thereby preventing approximately 1 million deaths in children annually (de Zoysa and Feachen, 1986).

II. ROTAVIRUS ANTIGENIC COMPOSITION

The rotavirus genome segments code for 11 proteins, several of which are posttranslationally modified through cleavage, glycosylation, or phosphorylation, to produce a series of proteins ranging in molecular weight from 21,700 to 125,005 daltons. Three of these proteins, VP4, VP6, and VP7, form the wheel-like structure characteristic of rotaviruses (Figs. 1 and 2). The inner capsid is composed primarily of VP6 (SA-11 molecular weight 44,816) and makes up 51% of the total viral protein. The outer capsid is composed of VP7 (molecular weight 37,247), which is normally glycosylated at one or two sites to produce a mature glycoprotein (molecular weight ~41,000). The carbohydrate composition and the extent of glycosylation have been reported to be strain dependent (Estes, 1990). The VP4 protein (molecular weight 86,719) functions as the viral hemagglutinin and forms the spikelike projections protruding from the surface of the virus. Prasad et al. (1988) have studied the structure of rotavirus by cryoelectron microscopy and have shown the presence of 60 spikes, composed of VP4 dimers, on each particle. In a subsequent study, the same group reported that antibodies capable of neutralizing the virus bind to the tip of the spike (Prasad et al., 1990).

Infection by rotavirus is enhanced by proteolytic cleavage of VP4, which produced two proteins, VP5* and VP8*, which remain attached to the viral particle. Recent evidence suggests that VP4 plays a major role in viral attachment and evidence from our group and others (Fiore et al., 1991) attributes this activity to the VP8* region. The studies of Ruggeri and Greenberg (1991) have indicated that both hemagglutinating and attachment domains reside at the carboxyl terminus of VP8*. However, a role for other viral proteins, such as VP7 (Fukuhara et al., 1988; Sabara et al., 1985) or NS 35 (Bass et al., 1990), in the attachment phase of infection cannot be ruled out.

Analyses of immune sera indicate that VP6 is the major antigenic protein present in rotavirus. Although most prevalent in response, antibodies to VP6 are devoid of virus neutralization activity. In contrast, VP4 and VP7 independently induce neutralizing antibodies that protect against disease. Serologic studies indicate that the relative prevalence of antibodies toward either VP4 or VP7 varies with the strain of virus, the age

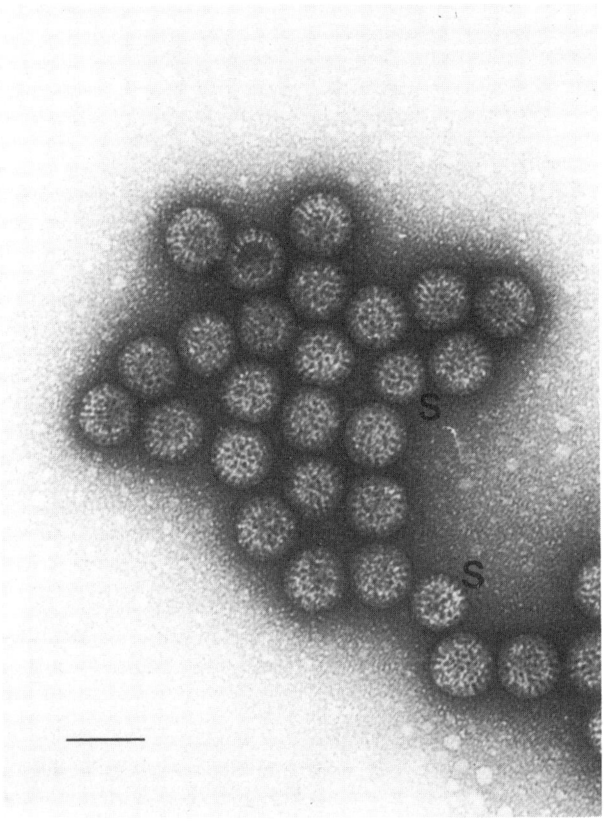

FIGURE 1 Electron micrograph of rotavirus particles negatively stained with uranyl acetate. Intact particles are composed of an inner capsid of VP6 onto which the outer shell of VP7 is layered. The spherical single-shelled particle (s) is a viral particle from which VP7 was lost. Bar represents 100 nm.

at which the individual is exposed to the virus, as well as the route of exposure (Greenberg et al., 1981; Shaw et al., 1987; Ward et al., 1988).

Immunologic reactivity with monoclonal antibodies specific to VP6 has been used to differentiate between two subgroups of rotavirus and forms part of the basis for virus characterization. Human strains of rotavirus belong to both subgroup I and II whereas animal rotaviruses with few exceptions belong to subgroup I. In addition to subgroups, rotaviruses are classified by serotypes based on the VP4 and VP7 protein (Kapikian and Chanock, 1990). At least 11 serotypes

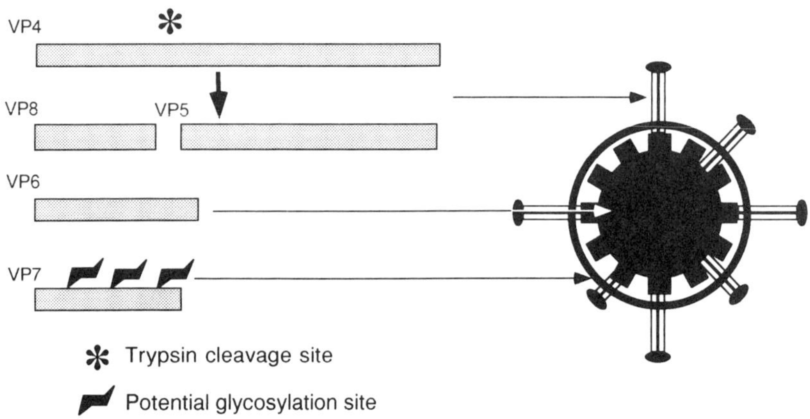

FIGURE 2 Schematic diagram of rotaviral proteins and viral particle composition. The inner capsid is formed from VP6. Surrounding the capsid is a layer of VP7. Sixty spikes of VP4 protrude from the particle's surface.

based on VP7 and three based on VP4 have been described (Larralde et al., 1991). Studies also suggest that the combination of VP7 and VP4 proteins can alter the configuration of these proteins such that a specific serotype may be altered. Sequence analysis shows nine regions of VP7 in which the sequence is highly divergent and probably responsible for serotype differences (Fig. 3). The sequence of VP4 also shows considerable strain divergence, an exception being the trypsin cleavage site, which is conserved in every VP4 sequenced to date. The diversity of the VP4 and VP7 proteins presents a major problem in developing vaccines that would induce protection against multiple serotypes of virus. Thus one will either need to find crucial conserved regions, such as the VP4 trypsin cleavage site, or produce vaccines that contain multiple proteins or epitopes that recognize all the major serotypes.

Several factors must be considered when planning a rotavirus vaccination strategy: the need to induce a local, mucosal immune response (Welliver and Ogra, 1978); the presence of maternal antibody either-in colostrum or by transplacental transfer, as well as other nonspecific inhibitors in breast milk and serum that could interfere with the efficacy of the vaccine (Edelman et al., 1989); the presence of several rotavirus serotypes circulating in the population (Green et al., 1990; Kapikian et al., 1986; Lanata et al., 1989; Snodgrass et al., 1984); and the compatibility between various vaccination regimens implemented in young children.

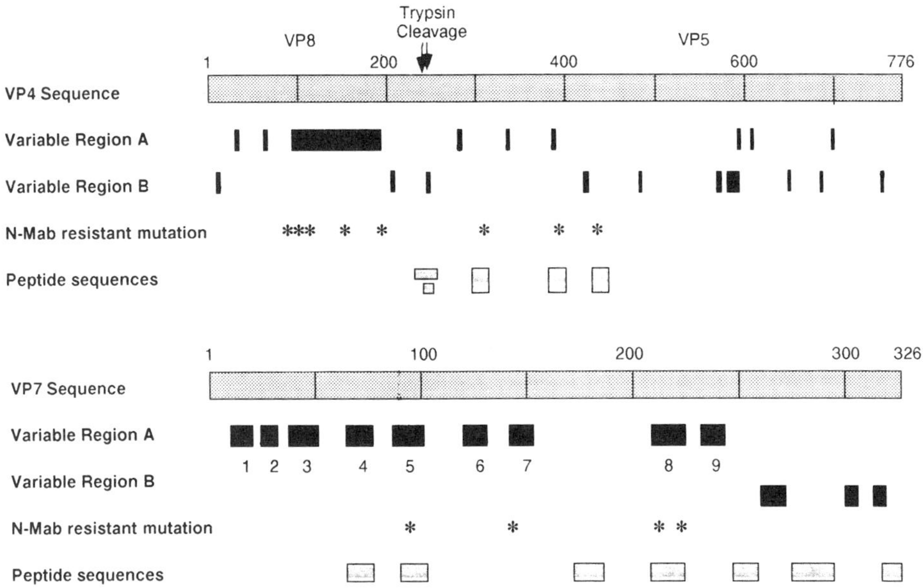

FIGURE 3 Schematic diagram of rotavirus proteins VP4 and VP7 illustrates important sequence variation and antigenic characteristics. Variable region A was compiled from references (Dyall-Smith et al., 1986; Green et al., 1989; Mackow et al., 1988a, Taniguchi et al., 1988a,b). Variable region B was produced by analysis of all rotavirus VP4 and VP7 sequences available on GenBank release 63. Neutralizing monoclonal antibody resistant mutations were compiled from work by Taniguchi et al. (1988a,b). Peptide sequences were from references (Gun et al., 1985; Ijaz et al., 1991; Taniguchi et al., 1988b).

To date, the method for vaccinating humans has been aimed at the target population, children less than 2 years of age, and is termed active immunization (Green et al., 1990). In other animals, where the young receive immunoglobulin from colostrum and milk instead of by transplacental transfer, dams are vaccinated in an attempt to raise protective antibody levels that can then passively immunize suckling neonates (Saif et al., 1983; Wyatt et al., 1983). This is possible since protection of animals is only required for the first month or 2 of life.

Several approaches have either been tested or have been proposed for rotavirus vaccine development. The first approach has been used almost exclusively for a human rotavirus vaccine while the last two approaches have applications to both human and animal vaccines.

A. Live Attenuated Virus Vaccines

A major research effort has been made in the development of live attenuated vaccines, since it was believed that they would have the best chance of stimulating local, mucosal immunity after oral administration. These vaccines would ideally retain the native viral antigenic characteristics, attach to and penetrate host cells, and persist long enough to elicit a strong immune response, while they are restricted in replication so that clinical disease is not produced. Three classes of live attenuated vaccine are currently under consideration: live attenuated or naturally avirulent strains; live attenuated, heterologous strains from nonhuman hosts; and attenuated, genetically reassorted (human × animal) strains.

One of the first live rotavirus vaccines ever produced was a calf rotavirus vaccine given orally to calves at birth (Mebus et al., 1973). This formed the foundation for the development of live rotavirus vaccine for other species including humans. One of the first live attenuated human vaccine candidates tested was a WA human rotavirus strain passaged in piglets and then cultured in primary African green monkey kidney cells. This virus proved to be attenuated and safe in initial studies using piglets. However, in a trial in 1983 using 12 adults, 10 days after challenge volunteers developed low-level elevations of serum transaminase levels. Testing of the vaccine was consequently discontinued (WHO, 1984).

A naturally attenuated rotavirus strain isolated from a nursery, with an altered VP4 protein, was developed as a candidate rotavirus vaccine in the United States (Flores et al., 1986). This strain, designated M37 was shown to be an intertypic virus that cross-reacted in vitro with human serotypes 1, 2, 3, and 4. The rationale for developing vaccines based on nursery rotavirus strains was that they infect neonates in maternity wards without causing illness (Bishop et al., 1983). These infants were subsequently protected, at least in part, against diarrhea associated with a virulent human rotavirus. To date this vaccine candidate has not demonstrated heterotypic protection and is presently being formulated with other live-attenuated candidates (Flores et al., 1990).

Live attenuated, heterologous strains of rotavirus from nonhuman hosts are also being evaluated for their potential as vaccines. This strategy involves the use of animal rotavirus strains such as the bovine strains, NCDV and WC3, or the rhesus strain, RRV, which can infect humans and evoke cross-protective immunity without inducing illness (Kapikian et al., 1986). The genesis of this approach was the observation that calves immunized in utero with NCDV were resistant to challenge with human rotavirus. To explain this heterotypic protection, sera from calves were tested for their ability to neutralize human rotavirus of serotypes 1, 2, and

3 (Wyatt et al., 1983). The results clearly demonstrated heterologous neutralization.

After several trials in developed countries, the RIT 4237 vaccine (isolate of bovine NCDV origin) was found to be safe and effective if given at a high dose (10^8 plaque-forming units) (Vesikari, 1985). However, its efficacy was easily blocked by maternally acquired serum antibodies. A reduced dosage or concurrent immunizations with poliovirus vaccines also appeared to reduce its efficacy. In developing countries the vaccine was much less effective, induced low rates of seroconversion (Hanlon et al., 1987), and did not reduce the severity of clinical infection or disease. Furthermore, it was also more effective against serotype 1 and possibly serotype 4 viruses than other serotypes (Lanata et al., 1989; Mutz et al., 1989). As a consequence the enthusiasm that prevailed during the early trials with this vaccine is waning.

Initial trials using the WC3 vaccine demonstrated good efficacy in developed countries, providing protection against disease by human serotype 1 virus (Clark et al., 1988). However, further testing in developing countries indicated a pattern of efficacy similar to that described for RIT 4237. A similar result was also obtained following the exhaustive testing of the RRV-derived MMU 18006 vaccine (Bennels et al., 1987; Ho et al., 1989). A major conclusion drawn from these studies was that the specificity of protection was towards the parental strain serotype and that heterologous protection would require a combination of serotypes in the vaccine formulation (Chanock et al., 1988; Gothefors et al., 1989).

Reassortants, which are attenuated, genetically engineered (human × animal) strains may be the solution to the problem of achieving heterotypic protection. Reassortants have been produced in which the VP7 antigens of serotype 1, 2, and 4 of human rotavirus were incorporated into the rhesus or bovine parent virus (Midthun et al., 1989). Several RRV and WC3 reassortants are currently in phase I clinical trial testing for safety and immunogenicity (Flores et al., 1989; Holsey et al., 1988). The major issues governing the success of these candidates are the "take" of individual strains and the immunogenicity of the protective antigens in single-gene reassortants in the context of the parental gene constellation (Tajima et al., 1990).

The interest in reassortants is not limited to the production of heterotypic immunity. Many human rotavirus isolates do not replicate sufficiently well in vitro to make vaccine production economical. Reassortants that combine strains such as WC3, which replicates well in culture, and the VP4 and VP7 from human strains may make it possible to produce economical vaccines that protect individuals against multiple serotypes of rotavirus.

B. Live Vectored Vaccines

The limited success in the development of live attenuated vaccines has led to the vigorous pursuit of alternative strategies for the production of vaccine candidates that are efficacious in both developed and developing countries. One such candidate is a live, bacterial vectored vaccine. Such vaccines are composed of bacterial vectors containing cloned rotavirus genes that express protective rotavirus antigens. Oral vaccines for human and animal rotavirus diarrhea are currently under development using attenuated enteric bacteria such as *Salmonella* or *E. coli* (WHO, 1986). There are several advantages to using bacterial carriers to present viral antigens to the gut lymphoid tissue, including the ability to attenuate bacteria in such a way that they colonize but do not cause disease, the possibility of reduced interference by other rotaviruses and enteroviruses (such as poliovirus vaccine), reduced chance of neutralization by antirotavirus antibodies in the gut, and the reduced chance of reversion or reassortment. However, the system is limited in its applicability to viral antigens. Prokaryotic expression systems cannot glycosylate or posttranslationally modify proteins and consequently protein folding is frequently incorrect. Since many functional epitopes, especially on VP7, are conformational, expression in prokaryotic systems may be of limited value. However, a linear epitope, the trypsin cleavage site of VP4, that can protect animals should be tried in live vectored bacterial vaccines.

An alternative vectoring system is a live virus vector. One candidate under consideration is adenovirus. Adenovirus types 4 and 7 have been safely used as vaccines in U.S. military personnel over the last 20 years. Since adenovirus, like many other viruses, has regions within the genome that are nonessential for replication (E3), it is possible to replace these sequences with foreign DNA. At present a large number of different genes have been inserted gene sequence is physically restricted, the vector is suitable for insertion of genes of the size of rotavirus VP4 or VP7. The system is also suited to enteric vaccination with the peptide sequences identified below (see section on synthetic peptide vaccines). With more knowledge regarding the enteric adenoviruses serotypes 40 and 41, it may be possible to develop a chimeric virus to protect infants against the enteric adenoviruses as well as rotaviruses. Whether such a vaccine will be licensed by the authorities remains to be seen.

C. Subunit Vaccines

Subunit vaccine candidates are based on individual rotavirus antigens, either produced in culture by cells containing cloned rotavirus DNA or prepared synthetically. In vaccine formulation these antigens may either be used individually or in combination to produce immunity to a broad spectrum of rotaviruses.

Both VP4 and VP7 have been cloned into prokaryotic and eukaryotic expression vectors. The use of prokaryotic expressed protein as vaccines has met with limited success: an *E. coli*-expressed protein containing 45% of VP4 (including the trypsin cleavage site) produced antibodies with 5% of the neutralizing capacity of the whole virus (Arias et al., 1987). Immunization with *E. coli*-expressed VP7, amino acids 50–265, also failed to produce neutralizing antibodies, although the recombinant protein was immunoreactive with neutralizing monoclonal antibodies (Francavilla et al., 1987). Arias et al. (1986) succeeded in producing a neutralizing immune response by cloning a larger genomic segment of VP7 encoding amino acids 63-300. However the titers produced in response to this protein were significantly lower than those induced by virus. It is believed that the folding and presentation of the recombinant protein are major factors in producing strong humoral immunity. This theory is supported by the mapping of major neutralization epitopes to discontinuous sequences in VP7 (Dyall-Smith et al., 1986). It is also significant to note that these domains are made up in part of variable regions 5 and 8, within which several point mutations have been found (Fig. 3).

Expression of rotavirus proteins has also been accomplished in other systems, such as vaccinia and baculovirus. A secreted form of VP7 produced by a vaccinia virus expression system only induced low levels of neutralizing antibodies (Andrew et al., 1987). However, higher neutralization titers were obtained when the VP7 gene was fused to the membrane spanning region from influenza virus hemagglutinin (Andrew et al., 1990), which reinforced the suggestion that proper membrane transport and posttranslational modification and presentation to the immune system are required for VP7 to be highly immunogenic. Other rotavirus genes have also been cloned into the vaccinia virus expression system and have proved to be valuable tools in investigations of cell-mediated responses to individual rotavirus proteins (Andrew et al., 1987; Poncet et al., 1990). There is mounting evidence that cell-mediated immunity is an important aspect of protection from rotavirus disease (Bridger and Oldham, 1987; Offit and Dudzik, 1988) and it has been reported that this type of protective immunity may be passively transferred from dam to offspring even when the dam has low or no serum antibody to rotavirus (Archambault et al., 1988). Cell-mediated immunity should certainly be considered in the formulation of vaccines.

Recently baculoviruses have been used to express several rotavirus proteins, most notably the inner capsid protein VP6 and the two outer shell proteins VP4 and VP7 (Estes et al., 1987; Mackow et al., 1989). A major advantage of this invertebrate virus expression vector over bacterial, yeast, and mammalian expression systems is the abundant expression of recombinant proteins that are often immunologically and functionally similar to their authentic counterparts. The baculovirus vector incorporates many of the protein modifications, processing, and transport systems that occur in higher eukaryotic cells and that may be essential for the complete function of a recombinant protein (Lucknow and Summers, 1988). Unfortunately protein glycosylation by baculovirus is not always identical to mammalian processed proteins; differences in carbohydrate composition may affect the folding and antigenic presentation of the recombinant molecules and so efficacy must be established based on the individual protein. An additional advantage is that baculoviruses are not pathogenic to vertebrates and do not use transformed cells or transforming elements, as do the mammalian expression systems. The baculovirus expression system is therefore well suited to producing antigens for human vaccines.

The cloning of VP6 into baculovirus was first reported by Estes et al. (1987). As expected, the recombinant protein in the form of cell lysates did not induce virus-neutralizing antisera. We likewise immunized animals with crude baculovirus-expressed VP7 and failed to obtain virus-neutralizing antisera. However, the offspring of immunized dams were partially protected from challenge with homologous virus. It may be possible to improve this protection by using purified VP7 antigen. In contrast, baculovirus-produced bovine C486 VP4 induced high levels of neutralizing antibody and exhibited a high degree of both homologous and heterologous protection (Redmond et al., 1992). The induction of heterologous protection by vaccination with recombinant VP4 is apparently dependent on the strain of rotavirus from which the gene 4 was isolated, since recombinant rhesus VP4 induces only homotypic immunity (Mackow et al., 1988a, 1989). However, recombinant rhesus VP8*, corresponding to the amino terminal side of the VP4 trypsin cleavage site, does induce heterologous neutralization (Fiore et al., 1991). Considering these findings, one may postulate that some strains of rotavirus conceal important epitopes (e.g., receptor binding sites) until after proteolytic cleavage and thereby evade the host's immune system. Based on this observation one should attempt to formulate vaccines with strains that do not conceal important epitopes or, as an alternative, engineer the virus protein so as to expose these epitopes.

Another approach to the development of a subunit rotavirus vaccine involves the identification and synthesis of protective epitopes. Several important epitopes have been identified using monoclonal antibodies and by analysis of protein sequences for surface probability or conservation/divergence amongst serotypes (Arias et al., 1989; Frenchick et al., 1988; Streckert et al., 1988). Neutralizing monoclonal antibodies to VP4 have been used to produce neutralization-resistant mutants; the point mutations produced were mapped to approximately eight sites on the mature protein. Taniguchi et al. (1988b) selected three of these sites (VP4, amino acids 296–313, 380–400, 428–447) as sequences for potential synthetic peptide vaccines. Only the VP4 peptide sequence at amino acids 296–313 reacted with neutralizing antisera, suggesting that only this sequence was contiguous on VP4 and that the other point mutations were contained in a discontiguous/structural epitope. We have studied peptides derived from the vicinity of the trypsin cleavage site (VP4, amino acids 232–255) and have reported that neutralizing antiserum was produced when this peptide was linked to a carrier protein and used to vaccinate mice. Furthermore, when challenged with either homologous or heterologous strains of rotavirus, the offspring of immunized dams were protected from clinical disease (Ijaz et al., 1991). Peptides from VP7 were selected by Gunn et al. (1985) using an algorithm for mapping protein hydrophobicity. Six sequences were synthesized (VP7, amino acids 66–76, 90–103, 174–183, 208–225, 247–259, 275–295) and chemically conjugated to a carrier protein. The conjugates, when injected into rabbits, failed to produce neutralizing antibody, although the antisera did react with denatured VP7. Ijaz et al. (1991) also synthesized VP7, amino acids 275–295 but, by linking the peptide to carrier proteins through alternative methods, showed that this converted sequence can elicit protective immunity against three of four serotypes of rotavirus (1, 2, and 6). Based on these studies it is evident that at least some of the crucial and potentially protective epitopes have been identified and now their effectiveness under field conditions needs to be determined. A mixture of these peptides may be required to induce a broad humoral and cellular immune response.

Although synthetic peptides are attractive candidates for use in vaccines, most do not produce acceptable antibody titers or cellular immunity when used in their unconjugated, monomeric form. Research has therefore centered on the development of methods for polymerizing or conjugating peptides to large carrier proteins or polymers suitable for human or veterinary applications. One such approach involves the construction of genetically engineered, self-assembling particles that contain epitopes engineered from foreign organisms (Burke et al., 1988; Haynes et al., 1986; Valenzuela et al., 1985). The major problem with this approach is the size of the epitope that can be expressed in the self-assembling particle without disrupting the ability of the particle to assemble. To overcome this limitation, a modification of this approach has involved the efficient attachment of rotavirus peptides to an assembled rotavirus spherical particle comprised of VP6. Baculovirus–produced VP6 retains its ability to assemble into trimers; the viruslike particles may then be used as carriers for peptides or carbohydrate antigens (Frenchick et al., 1989; Redmond et al., 1991). Furthermore, the VP6 carrier produces potent immunity with adjuvants suitable for human vaccines (e.g., aluminum hydroxide). The heterologous protection obtained by linking rotavirus peptides to VP6 (Ijaz et al., 1991) suggests that this combination may be a suitable candidate for a human vaccine. The rotavirus spherical particles described are also versatile in the range of antigens suitable for coupling. This presents an opportunity to vaccinate infants not only with rotavirus antigens but also protein or carbohydrate subunits derived from other prominent pediatric viral or bacterial pathogens (Figure 4).

The ability to assemble recombinant viral proteins into viruslike particles presents the opportunity of vaccination with multiple antigens

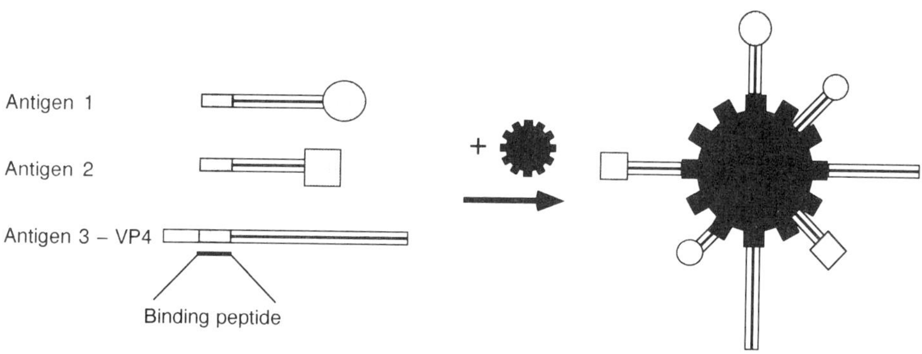

FIGURE 4 Schematic diagram represents the assembly of a multivalent vaccine for the protection of infants against prominent childhood diseases. Viral or bacterial antigens (protein or carbohydrate) may be linked to the VP6 spherical particle either directly using chemical means, or first synthesized with or coupled to a specific VP6-binding peptide, and then mixed with VP6 to produce the vaccine antigen. The proposed system would elicit protection against multiple diseases from a single vaccination.

presented in the correct structural format required to induce immunity. Support for this approach comes from the observation that immunization with empty capsids derived from an in vitro rotavirus infection protected against disease in an animal model (Brussow et al., 1990; Ready et al., 1988). We have succeeded in assembling recombinant VP4 and VP7 onto VP6 spherical particles and utilized these preparations to vaccinate mice in a challenge mode. Results indicate that heterologous protection could be achieved by vaccination with viruslike particles (Redmond et al., 1992). It may be expected that this vaccine would have advantages over the use of VP4 alone since it provides a more extensive repertoire of antigens to the immune system. Furthermore, these antigens are presented in the correct conformation. Another advantage is that is possible to decorate the VP6 spheres with many more VP4 molecules than are normally present on rotavirus, thus making it more immunogenic on a molar basis.

An advantage of subunit vaccines is the opportunity for vaccine administration by oral, parenteral, or a combination of both routes. The rationale for developing live-attenuated rotavirus vaccines has always been that they should be more effective against mucosal infections (Chanock et al., 1988). However, as mentioned previously, due to the presence of maternal antibodies and nonspecific inhibitors of virus replication in serum and milk the immunizing virus must be highly immunogenic but sufficiently attenuated to prevent adverse reactions to the vaccine. The proposed assembled subunit vaccine offers the opportunity to overcome some of these liabilities. If the antigens responsible for the attachment and penetration of virus particles to the target cell are present, they may facilitate the retention of the immunogen in the gut after oral administration (Redmond et al., 1991). The maintenance of antigen in the gut would, in turn, increase antigen-driven proliferation of rotavirus specific IgA-precursor cells (Bradtzarg, 1989). In addition, larger dosages of the immunogen could be administered without fear of side effects due to the inability of the antigen to replicate.

Despite these advantages it may still be necessary to combine an inactivated vaccine with an attenuated one to induce a protective response in the gut. Several studies done in animals demonstrate that a parenterally administered rotavirus vaccine can prime for a protective heterotypic response after a natural infection, thereby supporting this type of approach (Brussow et al., 1988). In addition, novel delivery systems and adjuvants are being investigated for enhancing an appropriate protective response. The current vaccine candidates and their respective stage of development are shown in Table 1.

TABLE 1 Summary of Rotavirus Vaccines Currently Under Development

Vaccine Type	Designation	Origin	Delivery	Development Phase	References
Live, attenuated	—	WA	Ent/Par	Discontinued	WHO, 1984
	M37	Nursery isolate	Ent/Par	Completed phase 1	Flores et al., 1986
	RIT 4237	NCDV	Ent/Par	Completed phase 1	Hanlon et al., 1987; Vesikari, 1985
		WC3	Ent/Par	Completed phase 1	Clark et al., 1988
	MMM 18006	RRV	Ent/Par	Completed phase 1	Bennels et al., 1987; Ho et al., 1989
Reassortments	—	RRV	Ent/Par	Early phase 1	Holsey et al., 1988
	—	WC3	Ent/Par	Early phase 1	Flores et al., 1989
Live bacterial vectored	—	*E. coli/Salmonella*	Ent	R/D	WHO, 1986
Live viral vectored	—	Adenovirus	Ent	R	Babiuk, 1991, unpublished
Recombinant protein	—	Baculovirus	Par	R	Mackow et al., 1990
Viruslike particle	—	Baculovirus	Ent/Par	R/D	Redmond, Ijaz et al., 1992
Peptide	—	—	Par	R	Ijaz et al., 1991

Ent, enteric, oral delivery; Par, parenteral delivery; R, research phase; D, preclinical development.

III. CONCLUSION

It is evident from the material presented here that a number of different promising approaches are available for producing future rotavirus vaccines. It is anticipated that new vaccines will be available to control animal rotavirus infections within 1–2 years. The exact time for licensing human vaccines cannot be determined at present, but the summary presented in Table 1 clearly demonstrates the number of these in clinical trials, depending on their success the vaccines could be moved along to licensing shortly. It is also clear that the numerous serotypes present in humans will make a universal human rotavirus vaccine much more difficult to produce than if only one serotype was responsible for the infection. Although one would expect that a vaccine delivered orally would be the most suitable for human immunization, the specific delivery system, whether live-vectored, reassortants, or subunit vaccines, still needs to be determined. It is also possible, as with many other diseases, that no one vaccine will gain universal acceptance. The progress in molecular biology and understanding of rotavirus epidemiology nevertheless provides us with optimism that an effective vaccine will become available in the near future.

REFERENCES

Andrew, M. E., Boyle, D. B., Couper, B. E. H., Whitfeld, P. L., Both, G. W., and Bellamy, A. R. (1987). *J. Virol. 61*:1054–1060.

Andrew, M. E., Boyle, D. B., Whitfeld, P. L., Lockett, L. J., Anthony, I. D., Bellamy, A. R., and Both, G. W. (1990). *J. Virol. 64*:4776–4783.

Archambault, D., Morin, G., Elazharg, Y., Roy, R. S., and Joncas, J. H. (1988). *Am. J. Vet. Res. 49*:1084–1981.

Arias, C. F., Ballado, T., Plebanski, M. (1986). *Gene 47*:211–219.

Arias, C. F., Lizano, M., and Lopez, S. (1987). *J. Gen. Virol. 68*:633–661.

Arias, C. F., Garcia, G., and Lopez, S. (1989). *J. Virol. 63*:5393–5398.

Bass, D. M., Mackow, E. R., and Greenberg, H. B. (1990). *J. Virol. 64*:322–330.

Bennels, M. B., Losonsky, G. A., Shindledecker, C. L., Hughes, T. P., Kapikian, A. Z., and Levine, M. M. (1987). *Pediatr. Infect Dis. J. 6*:260–264.

Bishop, R. F., Barnes, G. L., Cipriani, E., and Lund, J. S. (1983). *N. Engl. J. Med. 309*:72–76.

Black, R. E., Merson, M. H., Huq, L., Alim, A. R. M. A., and Ynus, M. (1981). *Lancet 1*:141–143.

Bradtzarg, P. (1989). *Curr. Top. Microbiol. Immunol. 146*:13–25.

Bridger, J. C., and Oldham, G. (1987). *J. Gen. Virol. 68*:2311–2317.

Brussow, H., Walther, I., Fryder, V., Sidoti, J., and Bruttin, A. (1988). *J. Gen. Virol. 69*:1647–1658.

Brussow, H., Bruttin, A., and Marc-Martin, S. (1990). *J. Virol. 64*:3635–3642.

Burke, K. L., Dunn, G., Ferguson, M., Minor, A. D., and Almond, J. W. (1988). *Nature (Lond.).* 332:81–82.

Chanock, R. M., Murphy, B. R., Collins, R. L., Coelingh, K. V. W., Olmstead, R. A., Snyder, M. H., Spriggs, M. K., Prince, G. A., Moss, B., Flores, J., Gorziglia, M., and Kapikian, A. Z. (1988). *Vaccinia* 6:129–133.

Clark, H. F., Borian, F. G., Bell, L. M., Modesto, K., Gouvea, V., and Plotkin, S. A. (1988). *J. Infect. Dis.* 158:570–587.

Davis, A. R., Kostek, B., Mason, B. B., Hsiao, C. L., Morin, J., Dheer, S. K., and Hung, P. P. (1985). *Proc. Natl. Acad. Sci. USA* 82:7560–7564.

de Zoysa, I., and Feachen, R. G. (1986). *Bull. WHO* 63:569–583.

Dyall-Smith, M. L., Lazdins, I., Tregear, G. W., and Holmes, I. H. (1986). *Proc. Natl. Acad. Sci. USA* 83:3465–3468.

Edelman, R., Flores, J., and Kapikian, A. Z. (1989). *Curr. Top. Microbiol. Immunol.* 146:123–135.

Estes, M. K. (1990). In *Virology*. B. N. Fields, et al. (Eds.). Raven Press, New York, pp. 1329–1352.

Estes, M. K., Crawford, S. E., Penaranda, M. E., Petrie, L., Burns, W. J., Chan, W. K., Ericson, G., Smith, E., and Summer, M. D. (1987). *J. Virol.* 5:1488–1494.

Fiore, L., Greenberg, H. B., and Mackow, E. R. (1991). *Virology* 181:553–563.

Flores, J., Midthun, K., Hoshino, Y., Green, K., Gorziglia, M., Kapikian, A. Z., and Chanock, R. M. (1986). *J. Virol.* 60:972–979.

Flores, J., Perez-Schall, I., Blanco, M., Vilar, M., Garcia, D., Perez, M., Daoud, N., Midthun, K., and Kapikian, A. Z. (1989). *J. Clin. Microbiol.* 27:512–518.

Flores, J., Perez-Schael, I., Blanco, M., White, L., Garcia, D., Vilar, M., Cunto, W., Mendez, M., and Kapikian, A. Z. (1990). *Lancet* 336:330–334.

Francavilla, M., Miranda, P., DiMatteo, A., Sarasini, A., Gerna, G., and Milanesi, G. (1987). *J. Gen. Virol.* 68:2975–2980.

Frenchick, P. J., Sabara, M. I., Ijaz, M. K., and Babiuk, L. A. (1988). In *Applied Virology Research*. 1. Kurstak et al. (Eds.). Plenum, New York, pp. 141–151.

Frenchick, P. J., Sabara, M. I. J., and Babiuk, L. A. (Eds.). (1989). *CSH Symp. Proc. Vaccine* 89:479–483.

Fukuhara, N., Yoshie, O., Kitakoa, S., and Konno, T. (1988). *J. Virol.* 62:2209–2218.

Gothefors, L., Wadwell, G., Juto, P., Taniguchi, K., Kapikian, A. Z., and Glass, R. I. (1989). *J. Infect. Dis.* 159:753–757.

Green, K. Y., Hoshino, Y., and Ikegami, N. (1989). *Virology* 168:429–433.

Green, K. Y., Taniguchi, K., Mackow, E., and Kapikian, A. Z. (1990). *J. Infect. Dis.* 61:667–679.

Greenberg, H. B., Kalica, A. R., Wyatt, R. G., Jones, R. W., Kapikian, A. Z., and Chanock, R. M. (1981). *Proc. Natl. Acad. Sci.* 78:420–424.

Gunn, P. R., Sata, F., Powell, K. F. H., Bellamy, A. R., Napier, J. R., Harding, D. R. K., Hancock, W. S., Siegman, L. J., and Both, G. W. (1985). *J. Virol.* 54:791–797.

Hanlon, P., Marsh, V., Shenton, F., Jobe, O., Hayes, R., Whittle, H. C., Hanlon, L., Bypass, P., Sillah, H., M'Boge, B. H., and Greenwood, B. M. (1987). *Lancet* 1:1342–1345.

Haynes, J. R., Cunningham, J., Von Selfriesh, A., Lennick, M., Garvin, R. T., and Shen, S. H. (1986). *Bio/Technology* 4:637–639.
Ho, M. S., Glass, R. I., Piasky, P. F., and Anderson, L. L. (1988). *J. Infect. Dis.* *158*:1112–1116.
Ho, M. S., Floyd, L. R., Glass, R. I., Pallansch, M. S., Jones, B., Hamby, B., Woods, P., Penaranda, M. E., Kapikian, A. Z., Bohan, G., Wilcox, W. D., and Blumberg, R. (1989). *Pediatr. Infect. Dis. J.* *8*:692–696.
Holsey, N. A., Andreson, E. L., Sears, S. D., Steinhoff, M., Wilson, M., Belshe, R. B., Midthun, K., Kapikian, A. Z., Burns, B., and Clements, M. L. (1988). *J. Infect. Dis.* *158*:1261–1267.
Ijaz, M. K., Attah-Poku, S. K., Redmond, M. J., Parker, M. D., Sabara, M. I., and Babiuk, L. A. (1991). *J. Virol.* *65*:3106–3113.
Institute of Medicine (1985). In *New Vaccine Development*. I. National Academy Press, pp. 410–423.
Institute of Medicine (1986). In *New Vaccine Development*. II. National Academy Press, pp. 308–318.
Kapikian, A. Z., and Chanock, R. M. (1990). In *Virology*, B. N. Fields et al. (Eds.). Raven Press, New York, pp. 1352–1404.
Kapikian, A. Z., Flores, J., Hoshino, Y., Glass, R. I., Midthun, K., Gorziglia, M., and Chanock, R. M. (1986). *J. Infect. Dis.* *153*:815–822.
Lanata, C. F., Black, R. E., del Aguila, R., Gil, A., Verastegui, H., Gerna, G., Flores, J., Kapikian, A. Z., and Andre, F. E. (1989). *J. Infect. Dis.* *159*:452–459.
Larralde, G., Li, B., Kapikian, A. Z., and Gorziglia, M. (1991). *J. Virol.* *65*:3213–3218.
Lucknow, V. A., and Summers, M. D. (1988). *Bio/Technology* *6*:1411–1418.
Mackow, E. R., Shaw, D., Matsui, S. M., Vo, P., Benfield, D. A., and Greenberg, H. B. (1988a). *Virology* *165*:511–517.
Mackow, E. R., Shaw, R. D., Matsin, S. M., Vo, P. T., Dang, M. N., and Greenberg, H. B. (1988b). *Proc. Natl. Acad. Sci. USA* *85*:645–649.
Mackow, E. R., Barnett, J., Chow, H., and Greenberg, H. B. (1989). *J. Virol.* *63*:1661–1668.
Mackow, E. R., Vo, P. T., Broom, R., Bass, D. M., and Greenberg, H. G. (1990). *J. Virol.* *64*:1698–1703.
Mebus, C. A., White, R. G., Bass, E. P., and Twiehaus, M. J. (1973). *J. Am. Vet. Med. Assoc.* *163*:880–887.
Midthun, K., Greenberg, H. B., Hoshino, Y., Kapikian, A. Z., Wyatt, R. G., and Chanock, R. M. (1989). *J. Virol.* *53*:949–954.
Mutz, I. D., Krainer, F., Dutsch, J., Kunz, C., and Terwan, D. E. (1989). *Eur. J. Pediatr.* *148*:6334–635.
Offit, P. A., and Dudzik, K. I. (1988). *J. Virol.* *62*:127–131.
Poncet, D., Corthier, G., Charpiliene, A., and Cohen, J. (1990). *Virus Res.* *15*:267–274.
Prasad, B. V. V., Wang, G. J., Clerx, J. P. M., and Chin, W. (1988). *J. Mol. Biol.* *199*:269–275.
Prasad, B. V. V., Burns, J. W., Marietta, E., Estes, M. K., and Chin, W. (1990). *Nature (Lond.)* *343*:476–479.
Ready, K. F. M., Sabara, M. I., and Babiuk, L. A. (1988). *Virology* *167*:269–273.

Redmond, M. J., Bielefeldt Ohmann, H., Hughes, H. P. A., Sabara, M. I., Frenchick, P. J., Attah-Poku, S. K., Ijaz, M. K., Parker, M. D., Laarveld, B., and Babiuk, L. A. (1991). *Mol. Immunol. 28*:269–278.
Redmond, M. J., Ijaz, M. K., Parker, M. D., Sabara, M. I., Dent, D., Gibbons, E., and Babiuk, L. A. (1992). Submitted.
Ruggeri, F. M., and Greenberg, H. B. (1991). *J. Virol. 65*:2211–2219.
Sabara, M., Gilchrist, J. E., Hudson, G. R., and Babiuk, L. A. (1985). *J. Virol. 53*:58–66.
Sack, D. A., Freij, L., and Holmgren, J. (1991). *J. Infect. Dis. 163*:503–506.
Saif, L. J., Redman, D. R., Smith, K. L., and Theil, K. W. (1983). *Infect. Immun. 41*:1118–1131.
Shaw, R. D., Fong, K. J., Losonsky, G. A., Levine, M. M., Maldonado, Y., Yolken, R., Flores, J., Kapikian, A. Z., Vo, P. T., and Greenberg, H. B. (1987). *Gastroenterology 93*:941–950.
Snodgrass, D. R., Ojeh, C. K., Campbell, I., and Herring, A. J. (1984). *J. Clin. Microbiol. 20*:342–346.
Streckert, H. J., Brussow, H., and Uterchari, H. (1988). *J. Virol. 62*:4265–4269.
Tajima, T., Thompson, J., Wright, P. F., Kando, Y., Tollefson, S. J., King, J., and Kapikian, A. Z. (1990). *Vaccine 8*:7075.
Taniguchi, K., Hoshino, Y., Nishikawa, K., Green, K. Y., Maloy, W. L., Morta, Y., Urasawa, S., Kapikian, A. Z., Chanock, R. M., and Gorziglia, M. (1988a). *J. Virol. 62*:1870–1874.
Taniguchi, K., Maloy, W. L., Nishikawa, K., Green, K. Y., Hoshino, Y., Urasawa, S., Kapikian, A. Z., Chanock, R. M., and Gorziglia, M. (1988b). *J. Virol. 62*:2421–2426.
Valenzuela, P., Coit, D., Medina-Selby, M. A., Kuo, C. H., Van Nest, G., Burke, R. L., Bull, P., Urdea, M. S., and Graves, P. V. (1985). *Bio/Technology 3*:323–326.
Vesikari, T. (1985). *J. Pediatr. 107*:189–194.
Ward, R. L., Knowlton, D. R., Schiff, G. M., Hoshino, Y., and Greenberg, H. B. (1988). *J. Virol. 62*:1543–1549.
Welliver, R. C., and Ogra, P. L. (1978). *J. Am. Vet. Med. Assoc. 173*:560–564.
WHO (1984). *Third Programme Report: World Health Organization Disease Control Programme*, Geneva.
WHO (1986). *Fifth Programme Report: World Health Organization Disease Control Programme*, Geneva.
Wyatt, R. G., Kapikian, A. Z., and Mebus, C. A. (1983). *J. Clin. Microbiol. 18*:505–508.

Part VII

Virus Vaccines and Biotechnology

17

ARE WE GOING TO PRODUCE ALL VIRUS VACCINES BY BIOTECHNOLOGY?

John Furesz, Gillian Chaloner-Larsson,* Guillermo Contreras, Daniel Hazlett, Laszlo Palkonyay, and Changgao Yang
Health and Welfare Canada, Ottawa, Ontario, Canada

Biotechnology is defined as the use of biological systems for the production of goods and services. Using this definition, it is clear that all commercially produced vaccines are made by biotechnology. What we really mean today when we speak of vaccines and biotechnology are the *new* biotechnologies: the genetic engineering techniques that permit the recombining of genes from different organisms or the fusing of cells to create useful cells or organisms that do not exist in nature. We shall use the word *bioengineering* when referring to these new biotechnologies. Much research has been done in the past 10 years so that the techniques of recombinant DNA and hybridoma formation that amazed us in the 1970s have become commonplace in the 1980s.

The question "Are we going to produce all virus vaccines by bioengineering?" should really be divided into two subquestions. First, "*Can* we produce all virus vaccines by bioengineering?" and, second, "*Should* we produce all virus vaccines by bioengineering?"

In this chapter, we shall try to answer both questions by reviewing the main features of both conventional and bioengineered vaccines and by looking at the economical, ethical, and regulatory aspects of the introduction of these new vaccines.

---

*Retired

I. EXISTING VIRUS VACCINES

Human virus vaccines at present licensed in Canada are shown in Table 1. The inactivated virus vaccines are against poliomyelitis, rabies, influenza, and hepatitis B virus (HBV) infections. The live, attenuated virus vaccines are against poliomyelitis, measles, mumps, rubella, yellow fever, and adenovirus types 4 and 7. In addition, inactivated Japanese B encephalomyelitis vaccine is available for administration to travelers to endemic areas. All are administered parenterally, with the exception of the live poliomyelitis and adenovirus vaccines, which are given orally. Most of these existing vaccines have very well-proven efficacy and safety records and, in fact, some have been so outstandingly successful that it will be difficult to improve upon them. However, it is possible that vaccines developed by bioengineering techniques could have advantages over existing vaccines or could provide the technology to develop vaccines that are unavailable at present.

II. NEW BIOTECHNOLOGIES

The remarkable technological breakthroughs in molecular biology made it possible to produce vaccines in several ways. Some examples of virus vaccines at different stages of development using various biotechnological approaches are shown in Table 2. The first approach deals with producing immunogenic polypeptides; this can be obtained by using recombinant

TABLE 1 Human Viral Vaccines Licensed in Canada[a]

Inactivated	Live, Attenuated
Poliomyelitis	Poliomyelitis
Rabies	Measles
Influenza	Mumps
Hepatitis B	Rubella
	Yellow fever
	Adenovirus (types 4 and 7)[b]
	Smallpox[c]

[a]All vaccines are administered parenterally, with the exception of the live polio and adenovirus vaccines, which are given orally.
[b]Licensed but used only by the Canadian Armed Forces.
[c]Licensed but available only through the Laboratory Centre for Disease Control, Health and Welfare Canada.

DNA (rDNA) technology or chemical synthesis or by using anti-idiotypic monoclonal antibodies. The second approach makes use of virus or other vectors that have been bioengineered to carry genetic information for the synthesis in the vaccine recipient of viral immunogenic polypeptides. The third approach applies various new technologies to the creation of live virus vaccines similar to conventionally attenuated live vaccines. Gene segment reassortment takes advantage of the natural ability of certain viruses to make genetic recombination between different strains in the host cell during coinfection (e.g., rotavirus). Directed mutagenesis relies on direct alteration or deletion of viral genes responsible for virulence. Monoclonal antibodies serve as highly specific tools for the analysis of microbial antigens and allow selection of those that are of relevance to immunity and hence may be candidates for inclusion in vaccines. One special kind of virus vector, in which one genetically stable and harmless virus carries information for other virus immunogenic proteins, has been called a virus chimera in recent literature.

A. Immunogenic Polypeptides

Recombinant DNA–Derived Polypeptides

One example of the first approach is an rDNA acquired immunodeficiency syndrome (AIDS) virus subunit (gp160) vaccine made in a genetically engineered insect cell line (La Montagne, 1989). At present, phase I clinical trials are being conducted in the United States and elsewhere with a number of different human immunodeficiency virus (HIV) vaccines, including the one above. Recombinant DNA technology has also been used for the production of poliovirus polyprotein and VP1 capsid protein in *Escherichia coli (E. coli)* and insect cells; herpes simplex virus (HSV) glycoprotein D (gpD) subunits in bacterial and Chinese hamster ovary (CHO) cells; the hepatitis B surface antigen (HBsAg) of HBV in yeast, insect, and CHO cells; hepatitis A virus (HAV) proteins in *E. coli, Salmonella typhi (S. typhi)*, yeast, and insect cells; the hemagglutinin (HA) of influenza virus also in bacterial, yeast, and insect cells; rabies and respiratory syncytial virus (RSV) glycoproteins in insect cells; and rotavirus surface subunits in *E. coli* and insect cells. Of all these viruses, to date only HBV vaccine prepared in yeast cells has been licensed in Canada. The fear that HIV, transmitted by blood (the source of the first HBV vaccine), might have survived in the inactivated vaccine was partly responsible for the impetus behind the development and licensing of the rDNA HBV vaccine.

TABLE 2 Biotechnologic Approaches to Viral Vaccine Development

	HIV	Polio	HSV	HBV	HAV	Cox	Flu	Rabies	PIV	RSV	Mum	Rota	Dengue	CMV
Polypeptides														
Genetic expression	X	X	X	X	X		X	X	X	X		X	X	X
Chemical synthesis	X	X	X	X	X		X							
Anti-idiotypes	X	X	X	X		X		X						
Vectors														
Viral	X	X	X	X	X		X	X		X			X	
Bacterial		X		X	X		X	X						
Other approaches														
Gene segment reassortment							X					X		
Directed mutations	X	X	X											
Mutants selected with monoclonal antibodies			X			X		X			X			
Virus chimeras	X	X			X									

HIV, human immunodeficiency virus; Polio, poliovirus; HSV, herpes simplex virus; HBV, hepatitis B virus; HAV, hepatitis A virus; Cox, coxsackievirus; Flu, influenza virus; Rabies, rabies virus; PIV, parainfluenza virus; RSV, respiratory syncytial virus; Mum, mumps virus; Rota, rotavirus; Dengue, dengue virus; CMV, cytomegalovirus.

Chemically Synthesized Peptide Vaccines

Recent progress in methods for determining nucleic acid sequences and the corresponding amino acid composition of the related proteins, and improvements in oligonucleotide and peptide synthesis, have made possible the construction of synthetic peptide vaccines (Barteling, 1988). Thus, detailed knowledge of the antigenic structure of protective immunogens may facilitate the production of vaccines by incorporating as immunogens only the essential structures. However, for many viruses, we are still limited by our lack of knowledge of the epitope(s) required for the induction of a protective immune response. Nevertheless, this approach has been pursued, with varying degrees of success, for a wide range of viruses. Phase I clinical trials with an HIV vaccine based on a synthetic peptide are already under way (Goldstein et al., 1991) and other groups are also pursuing this approach with a number of other viruses. Synthetic peptides containing the amino acid sequences of a major neutralization epitope in the VP1 capsid protein of poliovirus types 1 and 3 have been shown capable of inducing the production of neutralizing antibodies in rabbits (Emini et al., 1983; Ferguson et al., 1985). An N-terminal fragment of gpD of HSV can also induce the production of neutralizing antibodies, but these only partially protected mice against virus challenge (Eisenberg et al., 1985). Synthetic peptides composed of amino acid sequences from various regions of the HBsAg of HBV, the VP1 major surface protein of HAV, and the HA of influenza virus have all been shown to be capable of inducing an immune response in mice or rabbits, but in general the antibodies were not neutralizing and, at best, only partly protective (Barteling, 1988).

A new approach for producing synthetic peptides called mimotypes is based on the three-dimensional conformation of many antigenic epitopes. This technique, designated as repeated amino acid replacement, operates through continuous replacement of amino acid residues within a synthetic peptide until a primary structure, not necessary identical with the native protein, will mimic a natural three-dimensional epitope (Geysen et al., 1984, 1985).

Anti-Idiotypic Monoclonal Antibodies Used as Viral Vaccines

Anti-idiotypic monoclonal antibodies (AIMA) whose combining sites mimic viral antigens can induce the production of antiviral antibodies in the absence of infectious virus particles. One group of investigators has had some success in developing in mice AIMA that specifically recognize the CD4-binding site for HIV as well as simian immunodeficiency virus (Dalgleish et al., 1987). The same group had shown earlier that another

AIMA was able to protect chimpanzees from infectious HBV challenge (Kennedy et al., 1986). As shown in Table 2, research based on AIMA is also proceeding in an effort to develop vaccines against several other viruses. Neutralizing antibodies were developed in mice by inoculating them with mouse monoclonal anti-idiotypic antibodies against murine monoclonal antipoliovirus type 2 antibodies, but these provided only partial protection against lethal challenge (Uytdehaag and Osterhaus, 1985). Mice immunized with rabbit anti-idiotypic antibodies to mouse monoclonal antibodies against HSV type 1 developed a cell-mediated immune response after challenge with homologous viral antigen, but protection did not necessarily ensue (Gell and Moss, 1985). In fact, in some cases susceptibility to infection may have actually increased (Kennedy et al., 1984). Mice immunized with rabbit polyclonal antibodies that mimic rabies virus surface glycoprotein developed neutralizing antibodies but were not protected against intracerebral rabies virus challenge (Reagan et al., 1983). The general lack of success in inducing with AIMA a sustained and protective immunologic response in animals has not been encouraging. Nevertheless, it has been proposed that AIMA may be useful for priming or boosting a response to another vaccine preparation against the same virus (Stein and Söderström, 1984).

B. Vectors

Viral Vectors

Another successful approach is to incorporate the genes coding for one or more immunogens into the genomes of large carrier viruses, or into non-pathogenic bacteria, which can then be administered to humans. Development of virus vector vaccines has concentrated on exploiting the use of pox-, adeno-, or herpes viruses as the vector. Members of each of these three virus groups have been shown to be capable of accepting an inserted gene, producing the desired gene product, and presenting the peptide on the surface of the recombinant virus or infected cell. Already, an AIDS vaccine in which vaccinia virus serves as the vector is undergoing clinical trials in the United States (Koff et al., 1990). Work is also being carried out to develop vector virus vaccines against HSV, HBV, HAV, influenza, rabies, respiratory syncytial, and dengue viruses using various strains of vaccinia virus as the vector (Jordan, 1988; Piccini and Paoletti, 1988); against HSV, HBV, and rabies virus using adenovirus as the vector (Morin et al., 1987; Johnson et al., 1988; Prevec and Graham, 1989); against HBV using HSV as the vector (Shih et al., 1984); against Epstein-Barr virus using herpes varicella zoster as vector (Lowe et al., 1987); and against rabies virus using raccoon poxvirus as the vector (Esposito et al., 1988). Recent experiments demonstrated that one virus vector (vaccinia) could express simultaneously genes of two viruses, such as influenza and HSV type 1 (Flexner et al., 1988).

At least two problems could be encountered when vaccinia is used as a vector. Existing immunity of the host to either the vector virus or the recombinant viruses may restrict the replication of the vector virus. Clinical trials with a vaccinia vector expressing the gp 160 HIV envelope glycoprotein demonstrated a stronger response in vaccinia-naive than vaccinia-primed subjects (Cooney et al., 1991). It is also well known that vaccinia virus used for the eradication of smallpox was found occasionally highly reactogenic in humans, causing some severe adverse reactions. Attempts are made to reduce or eliminate these characteristics of vaccinia by molecular manipulation of the virus, such as insertional or deletional mutations in the genes of thymidine kinase, growth factor, or hemagglutinin or incorporation of the interleukin-2 gene into the viral genome (Moss et al., 1988).

Bacterial Vectors

Bacterial vectors may be used in a manner similar to that in which viral vectors could be used. This approach is already under study for the development of poliovirus vaccines in which *E. coli* (Hoatlin et al., 1987; Charbit et al., 1988) and attenuated *S. typhimurium* (Charbit et al., 1988) are used as vectors via the oral or parenteral routes. Thus, using *E. coli* as vector for the viral RNA encoding parts of the VP1 capsid region of poliovirus, two groups of investigators have recently reported success in inducing the production of poliovirus-neutralizing antibodies in rabbits following parenteral administration of the recombinant bacteria (Hoatlin et al., 1987; Charbit et al., 1988).

Bacteria harboring recombinant expression vectors (e.g., plasmids) are prone to lose some of their extrachromosomal DNA constructs when the selective pressure of antibiotics disappears in vivo, which leads to suboptimal antigen delivery to the preferred site. One possible approach to overcoming this disadvantage could be the integration of expression sequences into the bacterial chromosome (Strugnell et al., 1990).

C. Other Biotechnologic Approaches to Viral Vaccine Development

Vaccines Produced by Gene Segment Reassortment

Viruses with segmented genomes (e.g., rotavirus, influenza) are able to form hybrid virus particles during coinfection. Rhesus or bovine rotavirus strains can be used as donors of attenuating genes during coinfection with virulent human serotypes to produce single-gene substitution hybrids under selective pressure of antibodies to the animal rotavirus. Such reassortants are available for three of the four human serotypes expressing the major neutralization protein (VP7) of the human serotypes (Midthun et al., 1985, 1986). It might be feasible to form reassortants that express the broadly reactive VP3 (another capsid protein with the ability to induce neutralizing antibodies in animal models) and the VP7 protein of a human rotavirus (Kapikian et al., 1989). This strategy was successful in colostrum-deprived gnotobiotic piglets using porcine rotavirus recombinants (Hoshino et al., 1988). This approach might also be useful for producing potentially effective influenza recombinants in the near future. Intranasally administered reassortant influenza vaccines are considered satisfactorily attenuated, immunogenic, nontransmissible, and phenotypically stable in adults and children (Sears et al., 1988).

Directed Mutations

Deletion or alteration of virulence genes by site-directed mutation has been used to attenuate HIV (Lasky, 1989), poliovirus (Melnick, 1988), and herpesviruses (Kit et al., 1987). In animal herpesvirus studies, synergistic attenuation was described with multiple deletion in genes of pseudorabies virus glycoproteins (Mettenleiter et al., 1988). Genetic manipulation in noncoding regions also can produce viable mutants (Kuge and Nomoto, 1987). The great potential of directed mutagenesis is based on the fact that attenuation can be achieved by partial deletion within one gene (including point mutation), deletion of an entire gene, synergistic interaction between two deleted genes, and deletion within noncoding regions (Murphy and Chanock, 1990).

Another successful approach to achieving attenuation was the use of insertional mutagenesis. A lymphokine gene (interleukin-2) was inserted into the vaccinia genome and the modified virus was found not to be lethal for immunodeficient mice that otherwise would have been killed by the unmodified virus (Ramshaw et al., 1987). This favorable method of immune response modification could reduce the risk of immunization with live viruses in immunocompromised subjects. Similar beneficial effect may be anticipated from other cytokines (e.g., interferon).

Mutants Selected with Neutralizing Monoclonal Antibodies

Missense mutations can occur in viral genomes spontaneously and nucleotide substitution(s) might result in amino acid change in the expressed protein, with the possible consequence of detectable phenotypic changes (e.g., temperature sensitivity, altered tissue tropism and/or decreased virulence, etc.). Stable mutations affect surface glycoproteins, resulting in decreased virulence and target cell tropism but maintained immunogenicity, which are characteristics desirable for live vaccines.

Neutralizing monoclonal antibodies might be used to select mutants that could serve as candidate vaccines. When HSV was cultivated under the selective presence of monoclonal antibodies, monoclonal antibody-resistant (*mar*) mutants were obtained that maintained resistance to the neutralizing effect of the selective agent (Holland et al., 1983). HSV type 1 *mar* mutants that showed single or multiple point mutations in the genome coding for different surface glycoproteins were less pathogenic for mice and vaccination with these mutants resulted in resistance to "wild" virus challenge (Kümel et al., 1985). Similar strategy was used to select attenuated picornavirus mutants (Coxsackievirus B4), in which multiple mutations lead to a gradual decrease in mortality in intraperitoneally inoculated suckling mice (Prabhakar et al., 1987). These mutants were stable. Similar results were also obtained with other viruses. These findings are promising if we consider the extreme instability of natural missense mutants.

Chimeric Viral Vaccines

It is possible to produce chimeric viruses that express surface epitopes and other desirable characteristics of two or more viruses. Laboratory tests have shown encouraging results using poliovirus chimeras that possess the genetic stability of poliovirus type 1 and surface antigens of poliovirus type 2 (Martin et al., 1988) or type 3 (Burke et al., 1988). These intertypic RNA virus hybrids were obtained via infectious, cloned, complementary DNA. The combination of a greater stability of Sabin type 1 poliomyelitis strain with the entire type 3 surface region was suggested as a possible candidate for a new, probably safer, type 3 live vaccine (Kohara et al., 1988). In a recent publication Evans and co-workers (1989) demonstrated that a bioengineered polio type 1 virus containing an epitope from the transmembrane glycoprotein (gp41) of HIV 1 elicited the production of broadly reactive HIV-neutralizing antibodies in rabbits. The latter observation opens up the possibility of immunizing against HIV by the oral route using enteroviruses as vectors. The choice of Sabin poliovirus type 1, with its excellent vaccine field record, is possibly the best option. Other enteric viruses, such as adeno-, echo-, and coxsackieviruses, could also be candidates but they do not have the long successful history of the Sabin poliovirus type 1 vaccine strain and would require extensive testing to determine their safety and stability.

New Assays in Molecular Biology for Vaccine Development

Recently discovered new techniques in molecular biology will undoubtedly accelerate further the development of engineered vaccines. For instance, the polymerase chain reaction (PCR) technique allows a given sequence of DNA or RNA to be amplified to the extent that it may be analyzed directly even from minute amounts of starting material. In the case of RNA, a preliminary reverse transcription step is needed to produce complementary DNA molecules required for the method. The PCR technology is based on the repetitions of three steps conducted in succession under controlled temperature and time conditions: melting of double-stranded DNA molecules at 92°–96°C (denaturation), annealing of a pair of primer DNAs to sites flanking the region to be amplified, and DNA synthesis catalyzed by a thermostable DNA polymerase enzyme.

PCR technology may soon replace the present procedures of gene cloning (cultivation of large quantities of virus, extraction of viral RNA or DNA, addition of linkers, cloning into vectors, etc.) as the amplification of choice due to the minute amount required as the starting material. This technique shows great promise for the production of recombinant molecules of viruses that are slow growers or noncultivable.

Another technologic advance is the development of an "epitope library" by the use of fusion phage (Scott and Smith, 1990). Fusion phage is a bacteriophage vector capable of displaying foreign antigenic determinants cloned into the so-called gene III of the phage genome. An epitope library can be applied as a tool for epitope mapping and for identifying peptides that can be useful for future vaccines.

III. CHARACTERISTICS OF CONVENTIONAL AND BIOENGINEERED VACCINES

A. Inactivated Vaccines

The production of conventional inactivated vaccines requires large quantities of virulent virus antigens. Mass production of antigen taxes the logistics of handling large volumes and requires special precautions to prevent exposure of laboratory personnel to the virulent virus and the possible escape of the virus from the production area. The selection of the inactivating agent is crucial to preserve the structure of the virus antigens. Purification of virus harvests is essential to reduce or eliminate host cell impurities, thus avoiding possible short- or long-term adverse reactions in vaccine recipients.

To assess the advantages and disadvantages of the use of conventional and bioengineered vaccines, we classified the major characteristics of these vaccines into the following groups (Table 3): product, immunogenicity, efficacy, clinical adverse reactions, and production costs. Since the bioengineered vaccines contain only part(s) of the virus genome, no inactivating agent is required; consequently, no risk of incomplete inactivation occurs. Although purification of either type of vaccine is necessary, some impurities from the cell substrate still will be present in

TABLE 3 Comparison of Inactivated Conventional and Bioengineered Virus Vaccines

	Vaccine	
	Conventional	Bioengineered
Product		
Inactivating agent required	Yes	No
Risk of incomplete inactivation	Yes	No
Impurities from cell substrate	Yes	Yes
Stability during storage	Yes	May be a problem
Immunogenicity, Efficacy		
Adjuvant required	No	Yes
Number of antigens or epitopes	Multiple	One or few ("cocktail" may be required)
Immunogen elicits protective antibody in recipient	Yes	May be a problem
IgG production	Yes	Yes
IgA, IgM production	Limited	Limited (?)
CMI response	Limited	Limited (?)
Multiple vaccine doses	Yes	Yes
Booster vaccine dose(s)	Yes	Yes
Possible combination with other vaccines	Yes	Probably
Clinical Adverse Reactions		
Local and systemic reactions	Minimal	Adjuvant-dependent
Delayed hypersensitization to "wild" virus	Occasionally	Not yet known
Production Costs	High	High

both products. Stability during storage may also be a problem with the new vaccines.

It is well known that the immunity conferred by conventional inactivated vaccines is often brief. Multiple doses, and often booster doses, are required to ensure continuous protection of the vaccine recipient. Parenteral administration of an inactivated vaccine, even when it stimulates circulating antibody (IgM, IgG) to satisfactory levels, has sometimes given limited protection because local resistance (IgA) is not induced adequately and because the cell-mediated immune (CMI) response is generally poor. In view of the limited immunogenicity of the purified proteins prepared either by genetic expression or chemical synthesis, the problems described above for the conventional inactivated vaccines become even more relevant. Many of these newly developed epitopes act more like haptens than like complete antigens; therefore, they have to be enhanced immunologically by various methods. Aggregation into clumps (micelles), incorporation into phospholipids to form liposomes (immunosomes), coupling with longer-chain carrier proteins, and incorporation into a safe and effective new immunological adjuvant are promising methods for overcoming the limited immunogenicity of these antigens. There are numerous compounds in the process of being developed as adjuvants, some of which might have a potential for human use (Warren and Chedid, 1988). One example of these experimental compounds is a lipophylic derivative of muarmyl tripeptide (MTP-PE), a mycobacterial cell wall component, which is covalently linked to a recombinant vaccine. It was found in animal studies as immunogenic as the complete Freund adjuvant (Sanchez-Pescador et al., 1988). The new immune enhancers ideally should stimulate both humoral and cell-mediated immunity with acceptable toxicity, such as gamma inulin, a nontoxic plant storage carbohydrate. In a mouse model gamma inulin was found to be an effective adjuvant for humoral immune response, however, more investigation is needed for assessing its ability to boost the cell-mediated immunity (Leslie et al., 1990). The simultaneous application of the newly developed immunomodulators (interferons, interleukins), prepared with rDNA techniques, in recipients of bioengineered or conventional vaccines, appears to be another promising approach in this field (Hibberd and Rubin, 1989).

As far as clinical adverse reactions are concerned, only minimal reactions may be anticipated following the administration of either type of vaccine. However, since past experience has shown that some inactivated virus vaccines (measles, RSV) induced hypersensitivity to a subsequent "wild" virus infection (Fulginiti et al., 1967; Kim et al., 1969), careful long-term clinical follow-up of recipients of the new bioengineered vaccines is highly desirable.

It is well known that the cost of production and administration of conventional inactivated virus vaccines, used in multiple doses, is high. There is no reason to believe that these costs will be reduced for the new vaccines.

In view of these facts, one may conclude that new vaccines prepared by rDNA technology in various host cells could be viable alternatives to conventional inactivated vaccines. The elimination of the virus genome regions responsible for multiplication and virulence makes the inactivation step unnecessary, which greatly simplifies the production procedures. However, we should not underestimate the problems in identifying the proper protective immunogens and the methods to be used for their immunologic enhancement in the vaccine recipient. Past experience has shown that some conventional subunit vaccines, albeit well-purified and less reactogenic, were not as immunogenic as whole virion vaccines. Therefore, we believe that a careful "case-by-case" analysis for each new candidate vaccine will be required to assess all parameters before any such vaccine is accepted for use.

B. Live Vaccines

In the past, development of conventional live virus vaccines was achieved either by selecting naturally attenuated virus strains or by cultivating "wild" viruses serially in various hosts and/or cell cultures. The goal was to obtain a modified virus that had lost its pathogenicity in humans but retained its ability to multiply in certain target cells of the host. Recombinant DNA technology provides two approaches for developing live virus vaccines. First, viral genes can be deleted or altered to eliminate the disease-causing potential without impairing immunogenicity. This approach so far has had limited use, as described earlier. Second, gene cloning and rDNA technology can be employed to insert a gene from the vaccine candidate virus into large vector viruses such as vaccinia or into bacteria (Table 2). To assess the advantages and disadvantages of the use of conventional live and bioengineered live vector vaccines, we used the same approach as described earlier in Table 3 for inactivated vaccines and classified the major characteristics of these vaccines into the same groups (Table 4). If the vaccines are produced in primary cell cultures or eggs, known or unknown adventitious agents may be present in either vaccine. Chemical impurities (proteins, nucleic acids, etc.) derived from cells will also be detected. It has been established that with some conventional vaccines (polio, rubella, mumps) there is an occasional risk of reversion to

TABLE 4 Comparison of Conventional Live and Bioengineered Live Vector Virus Vaccines

	Vaccine	
	Conventional	Bioengineered Vector
Product		
Adventitious agents from cell substrate	Yes	May be present
Impurities from cell substrate	Yes	Yes
Genetic stability	Risk of reversion	No risk of reversion but potential loss of gene insert during production
Stability during storage	May be a problem	Possible increased stability
Immunogenicity, Efficacy		
Number of antigens or epitopes	Multiple	One or few (?)
Immunogens elicit protective antibodies in recipient	Yes	May be a problem
CMI response	Yes	Very likely
Lasting immunity	Yes	Not yet known
Multiple doses required	Occasionally	Yes
Booster doses required	No	Not yet known
Simulates natural infection	Yes	Partially yes
Produces resistance at portal of entry	Yes	Occasionally
Possible combination with other vaccines	Yes	Yes
Interference with other viruses	Occasionally	Occasionally
Clinical Adverse Reactions		
Local and systemic reactions	Occasionally	Occasionally
Vaccine-associated disease	Occasionally[a]	No
Produces persistent infection	Occasionally	No
Production Costs	Low	Low

[a]Particularly in immunocompromised recipients.

virulence during multiplication in the vaccine recipient. Such reverted viruses can cause disease either in the recipient or in the susceptible person in contact with the recipient. Although the risk of such reversion is nonexistent in vaccines prepared in virus vectors, there is a possibility that the inserted gene could be lost during virus multiplication. During storage, the bioengineered vector vaccine appears to be more stable than some conventional ones.

The conventional live vaccines do multiply in the host, simulating natural infection, and consequently induce long-lasting humoral and cell-mediated immunities and elicit antibody production and resistance at the portal of entry. Since the inserted immunogens multiply in the recipient of the vector virus, bioengineered live vaccines also induce humoral and cell-mediated immunities. However, the portal of entry may be different from the natural route of infection and the induced immunity may last for a shorter period of time; thus, the administration of multiple doses may be required.

Local and systemic adverse reactions do occur occasionally in recipients of either vaccine. Bioengineered vector vaccines do not cause vaccine-associated "natural" disease and cause no persistent infections, as observed occasionally in recipients following the administration of conventional live vaccines. However, these new vaccines may fall behind conventional live vaccines in producing long-lasting protective immunity. It is noteworthy that the production costs of both types of vaccine are lower than those observed with inactivated vaccines.

IV. ETHICAL AND REGULATORY ISSUES OF BIOENGINEERED VACCINES

The past four decades can be described as the "coming of age" of virology and the birth of modern virus vaccine technology. The safety and efficacy records of the existing conventional virus vaccines are outstanding and the major problem today in the world is not the lack of good vaccines but failure to deliver them to susceptible populations. The question then arises: Should we replace these vaccines with new bioengineered vaccines? The obvious answer is that one does so only if the new vaccines are considerably safer, more efficacious, and more stable during storage and if production costs are lower.

Since there is an occasional risk of reversion to virulence of some conventional live virus vaccines either in the vaccine recipient or in susceptible contacts, attempts are made to develop genetically more stable vaccines with bioengineering techniques. Deletional mutations introduced into the 5′ noncoding region of type 1 polioviruses resulted in strains with decreased monkey neurovirulence (Nomoto et al., 1988). This observation provides a promising general strategy for the construction of new live poliovirus vaccines. The combination of Sabin type 1 vaccine strain with the type 3 virus surface region as a chimeric vaccine was mentioned above (Kohara et al., 1988).

Seronegative women of childbearing age not infrequently develop arthritis following administration of live rubella virus vaccine. In some cases this vaccine-associated arthritis becomes chronic, with up to 5 year persistence of the vaccine virus in the recipient (Chantler et al., 1982). Therefore, genetically manipulated live rubella strains might be considered as future vaccine alternatives for adult women.

Several investigators found that the Urabe live mumps virus vaccine may cause meningitis in children within 30 days of administration (Forsey et al., 1990, Furesz and Contreras, 1990; Takahasi et al., 1990; Brown et al., 1991). Selection of mumps virus *mar* mutants might lead to alternative vaccines (Löve et al., 1985).

Recent analysis of the nucleotide sequences of the live 17D yellow fever vaccine strain and its "wild" parent strain may further improve this vaccine (Hahn et al., 1987). Its genomic organization is similar to polioviruses and many of the nucleotide changes are located in the envelope glycoprotein gene (protective antigen).

The yeast-derived HBV vaccine was the first vaccine produced in recombinant cells and at present is the only type of recombinant vaccine licensed in North America for human use. Rabies virus glycoprotein expressed in vaccinia virus was successfully used for the oral immunization of foxes, dogs, and cats (Blancou et al., 1989). Such recombinant vaccines prepared at low cost could eventually replace the conventional, high-cost, inactivated human rabies vaccines prepared in diploid cell cultures.

How does one design the clinical studies so that participants will not be deprived of the benefits of existing vaccines? What should be the size of such studies to obtain meaningful data on the rare occurrence of severe adverse reactions and the real efficacy of the new vaccine? These issues will have to be carefully considered by manufacturers and various health and regulatory authorities in the decision-making process.

The situation is different when no vaccines are available for the prevention of a virus disease. Bioengineering techniques could provide the means to produce vaccines, perhaps more readily than conventional methods, to protect against the so-called "emerging viruses" (Morse, 1989). At a meeting held in May, 1989, in Washington, D.C., the concept of emerging viruses was analyzed and defined and its public health implications discussed. Examples of emerging viruses (and their associated diseases) presented included HIV, non-A/non-B hepatitis, Hantaan, Seoul, dengue, arena (Junin, Machupo), Marburg, Ebola, and monkey pox viruses (Kilbourne, 1990). It was emphasized that it is essential to build a worldwide surveillance network to detect early the appearance of emerging infectious diseases. Once the causative agents are isolated, bioengineering techniques might be useful in the development of specific preventive vaccines.

The usual cautious approach for the introduction of any new vaccine should apply: following the establishment of consistent manufacturing procedures and solid animal data, clinical studies will have to go through various phases until the safety and efficacy of the vaccine have been clearly demonstrated. Since society expects new vaccines to cause mild or no adverse reactions in recipients, the establishment of an active postmarketing surveillance system will be essential to monitor the performance of these vaccines.

While new bioengineering approaches are being pursued, efforts to develop vaccines along the old, conventional lines should also continue. Considerable success has been achieved in the development of a number of vaccines such as HSV (Skinner et al., 1987), varicella zoster (Gershon, 1987), cytomegalovirus (Plotkin et al., 1991), hepatitis A (Siegl and Lemon, 1990), and rotavirus (Vesikari et al., 1986) vaccines, to mention a few.

V. CONCLUSIONS

In this chapter we attempted to give an overall review of future vaccines in light of the remarkable technologic breakthroughs in molecular biology and rDNA technology. Are we going to produce all virus vaccines by bioengineering? Our answer is "no" in the 1990s and probably "yes" at the turn of the next century. In the introductory remarks the above question was divided into two subquestions. First, "*Can* we produce all virus vaccines by bioengineering?" and second, "*Should* we produce all virus vaccines by bioengineering?" To answer the first question: although we do have the modern tools to develop new vaccines, we have not yet defined a number of important factors essential for the production of safe and effective vaccines against a number of viral diseases. We have to identify and produce the epitope(s) of many viruses that may act as protective immunogen(s) in the recipient. New and safe methods are required to enhance the limited immunogenicity of these epitopes. Improved and safer virus or other vectors are needed to "manufacture" these new epitopes in the human recipients. In addition to these factors, laboratory manipulations aimed at specific genetic alterations in the virus will result in genetically more stable live virus vaccines.

As far as the second question is concerned, the rationale is that existing conventional vaccines that have served us well should only be replaced if the bioengineered vaccines demonstrate a distinct advantage over the existing vaccines. In the case of viruses for which there are no existing vaccines, bioengineering is the obvious answer. Even if bioengineered vaccines for all viral diseases do not become available, the increased knowledge of viral pathogenesis gained from the use of biotechnological methods may provide us with information useful in the development of improved methods of treatment or control of viral diseases. The new knowledge will pave the way for the development of chemically synthesized (protein-engineered) vaccines that will not carry the limited risks associated with vaccines produced by bioengineering.

REFERENCES

Barteling, S. J. (1988). In *Synthetic Peptides in Biotechnology*, A. Mizrahi (Ed.). Alan R. Liss, New York, pp. 25–60.

Blancou, J., Artois, M., Brochier, B., Thomas, I., Pastoret, P. P., Desmettre, P., Languet, B., and Kiény, M. P. (1989). *Ann. Rech. Vet.* *20*:195–204.

Brown, E. G., Furesz, J., Dimock, K., Yarosh, W., and Contreras, G. (1991). *Vaccine* *9*:840–842..

Burke, K. L., Dunn, G., Ferguson, M., Minor, P. D., and Almond, J. W. (1988). *Nature (Lond.)* *332*:81–82.

Chantler, J. K., Ford, D. K., and Tingle, A. J. (1982). *Lancet* *1*:1323–1325.

Charbit, A., Van der Werf, S., Mimic, V., Boulain, J. C., Girard, M., and Hofnung, M. (1988). *Ann. Inst. Pasteur/Microbiol.* *139*:45–58.

Cooney, E. L., Collier, A. C., Greenberg, P. D., Coombs, R. W., Zarling, J., Arditti, D. E., Hoffman, M. C., Hu, S.-L., and Corey, L. (1991). *Lancet* *337*:567–572.

Dalgleish, A. G., Thomson, B. J., Chanh, T. C., Malkovsky, M., and Kennedy, R. C. (1987). *Lancet* *2*:1047–1050.

Eisenberg, R. J., Cerini, C. P., Heilman, C. J., Joseph, A. D., Dietzschold, B., Golub, E., Long, D., Ponce de Leon, M., and Cohen, G. H. (1985). *J. Virol.* *56*:1014–1017.

Emini, E. A., Jameson, B. A., and Wimmer, E. (1983). *Nature* (Lond.) *304*:699–703.

Esposito, J. J., Knight, J. C., Shaddock, J. H., Novembre, F. J., and Baer, G. M. (1988). *Virology* *165*:313–316.

Evans, D. J., McKeating, J., Meredith, J. M., Burke, K. L., Katrak, K., John, A., Ferguson, M., Minor, P. D., Weiss, R. A., and Almond, J. W. (1989). *Nature* (Lond.) *339*:385–388.

Ferguson, M., Evans, D. M. A., Magrath, D. I., Minor, P. D., Almond, J. W., and Schild, G. C. (1985). *Virology* *143*:505–515.

Flexner, C., Murphy, B. R., Rooney, J. F., Wohlenberg, C., Yuferov, V., Notkins, A. L., and Moss, B. (1988). *Nature* (Lond.) *335*:259–262.

Forsey, T., Mawn, J. A., Yates, P. Y., Bentley, M. L., and Minor, P. D. (1990). *J. Gen. Virol. 71*:987–990.

Fulginiti, V. A., Eller, J. J., Downie, A. W., and Kempe, C. H. (1967). *JAMA 202*:1075–1080.

Furesz, J., and Contreras, G. (1990). *Canada Dis. Wkly. Rep. 16*:253–254.

Gell, P. G. H., and Moss, P. A. H. (1985). *J. Gen. Virol. 66*:1801–1804.

Gershon, A. A. (1987). *J. Pediatr. 110*:154–157.

Geysen, H. M., Meloen, R. H., and Barteling, S. J. (1984). *Proc. Natl. Acad. Sci. USA 81*:3998–4002.

Geysen, H. M., Barteling, S. J., and Meloen, R. H. (1985). *Proc. Natl. Acad. Sci. USA 82*:178–182.

Goldstein, A. L., Naylor, P. H., Sarin, P. S., Kirkley, J. E., Stambuk, D., Rios, A., Zagury, D., Achour, A., Gazzard, B., and Youle, M. (1991). *AIDS Res. Hum. Retroviruses 7*:154.

Hahn, C. S., Dalrymple, J. M., Strauss, J. H., and Rice, C. M. (1987). *Proc. Natl. Acad. Sci. USA 84*:2019–2023.

Hibberd, P. L., and Rubin, R. H. (1989). *Ann. Intern. Med. 110*:955–956.

Hoatlin, M. E., Kew, O. M., and Renz, M. E. (1987). *J. Virol. 61*:1442–1447.

Holland, T. C., Marlin, S. D., Levine, M., and Glorioso, J. (1983). *J. Virol. 45*:672–682.

Hoshino, Y., Saif, L. J., Sereno, M. M., Chanock, R. M., and Kapikian, A. Z. (1988). *J. Virol. 62*:744–748.

Johnson, D. C., Ghosh-Choudhury, G., Smiley, J. R., Fallis, L., and Graham, F. L. (1988). *Virology 164*:1–14.

Jordan, W. S., Jr. (1988). *Prog. Med. Virol. 35*:1–20.

Kapikian, A. Z., Flores, J., Hoshino, Y., Midthun, K., Gorziglia, M., Green, K. Y., Chanock, R. M., Potash, L., Sears, S. D., Clements, M. L., Halsey, N. A., Black, R. E., and Perez-Schael, I. (1989). *Rev. Infect. Dis. 11* (Suppl. 3):S539–S546.

Kennedy, R. C., Adler-Storthz, K., Burns, J. W., Sr., Henkel, R. D., and Dreesman, G. R. (1984). *J. Virol. 50*:951–953.

Kennedy, R. C., Eichberg, J. W., Lanford, R. E., and Dreesman, G. R. (1986). *Science 232*:220–223.

Kilbourne, E. D. (1990). *JAMA 264*:68–70.

Kim, H. W., Canchola, J. G., Brandt, C. D., Pyles, G., Chanock, R. M., Jensen, K., and Parrott, R. H. (1969). *Am. J. Epidemiol. 89*:422–434.

Kit, S., Sheppard, M., Ichimura, H., and Kit, M. (1987). *Am. J. Vet. Res. 48*:780–793.

Koff, W. C., Weskott, S. L., and Hoth, D. F. (1990). In *AIDS Vaccine Research and Clinical Trials*, S. D. Putney and D. P. Bolognesi (Eds.). Marcel Dekker, New York, pp. 425–438.

Kohara, M., Abe, S., Komatsu, T., Tago, K., Arita, M., and Nomoto, A. (1988). *J. Virol. 62*:2828–2835.

Kuge, S., and Nomoto, A. (1987). *J. Virol. 61*:1478–1487.

Kümel, G., Kaerner, H. C., Levine, M., Schröder, C. H., and Glorioso, J. C. (1985). *J. Virol. 56*:930–937.

La Montagne, J. R. (1989). *Rev. Infect. Dis. 11*(Suppl. 3):S639–S643.

Lasky, L. A. (1989). *Crit. Rev. Immunol. 9*:153–172.
Leslie, D. E., Nicholson, S., Dimitrakakis, M., Johnston, N., and Gust, I. D. (1990). *Immunol. Cell Biol. 68*:107–112.
Löve, A., Rydbeck, R., Kristensson, K., Orvell, C., and Norrby, E. (1985). *J. Virol. 53*:67–74.
Lowe, R. S., Keller, P. M., Keech, B. J., Davison, A. J., Whang, Y., Morgan, A. J., Kieff, E., and Ellis, R. W. (1987). *Proc. Natl. Acad. Sci. USA 84*:3896–3900.
Martin, A., Wychowski, C., Benichou, D., Crainic, R., and Girard, M. (1988). *Ann. Inst. Pasteur/Virol. 139*:79–88.
Melnick, J. L. (1988). *Am. J. Public Health 78*:304–305.
Mettenleiter, T. C., Schreurs, C., Zuckermann, F., Ben-Porat, T., and Kaplan, A. S. (1988). *J. Virol. 62*:2712–2717.
Midthun, K., Greenberg, H. B., Hoshino, Y., Kapikian, A. Z., Wyatt, R. G., and Chanock, R. M. (1985). *J. Virol. 53*:949–954.
Midthun, K., Hoshino, Y., Kapikian, A. Z., and Chanock, R. M. (1986). *J. Clin. Microbiol. 24*:822–826.
Morin, J. E., Lubeck, M. D., Barton, J. E., Conley, A. J., Davis, A. R., and Hung, P. P. (1987). *Proc. Natl. Acad. Sci. USA 84*:4626–4630.
Morse, S. S. (1989). *Am. Soc. Microbiol. News 55*:358–360.
Moss, B., Fuerst, T. R., Flexner, C., and Hugin, A. (1988). *Vaccine 6*:161–163.
Murphy, B. R., and Chanock, R. M. (1990). In *Virology*, B. N. Fields and D. M. Knipe (Eds.). Raven Press, New York, pp. 469–502.
Nomoto, A., Iizuka, N., Kohara, M., and Arita, M. (1988). *Vaccine 6*:134–137.
Piccini, A., and Paoletti, E. (1988). *Adv. Virus Res. 34*:43–64.
Plotkin, S. A., Starr, S. E., Friedman, H. M., Brayman, K., Harris, S., Jackson, S., Tustin, N. B., Grossman, R., Dafoe, D., and Barker, C. (1991). *Ann. Intern. Med. 114*:525–531.
Prabhakar, B. S., Srinivasappa, J., and Ray, U. (1987). *J. Gen. Virol. 68*:865–869.
Prevec, L., and Graham, F. L. (1989). Paper presented at the VIth International Conference on Comparative Virology, October 15–19, Banff, Alberta, Canada.
Ramshaw, I. A., Andrew, M. E., Phillips, S. M., Boyle, D. B., and Coupar, B. E. H. (1987). *Nature (Lond.) 329*:545–546.
Reagan, K. J., Wunner, W. H., Wiktor, T. J., and Koprowski, H. (1983). *J. Virol. 48*:660–666.
Sanchez-Pescador, L., Burke, R. L., Ott, G., and van Nest, G. (1988). *J. Immunol. 141*:1720–1727.
Scott, J. K., and Smith, G. P. (1990). *Science 249*:386–390.
Sears, S. D., Clements, M. L., Betts, R. F., Maassab, H. F., Murphy, B. R., and Snyder, M. H. (1988). *J. Infect. Dis. 158*:1209–1219.
Shih, M.-F., Arsenakis, M., Tiollais, P., and Roizman, B. (1984). *Proc. Natl. Acad. Sci. USA 81*:5867–5870.
Siegl, G., and Lemon, S. M. (1990). *Virus Res. 17*:75–92.
Skinner, G. R. B., Fink, C. G., Cowan, M., Buchan, A., Fuller, A., Hartley, C. E., Durham. J., Wiblin, C., and Melling, J. (1987). *Med. Microbiol. Immunol. 176*:161–168.

Stein, K. E., and Söderström, T. (1984). *J. Exp. Med. 160*:1001–1011.
Strugnell, R. A., Maskell, D., Fairweather, N., Pickard, D., Penn, C., and Dougan, G. (1990). *Gene 88*:57–63.
Takahasi, M., Ono, S., Shimuzu, T., Tasawa, M., Shimohara, M., Homma, T., Fukazawa, N., Suzuki, M., Tokodoro, M., Fujinaga, T., and Kuroume, T. (1990). *Jpn. Med. J. 3441*:43–45.
Uytdehaag, F. G. C. M., and Osterhaus, A. D. M. E. (1985). *J. Immunol. 134*:1225–1229.
Vesikari, T., Kapikian, A. Z., Delem, A., and Zissis, G. (1986). *J. Infect. Dis. 153*: 832–839.
Warren, H. S., and Chedid, L. A. (1988). *CRC Crit. Rev. Immunol. 8*:83–101.

Index